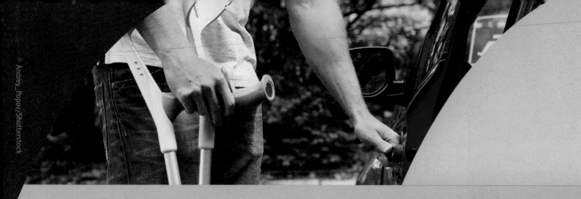

Epidemiology 101

SECOND EDITION

Robert H. Friis, PhD

Professor Emeritus and Chair Emeritus
Health Science Department
California State University
Long Beach, California
and
Retired Professor
Department of Medicine
University of California, Irvine
Irvine, California

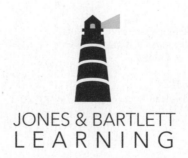

JONES & BARTLETT
LEARNING

D1209369

World Headquarters
Jones & Bartlett Learning
5 Wall Street
Burlington, MA 01803
978-443-5000
info@jblearning.com
www.jblearning.com

Jones & Bartlett Learning books and products are available through most bookstores and online booksellers. To contact Jones & Bartlett Learning directly, call 800-832-0034, fax 978-443-8000, or visit our website, www.jblearning.com.

13193-2

Production Credits
VP, Executive Publisher: David D. Cella
Publisher: Michael Brown
Associate Editor: Lindsey Mawhiney Sousa
Production Manager: Carolyn Rogers Pershouse
Associate Production Editor: Alex Schab
Senior Marketing Manager: Sophie Fleck Teague
Manufacturing and Inventory Control Supervisor: Amy Bacus
Composition: Integra Software Services Pvt. Ltd.
Cover Design: Kristin E. Parker
Rights & Media Specialist: Merideth Tumasz
Media Development Editor: Shannon Sheehan
Cover Image Clockwise from top left: © Andrey_Popov/Shutterstock,
 © Kateryna Kon/Shutterstock, © McIek/Shutterstock, © Oleg Baliuk/Shutterstock
Printing and Binding: LSC Communications
Cover Printing: LSC Communications

Library of Congress Cataloging-in-Publication Data
Names: Friis, Robert H., author.
Title: Epidemiology 101 / Robert H. Friis.
Other titles: Epidemiology one hundred and one | Epidemiology one hundred one
Description: Second edition. | Burlington, Massachusetts : Jones & Bartlett
 Learning, [2018] | Includes bibliographical references and index.
Identifiers: LCCN 2016054751 | ISBN 9781284107852
Subjects: | MESH: Epidemiology | Epidemiologic Methods
Classification: LCC RA651 | NLM WA 105 | DDC 614.4—dc23
LC record available at https://lccn.loc.gov/2016054751

6048

Printed in the United States of America
20 19 18   10 9 8 7 6 5 4

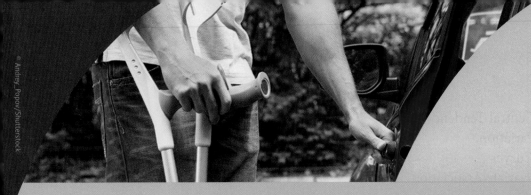
© Andrey_Popov/Shutterstock

Contents

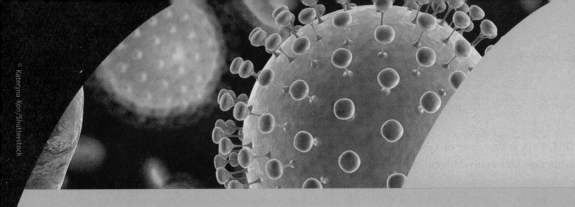

The Essential Public Health Series

Log on to www.essentialpublichealth.com *for the most current information on the series.*

Current and Forthcoming Titles in the *Essential Public Health* Series:

Public Health 101: Healthy People–Healthy Populations, Enhanced Second Edition*—Richard Riegelman, MD, MPH, PhD & Brenda Kirkwood, MPH, DrPH

Epidemiology 101, Second Edition*—Robert H. Friis, PhD

Global Health 101, Third Edition*—Richard Skolnik, MPA

Essentials of Public Health, Third Edition*—Bernard J. Turnock, MD, MPH

Essentials of Health Policy and Law, Third Edition*—Joel B. Teitelbaum, JD, LLM & Sara E. Wilensky, JD, MPP

Essentials of Environmental Health, Second Edition—Robert H. Friis, PhD

Essentials of Biostatistics in Public Health, Third Edition*—Lisa M. Sullivan, PhD

Essentials of Health Behavior: Social and Behavioral Theory in Public Health, Second Edition—Mark Edberg, PhD

Essentials of Health, Culture, and Diversity: Understanding People, Reducing Disparities—Mark Edberg, PhD

Essentials of Planning and Evaluation for Public Health Programs*—Karen Marie Perrin, MPH, PhD

Essentials of Health Information Systems and Technology*—Jean A. Balgrosky, MPH, RHIA

Essentials of Public Health Ethics—Ruth Gaare Bernheim, JD, MPH; James F. Childress, PhD; Richard J. Bonnie, JD; & Alan L. Melnick, MD, MPH, CPH

Essentials of Leadership in Public Health*—Louis Rowitz, PhD

Essentials of Management and Leadership in Public Health—Robert Burke, PhD & Leonard Friedman, PhD, MPH

Essentials of Public Health Preparedness—Rebecca Katz, PhD, MPH

Essentials of Global Community Health—Jaime Gofin, MD, MPH & Rosa Gofin, MD, MPH

Accompanying Case Books and Readings

Essential Case Studies in Public Health: Putting Public Health into Practice—Katherine Hunting, PhD, MPH & Brenda L. Gleason, MA, MPH

Essential Readings in Health Behavior: Theory and Practice—Mark Edberg, PhD

* These texts include Navigate 2 Advantage Access.

ABOUT THE EDITOR

Richard Riegelman, MD, MPH, PhD, is Professor of Epidemiology and Biostatistics, Medicine, and Health Policy, and founding dean of The George Washington University Milken Institute School of Public Health in Washington, D.C. He has taken a lead role in developing the Educated Citizen and Public Health Initiative, which has brought together arts and sciences and public health education associations to implement the Institute of Medicine of the National Academies' recommendation that "… all undergraduates should have access to education in public health." Dr. Riegelman also led the development of The George Washington University's undergraduate major and minor and currently teaches "Public Health 101" and "Epidemiology 101" to undergraduates.

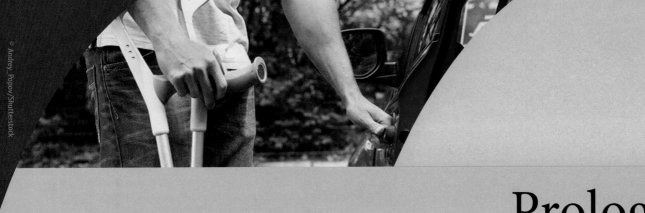

Prologue

Dr. Robert Friis' *Epidemiology 101*, Second Edition introduces you to the world of epidemiology, the basic science of public health, and shows you the many ways that epidemiology affects all of our lives. *Epidemiology 101* clearly conveys the key concepts of epidemiology with a minimum of mathematics. It presents epidemiology as a scientific way of thinking applicable to a wide range of fields, from basic and clinical sciences to public policy.

Epidemiology 101 builds upon Robert Friis' many years of teaching and writing about epidemiology and environmental health, bringing alive the excitement of these fields. You will come away from *Epidemiology 101* with enduring understandings that you can use and build upon in a wide range of careers for many years to come.

The first edition of *Epidemiology 101* set the standard for an undergraduate overview of epidemiology as expected for all public health majors and minors. Undergraduate epidemiology is increasingly serving the needs of many new types of students. These include students who seek to learn evidence-based thinking as a basic skill as recommended by the Association of American Colleges and Universities (AAC&U). These students include those who wish to prepare for the new MCAT® exam, which incorporates basic principles of study design and statistics as part of the Scientific Inquiry and Reasoning Skills (SIRS) component of the examination.

Epidemiology 101, Second Edition continues to serve as a core undergraduate epidemiology text. It also serves the needs of the rapidly expanding population of undergraduate students who are interested in learning about epidemiology. Dr. Friis has added two new chapters to the *Second Edition*. The first new chapter includes a look at how data can be analyzed and displayed. For those preparing for the MCAT® exam, this chapter is keyed to SIRS components, such as using statistical measures and drawing conclusions from quantitative relationships. The second new chapter is dedicated to screening tests within the context of the natural history of disease. In addition, exciting new topics presented in the *Second Edition* include "big data," Zika virus disease, and electronic cigarettes.

Robert Friis' *Epidemiology 101* was one of the first books to be published as part of our *Essential Public Health* series. It set a high standard for the series, which has now expanded to provide over 20 introductory textbooks that cover the full spectrum of public health.

In *Epidemiology 101, Second Edition,* Dr. Friis has done it again. Robert Friis brings to all his writing a lifetime commitment to teaching, a personal connection to students as they begin their study of epidemiology, and an impressive ability to clearly present complex subjects.

I know that you will enjoy and benefit from the second edition of *Epidemiology 101.* You will find the work of a true educator, a real pro. Take a look and see for yourself.

Richard Riegelman, MD, MPH, PhD
Series Editor—*Essential Public Health*

Acknowledgments

FOR THE FIRST EDITION

The concept for *Epidemiology 101* originated with Dr. Richard Riegelman, professor and founding dean of the School of Public Health and Health Services, at The George Washington University. I would like to thank Dr. Riegelman for his encouragement and support. This work is part of the *Essential Public Health* series, which offers a comprehensive curriculum in public health.

Writing textbooks and revising them requires considerable time and effort. Each project begins with enthusiasm, anxiety, and an ocean of blank pages. After several months—and sometimes years—the final manuscript emerges. From that point, additional months are required for production of the printed book.

From the author's perspective, the input of colleagues and students was essential in completing the first edition of this book. My colleagues and students were extremely helpful in providing comments. I wish to thank the following students from California State University, Long Beach: Sarah Long, Paula Griego, and Che Wankie. Students aided with literature searches, reviewed written text materials, and provided feedback. I also acknowledge the helpful comments and other contributions of Ibtisam Khoury-Sirhan, Claire Garrido-Ortega, Dr. Javier Lopez-Zetina, and Dr. Veronica Acosta-Deprez of California State University, Long Beach. These professional colleagues reviewed chapters that were relevant to their areas of expertise. Mike Brown, Publisher for Jones & Bartlett Learning, provided continuing encouragement and motivation for completion of the project; Jones & Bartlett Learning staff offered much helpful expertise. Finally, my wife, Carol Friis, was involved extensively with this project; for example, she critiqued the manuscript, typed final versions of the document, provided detailed editorial comments, verified the accuracy of the references, and helped with many other aspects of the book. Without her support and assistance, completion of the text would not have been possible.

FOR THE SECOND EDITION

For the second edition, I am especially indebted to Professor Riegelman, Publisher Mike Brown, and the editorial staff at Jones & Bartlett for their continuing support and encouragement for the revision of *Epidemiology 101*. The comments of anonymous reviewers aided me in updating and expanding the content of the *Second Edition*. I deeply appreciate their thoughtful comments. Throughout the process, my wife, Carol Friis, helped me to edit the various drafts. Her assistance was essential to the completion of a polished final manuscript.

R.H.F.

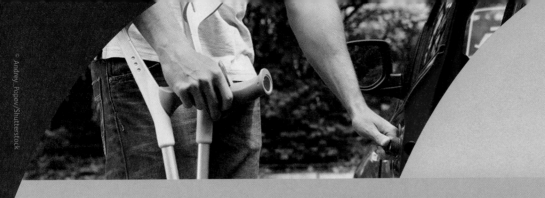

About the Author

Robert H. Friis, PhD, is Professor and Chair, emeritus, of the Department of Health Science at California State University, Long Beach (CSULB), and former Director of the CSULB-Veterans Affairs Medical Center, Long Beach, Joint Studies Institute. He is a past president of the Southern California Public Health Association and member of the governing council. He serves or has served on the advisory boards of several health-related organizations, including the California Health Interview Survey. He previously retired from the University of California, Irvine, where he was an Associate Clinical Professor in the Department of Medicine, Department of Neurology, and School of Social Ecology.

Dr. Friis has had a varied career in epidemiology. As a health department epidemiologist, he led investigations into environmental health problems such as chemical spills and air pollution. He has taught courses on epidemiology, environmental health, and statistics at universities in New York City and southern California. The topics of his research, publications, and presentations include tobacco use, mental health, chronic disease, disability, minority health, and psychosocial epidemiology.

Dr. Friis has been principal investigator or coinvestigator on grants and contracts from the University of California's Tobacco-Related Disease Research Program, the National Institutes of Health, and other agencies. This funding has supported investigations into topics such as tobacco control policies, geriatric health, depression in Hispanic populations, and infectious disease transmission in nursing homes. His academic interests have led him to conduct research in Mexico City and European countries. He has been a visiting professor at the Center for Nutrition and Toxicology, Karolinska Institute, Stockholm, Sweden; the Max Planck Institute, Munich, Germany; and the Medizinische Fakultät Carl Gustav Carus of the Dresden Technical University, Dresden, Germany. He frequently reviews articles for scientific journals, is on the international editorial board of *Public Health* (Elsevier Ltd.), and is an editor of the *Journal of Public Health* (Springer). Dr. Friis is a fellow of the Royal Society of Public Health, lifetime member of the governing council of the Southern California Public Health Association, member of the Society for Epidemiologic Research, and member of the American Public Health Association. His awards include a postdoctoral fellowship for study at the Institute for Social Research, University of Michigan, and the Achievement Award for Scholarly and Creative Activity from California State University, Long Beach.

He is author/coauthor of the following books published by Jones & Bartlett Learning:

- *Epidemiology for Public Health Practice*, with Thomas A. Sellers (editions one through five)
- *Essentials of Environmental Health*
- *Epidemiology 101*
- *Occupational Health and Safety for the 21st Century*

He is also the author/coauthor of textbooks on biostatistics and community/public health and is the editor of the *Praeger Handbook of Environmental Health* (Praeger).

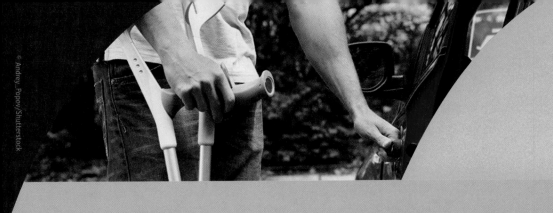

Preface

I wrote *Epidemiology 101* in response to a call to increase the epidemiologic content of undergraduate programs. A growing movement advocates for incorporating epidemiology into undergraduate curricula as a liberal arts subject. Consequently, students in undergraduate liberal arts programs, as well as those with limited public health or mathematical backgrounds, are the target audience for *Epidemiology 101*. No extant epidemiologic textbook is tailored exactly for this audience.

Epidemiology is ideally suited as a topic for liberal arts because habits of mind, such as problem analysis, deductive and inductive reasoning, and applying generalizations to a larger context, are key features of epidemiology. The discipline provides reinforcement of basic skills acquired in the natural sciences, mathematics and statistics, and the social sciences. Thus, a course in epidemiology might be taken in order to fulfill a distribution requirement in one of the basic or applied sciences. Furthermore, knowledge of epidemiology equips citizens with informed opinions regarding crucial health issues that appear daily in the media.

In addition to covering basic epidemiologic concepts, the text demonstrates how these concepts can be applied to problems encountered in everyday life, e.g., hazards posed by the food supply, risks associated with lifestyle choices, and dangers associated with youth violence. One of the features of *Epidemiology 101* is its emphasis on socially related determinants of health and health disparities. This text is one in the *Essential Public Health* series published by Jones & Bartlett Learning and edited by Richard Riegelman.

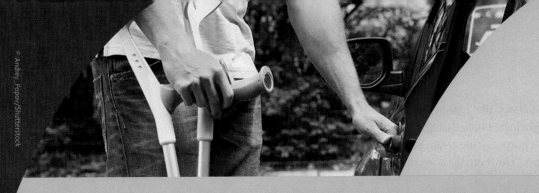

Introduction

Epidemiology 101 is written for students who have not had extensive backgrounds in health and biostatistics. The audience might include:

- Those seeking a simplified introduction to epidemiology. They could be nonmajors, people from allied fields, or students who are building a foundation for further work in epidemiology.
- Medical students who are preparing for the MCAT® exam. The textbook provides instruction relevant to Skill 4: Scientific Inquiry and Reasoning Skills: Data-Based Statistical Reasoning on the MCAT® exam. Chapter 2 provides content on basic statistical reasoning. The study questions and exercises section of this chapter contains sample questions for drilling for the MCAT®.
- Beginning statistics students. Chapter 2 provides a brief introduction to elementary statistics and preparation for a statistics course.
- Those who would like to study epidemiology in order to fulfill a requirement for a course in science.
- Advanced high school students who are enriching their educational experience.

Increasingly, curriculum designers recognize that as a discipline, epidemiology embodies many useful critical thinking skills, including gathering facts, forming hypotheses, and drawing conclusions. These processes are the hallmark of the scientific method and embody modes of thinking that benefit well-educated citizens even if they do not intend to become public health professionals.[1] In this respect, epidemiology resembles a liberal art.[2]

Epidemiology may be approached from a nontechnical point of view that students from a variety of backgrounds can appreciate. Examples of epidemiologic investigations into such problems as bird flu and studies of lifestyle and chronic disease are inherently appealing. Although epidemiology has strong quantitative roots, this text emphasizes the nonquantitative aspects of the discipline by creating a linkage with traditional liberal arts concepts, including social justice and health disparities. A background in mathematics and statistics is not required to use the book. The text incorporates numerous case studies, text boxes, vignettes, exhibits, photographs, figures, and illustrations to gain the interest of readers.

Epidemiology has evolved into a discipline that has applications in many fields. Once thought of as being confined to the investigation of infectious disease outbreaks, epidemiologic methods are used increasingly in such diverse health-related areas as traditional clinical medicine, healthcare administration, nursing, dentistry, and occupational medicine. In addition, the applications of epidemiologic methods are expanding to manufacturing processes, law, and control of international terrorism. *Epidemiology 101* will provide examples of many of these applications.

The content of this book follows the outline of the curriculum titled *Epidemiology 101*, recommended by the Consensus Conference on Undergraduate Public Health Education, November 7–8, 2006, Boston, Massachusetts.*

In some instances, for didactic purposes, the arrangement of the topics departs somewhat from the order presented in the conference's Working Group Reports. However, the content of this textbook is similar to the content shown in the curriculum suggested for *Epidemiology 101*.

This text contains a total of 12 chapters, which begin with coverage of basic epidemiologic principles and then increase in complexity. Chapters 11 and 12 illustrate current applications of epidemiology. The *Second Edition* has been updated extensively throughout, with two additional chapters and new tables, figures, and exhibits. Unique to this edition are expanded content on data presentation, basic statistical measures, policy, and screening. Examples chosen—such as the Ebola outbreak in Africa, Zika virus disease, and abuse of opioids—are recent and command the attention of students. The course content can be covered during an academic quarter or a semester. Jones & Bartlett Learning has developed an online course based on the first edition of *Epidemiology 101*. Instructors can adapt this textbook for online learning in their own educational settings.

Selected chapters are keyed to exercises from the College Board's Young Epidemiology Scholars (YES) Program. The Young Epidemiology Scholars: Competitions website provides links to teaching units and exercises that support instruction in epidemiology. The YES program, discontinued in 2011, was administered by the College Board and supported by the Robert Wood Johnson Foundation. The exercises continue to be available at the following website: http://yes-competition.org/yes/teaching-units/title.html.

A full set of supportive learning materials, e.g., slides in PowerPoint format, two sample syllabi, an instructor's manual, a *Second Edition* transition guide, and a test bank, is available online at www.jbpub.com/essentialpublichealth for students and instructors to access. Each chapter concludes with study questions and exercises for additional reinforcement. The study questions and exercises have been revised and expanded for the *Second Edition*. Students should be encouraged to use the supportive materials that are available on the website for this textbook. The interest level of students can be increased by using group exercises, lectures from public health experts, and field visits. The Robert Wood Johnson Foundation's YES exercises can be implemented as a laboratory component of an epidemiology course.

REFERENCES

1. Weed DL. Epidemiology, the humanities, and public health. *Am J Public Health*. July 1995;85(7):914-918.
2. Fraser DW. Epidemiology as a liberal art. *N Engl J Med*. February 5, 1987;316(6):309-314.

* Web address: www.aacu.org/sites/default/files/files/PublicHealth/Recommendations_for_Undergraduate_Public_Health_Education.pdf. (Accessed September 6, 2016.)

CHAPTER 1

History, Philosophy, and Uses of Epidemiology

LEARNING OBJECTIVES

By the end of this chapter you will be able to:

- Define the term epidemiology.
- Describe two ways in which epidemiology may be considered a liberal arts discipline.
- State the difference between description and analysis in epidemiology.
- Name three important landmarks in the history of epidemiology.
- List three uses of epidemiology.

CHAPTER OUTLINE

INTRODUCTION

As a member of contemporary society, you are besieged constantly with information about the latest health scare. One category of threats arises from infectious disease epidemics, including infection with the human immuno-deficiency virus (HIV), foodborne illness, Ebola disease, and Zika virus disease. Another threat is from chronic disease epidemics, such as the growing societal burdens of obesity and diabetes. Finally, we hear a great deal about conditions linked to adverse behaviors, such as the effects of smoking, binge drinking, and prescription drug abuse. In fact, threats such as these account for a devastating toll for the affected individual, our society, and the health-care system. Especially vexing is the stream of information from media reports of epidemiologic research. These pronouncements can be inconsistent and often are self-contradictory.

By exploring the aforementioned threats to society, you will learn how epidemiology is an exciting field with many applications that are helpful in solving today's health-related problems. (Refer to **Figure 1-1**.) For example, epidemiology can demonstrate the risks associated with smoking, as well as those related to exposure to secondhand cigarette smoke among nonsmokers. Currently, youth violence is an issue that confronts students, teachers, and administrators at both urban and suburban schools; epidemiologic research can identify factors related to such violence and suggest methods for its prevention. Other

FIGURE 1-1 Examples of the types of questions that can be answered by epidemiologic research.

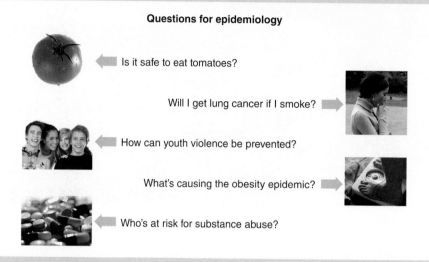

Questions for epidemiology

Is it safe to eat tomatoes?

Will I get lung cancer if I smoke?

How can youth violence be prevented?

What's causing the obesity epidemic?

Who's at risk for substance abuse?

Photo credits: © adsheyn/ShutterStock, Inc.; © Zdenka Micka/ShutterStock.com; © Yuri Areurs/ShutterStock, Inc.; Courtesy of Bill Branson/National Cancer Institute; © Photos.com.

contributions of epidemiology include the identification of factors associated with obesity and substance abuse, both of which, as noted, are major societal issues. Epidemiology has a track record of helping to investigate these problems as well. Refer to **Table 1-1** for a list of important terms used in this chapter.

EPIDEMIOLOGY AND RECENT EPIDEMICS

One of the more familiar applications of epidemiology is tracking down infectious disease epidemics. Consider three examples of infectious disease outbreaks and how they exemplify challenges to epidemiology. The examples are Ebola virus hemorrhagic fever, Zika virus disease, and foodborne illnesses.

Ebola Virus Hemorrhagic Fever

Infection with the Ebola virus is spread through direct contact with blood or bodily fluids; it is not an airborne condition nor is it transmitted through indirect means, such as food and water. The infection—which can produce severe headaches, gastrointestinal symptoms, and bleeding—causes a high proportion of fatalities. The largest outbreak in history descended upon West Africa in 2014. (See infographic in **Figure 1-2**.) By April 13, 2016, a total of 28,652 cases had been reported in Africa. Approximately two out of five people infected with Ebola virus died. When the Ebola outbreak exploded in 2014, public health officials scrambled to meet

TABLE 1-1 List of Important Terms Used in This Chapter

Analytic epidemiology	Miasmic theory of disease
Descriptive epidemiology	Morbidity
Demographic transition	Mortality
Determinant	Natural experiment
Disease management	Observational science
Distribution	Operations research
Epidemic	Outcome
Epidemiologic transition	Pandemic
Epidemiology	Population
Exposure	Quantification
Interdisciplinary science	Risk
John Snow	Risk factor

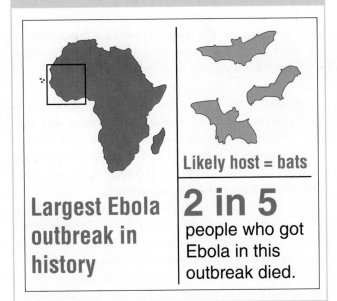

FIGURE 1-2 Ebola outbreak in West Africa.

Largest Ebola outbreak in history

Likely host = bats

2 in 5
people who got Ebola in this outbreak died.

Reproduced From: Centers for Disease Control and Prevention. Infographic: West Africa Ebola Outbreak. Available at: http://www.cdc.gov/vhf/ebola/pdf/west-africa-outbreak -infographic.pdf. Accessed July 26, 2016.

the challenge. Epidemiologic methods contributed to bringing this massive outbreak under control.

Zika Virus Disease

The mosquito-borne Zika virus, linked with development of a febrile rash, has been associated with adverse birth outcomes among pregnant women who become infected. The Centers for Disease Control and Prevention (CDC) asserts that congenital infection with the Zika virus is capable of producing microcephaly and abnormalities of the brain among infants born to infected pregnant women.[1] Since late 2014, health officials in Brazil observed increased Zika virus transmission that accompanied increased reports of microcephaly. As of January 2016, the total number of reports of suspected cases in Brazil reached 3,520.

Cases of Zika infection have also been reported in the U.S.—279 reports as of early May 2016. Most of these were associated with travel to areas where local transmission of Zika had taken place. However, by mid-summer of 2016, some cases were related to local occurrence in the continental United States (e.g., Florida and California) and U.S. territories. In addition to being mosquito-borne, the virus is sexually transmitted. Epidemiologic techniques, such as surveillance programs, have helped to track the Zika virus and reduce transmission risks.

Foodborne Illness

Foodborne illness outbreaks associated with *Escherichia coli* and *Salmonella* bacteria are excellent examples of conditions that can be researched and brought under control though the application of epidemiologic methods.

E. coli Infections

This bacterial agent produces mild to severe diarrhea with bloody stools. Severe infections can cause acute kidney dysfunction. Two outbreaks of foodborne infection with *E. coli* bacteria were linked to Chipotle Mexican Grill restaurants. The first, in October 2015, resulted in 55 reported cases. In December 2015, a second episode was associated with 5 reported cases. The CDC used genetic fingerprinting techniques to type the strain of *E. coli* that was involved.[2]

Salmonellosis

Foodborne salmonellosis is an infection caused by *Salmonella* bacteria. This agent can produce gastrointestinal symptoms (cramping, diarrhea, and fever) that begin 12 to 72 hours after the onset of infection. The majority of patients recover without treatment, although some endure life-threatening consequences.

A major outbreak that occurred in 2008 is particularly interesting. It affected more than 1,400 people and is believed to have contributed to two deaths.[3] Cases appeared in 43 states, most frequently in Texas, Arizona, and Illinois. The source of contamination was mysterious. All patients were affected with an uncommon strain of *Salmonella* Saintpaul, which had a distinctive genetic fingerprint. Initially, epidemiologic investigations implicated raw tomatoes. The public was advised not to eat red plum (red Roma) and round red tomatoes, which were suspected of being the implicated vehicle of infection. This news was indeed disturbing; tomatoes generally are considered to be healthful. They are used extensively in many popular items of the American diet, including salads, ketchup, spaghetti sauce, pizza, and salsa. Despite this diligent work, the origin of the bacteria that sickened so many people was never definitively linked to tomatoes. Eventually, the CDC discovered that the source of the *Salmonella* outbreak was jalapeño and serrano peppers from Mexico.

THE CONCEPT OF AN EPIDEMIC

What is meant by the term *epidemic*? An **epidemic** refers to "[t]he occurrence in a community or region of cases of an illness, specific health-related behavior, or other health-related events clearly in excess of normal expectancy."[4] The aforementioned *Salmonella* outbreak illustrates a foodborne-disease episode that reached epidemic proportions. Individual

Salmonella cases may arise sporadically; usually such occurrences are not epidemics but instead represent background cases. However, because in this instance a large number of people across the United States were affected with an unusual strain of *Salmonella* bacteria, the *Salmonella* outbreak could be considered an epidemic. Similarly, the Zika virus epidemic in Brazil, the Ebola virus scare in West Africa, and the *E. coli* outbreak associated with a U.S. chain restaurant are additional examples of epidemics.

Figure 1-3 demonstrates the concept of an epidemic in the case of the annual occurrence of a hypothetical disease. The "normal expectancy" is six cases per year. In three years, 2016, 2019, and 2020, the occurrence of the disease was in excess of normal expectancy. For these conditions (for example, influenza mortality), when the number of cases exceeds the background rate, an epidemic may be suspected.

You should be aware that in some instances a single case of a disease represents an epidemic. With respect to a new occurrence of an infectious disease not previously found in an area or the occurrence of an infectious disease that has long been absent, a single or small number of cases of that disease would be regarded as an epidemic. At present, examples of infrequently occurring diseases in the United States are measles and polio. A small outbreak of measles, polio, or other infrequently occurring infectious disease requires the immediate attention of public health officials and would be treated as an epidemic. As a matter of fact, an outbreak of 125 cases of measles occurred at a California Disney theme park between December 2014 and February 2015.

The use of the word "epidemic" is not limited to communicable diseases. The term is applied to chronic diseases and other conditions as well. Illustrations are the "epidemic of obesity," the "epidemic of diabetes," or the "epidemic of heart disease."

Related to the term epidemic is **pandemic**, defined as "[a]n epidemic occurring worldwide, or over a very wide area, crossing international boundaries, and usually affecting a large number of people."[4] The 1918 influenza pandemic discussed later in the chapter and periodic less-severe global influenza epidemics illustrate this concept.

The previous discussion leads to the question: What is the scope of epidemiology? This chapter will begin with a definition of the term epidemiology and illustrate how the study of epidemiology imparts skills that are useful in a variety of pursuits. As part of this exploration, the author will highlight the key historical developments in epidemiology and demonstrate how these developments have influenced the philosophy and practice of epidemiology. Some of these historical developments include concerns of the ancient Greeks about diseases caused by the environment, the observations of Sir Percival Pott on scrotal cancer among chimney sweeps in England, the work of John Snow on cholera, and modern work on the etiology of chronic diseases.

FIGURE 1-3 Annual occurrence, normal expectancy, and epidemic frequency of a hypothetical disease.

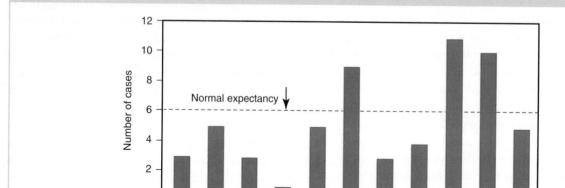

Epidemiology is one of the basic sciences of public health. Epidemiologic methods are applied to a variety of public health-related fields: health education, healthcare administration, tropical medicine, and environmental health. Epidemiologists quantify health outcomes by using statistics. They formulate hypotheses, and they explore causal relationships between exposures and health outcomes. A special concern of the discipline is causality: Do research findings represent cause-and-effect associations or are they merely associations? A simple example of a causal association would be whether a specific contaminated food such as tomatoes caused an outbreak of gastrointestinal disease; a more complex example is whether there is a causal association between smoking during the teenage years and the subsequent development of lung cancer later in life.

Although the foregoing examples of the applications of epidemiology are primarily health related, epidemiology is a body of methods that have general applicability to many fields. Two examples that are not disease related are mass shootings in schools and universities and bullying in high schools. A mass shooting on a school or university campus represents a tragic event that all too frequently rivets the attention of the national media.

Figure 1-4 summarizes information about mass shootings at U.S. schools. Since the mid-1960s, numerous fatal shootings have occurred on U.S. college campuses. Among the most deadly were shootings at the University of Texas at Austin in 1966 and at Virginia Tech in 2007.

At the secondary-school level, highly publicized shootings also have grabbed the headlines. One of these was the 1999 violence at Columbine High School in Littleton, Colorado, and the tragic shooting in 2012 at Sandy Hook Elementary School in Newtown, Connecticut. Although they command our attention, violent episodes that cause multiple homicides on school premises are actually highly unusual. Nevertheless, the National Academy of Sciences declared that youth violence "reached epidemic levels" during the

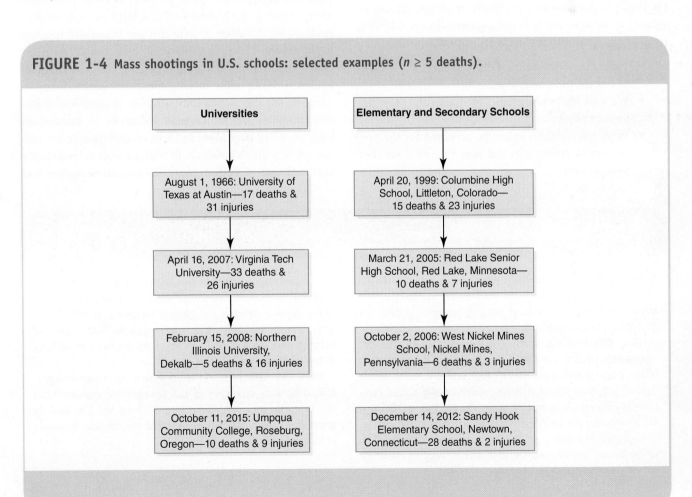

FIGURE 1-4 Mass shootings in U.S. schools: selected examples ($n \geq 5$ deaths).

Universities

August 1, 1966: University of Texas at Austin—17 deaths & 31 injuries

April 16, 2007: Virginia Tech University—33 deaths & 26 injuries

February 15, 2008: Northern Illinois University, Dekalb—5 deaths & 16 injuries

October 11, 2015: Umpqua Community College, Roseburg, Oregon—10 deaths & 9 injuries

Elementary and Secondary Schools

April 20, 1999: Columbine High School, Littleton, Colorado—15 deaths & 23 injuries

March 21, 2005: Red Lake Senior High School, Red Lake, Minnesota—10 deaths & 7 injuries

October 2, 2006: West Nickel Mines School, Nickel Mines, Pennsylvania—6 deaths & 3 injuries

December 14, 2012: Sandy Hook Elementary School, Newtown, Connecticut—28 deaths & 2 injuries

1990s. A total of 35 shooting incidents transpired at secondary schools or school-sponsored events from 1992 to 2001.

In what sense can school violence be regarded as an epidemic? Who is most likely to be targeted? Perhaps the answer is that any incident of violence (especially shootings) on school premises is significant. The CDC produced epidemiologic data on school-associated student homicides that occurred during the years 1992 to 2006. These data suggest that the preponderance of homicide victims were male students and students in urban areas.

As a second example of school violence, **Exhibit 1-1** provides information regarding school-related bullying, a topic of increasing public health and societal concern. Bullying can take the form of cyberbullying and physical bullying. Alarmingly, about 15% and 20% of high school students experience cyber-and physical bullying, respectively.

The foregoing exhibit regarding violence in schools, specifically bullying, illustrates the potential applications of epidemiology for solving a broad range of problems that affect the health of populations. Specifically, epidemiology can be used as a research tool that seeks answers to the following types of questions with respect to violence in schools:

- Violent episodes are most likely to affect which types of schools and universities?
- What are the characteristics of victims and perpetrators of violent acts?
- What interventions might be proposed for the prevention of violent acts and how successful are they likely to be?

DEFINITION OF EPIDEMIOLOGY

"**Epidemiology** is concerned with the distribution and determinants of health and diseases, morbidity, injuries, disability, and mortality in populations. Epidemiologic studies are applied to the control of health problems in populations."[5(p6)] The term epidemiology originates from the Greek: *epi* (upon) + *demos* (people) + *logy* (study of). The key characteristics of epidemiology are discussed next.

Population Focus

The unique focus of epidemiology is on the occurrence of health and disease in the population. The definition of a **population** is "[a]ll the inhabitants of a given country or area considered together…."[4] The approach of focusing on the population contrasts with clinical medicine's concern with the individual; hence epidemiology is sometimes called population medicine. Given examples of the *Salmonella* outbreak and violence in schools demonstrated epidemiologic investigations that were focused on entire population groups (such as the United States). A third example involves epidemiologic studies of lung disease; these investigations might examine the occurrence of lung cancer mortality across counties or among regional geographic subdivisions known as census tracts. Investigators might want to ascertain whether lung cancer mortality is higher in areas with higher concentrations of "smokestack" industries in comparison with areas that have lower levels of air pollution or are relatively free from air pollution. In contrast with the population approach used in epidemiology, the alternative approach of

---

EXHIBIT 1-1   What Is Epidemiology About? The Example of Bullying in Schools

Bullying occurs with alarming frequency in the nation's schools. (Refer to **Table 1-2**) It can take the form of cyberbullying and physical bullying. Any form of bullying torments victims and contributes to school avoidance.

Using data from the Youth Risk Behavior Survey, the CDC assessed the frequency of electronic bullying and also bullying on school property among the nation's high school students. Nearly 15% of U.S. high school students reported being bullied electronically during the 12 months before the 2013 survey. Bullying tactics included the use of email, instant messaging, and texting.

A greater percentage of females than males were bullied; white females experienced the highest frequency of electronic bullying among ethnic/racial groups examined.

Approximately one-fifth of high school pupils stated that they were bullied on school property. As was the case for cyberbullying, white females reported the highest frequency of school bullying among sex and racial/ethnic groups. Both forms of bullying were most common among ninth graders and declined in the later high school years.

Table 1-2 demonstrates an approach of epidemiology—comparing data according to the demographic characteristics (for example, sex, race/ethnicity, and school year) to identify population subgroups that experienced the highest frequency of bullying.

EXHIBIT 1-1 What Is Epidemiology About? The Example of Bullying in Schools (Continued)

TABLE 1-2 Percentage of High School Students Who Were Electronically Bullied*† and Who Were Bullied on School Property* by Sex, Race/Ethnicity, and Grade—United States, Youth Risk Behavior Survey, 2013.

| | Electronically Bullied | | | | | |
| | Female | | Male | | Total | |
Category	%	CI§	%	CI	%	CI
Race/ethnicity						
White¶	25.2	(22.6–28.0)	8.7	(7.5–10.1)	16.9	(15.3–18.7)
Black¶	10.5	(8.7–12.6)	6.9	(5.2–9.0)	8.7	(7.3–10.4)
Hispanic	17.1	(14.5–20.1)	8.3	(6.9–10.0)	12.8	(10.9–14.9)
Grade						
9	22.8	(19.5–26.6)	9.4	(7.9–11.1)	16.1	(14.1–18.2)
10	21.9	(18.7–25.5)	7.2	(5.4–9.6)	14.5	(12.6–16.6)
11	20.6	(17.4–24.3)	8.9	(7.3–10.7)	14.9	(13.0–16.9)
12	18.3	(16.3–20.5)	8.6	(7.0–10.5)	13.5	(12.2–14.9)
Total	21.0	(19.2–22.9)	8.5	(7.7–9.5)	14.8	(13.7–15.9)
	Bullied on School Property					
	Female		Male		Total	
Category	%	CI§	%	CI	%	CI
Race/ethnicity						
White¶	27.3	(25.0–29.8)	16.2	(14.1–18.5)	21.8	(20.0–23.7)
Black¶	15.1	(12.7–17.8)	10.2	(8.4–12.2)	12.7	(11.3–14.2)
Hispanic	20.7	(18.5–23.2)	14.8	(12.2–17.8)	17.8	(16.3–19.4)
Grade						
9	29.2	(26.2–32.5)	20.8	(18.1–23.8)	25.0	(22.9–27.2)
10	28.8	(25.5–32.2)	15.8	(13.3–18.8)	22.2	(20.1–24.4)
11	20.3	(17.2–23.7)	13.1	(11.5–15.0)	16.8	(15.0–18.8)
12	15.5	(13.3–17.9)	11.2	(8.8–14.1)	13.3	(11.5–15.4)
Total	23.7	(22.3–25.2)	15.6	(14.2–17.0)	19.6	(18.6–20.8)

*During the 12 months before the survey.

†Including being bullied through email, chat rooms, instant messaging, websites, or texting.

§95% confidence interval (CI).

¶Non-Hispanic.

Adapted and reprinted from Centers for Disease Control and Prevention. Surveillance Summaries. *MMWR.* 2014:63(SS-4);66.

clinical medicine would be for the clinician to concentrate on the diagnosis and treatment of specific individuals for the sequelae of foodborne illnesses, injuries caused by school violence, and lung cancer.

Distribution

The term **distribution** implies that the occurrence of diseases and other health outcomes varies in populations, with some subgroups of the populations more frequently affected than others. Epidemiologic research identifies subgroups that have increased occurrence of adverse health outcomes in comparison with other groups. In our exploration of epidemiology, we will encounter many illustrations of differential distributions of health outcomes: for example, variations in the occurrence of cancer, heart disease, and asthma in populations. A higher prevalence of adverse health outcomes among some subgroups in comparison with the general population may be a reflection of a phenomenon known as health disparities.

Determinants

A **determinant** is defined as "[a] collective or individual risk factor (or set of factors) that is causally related to a health condition, outcome, or other defined characteristic."[4] The term *risk factor* (an exposure that increases the probability of a disease or adverse health outcome) is discussed later in the chapter. Examples of determinants are biologic agents (e.g., bacteria and viruses), chemical agents (e.g., toxic pesticides and cancer-causing substances known as chemical carcinogens), and less specific factors (e.g., stress and deleterious lifestyle practices).

Related to determinants are **exposures**, which pertain either to contact with a disease-causing factor or to the amount of the factor that impinges upon a group or individuals. Epidemiology searches for associations between exposures and health outcomes. Examples of exposures are contact with infectious disease agents through consumption of contaminated foods and environmental exposures to toxic chemicals, potential carcinogens, or air pollution. In other cases, exposures may be to biological agents or to forms of energy such as radiation, noise, and extremes of temperature. For the results of an epidemiologic research study to be valid, the level of exposure in a population must be defined carefully; the task of exposure assessment is not easily accomplished in many types of epidemiologic research.

Outcomes

The definition of **outcomes** is "[a]ll the possible results that may stem from exposure to a causal factor...."[4] The outcomes examined in epidemiologic research range from specific infectious diseases to disabling conditions, unintentional injuries, chronic diseases, and conditions associated with personal behavior and lifestyle. These outcomes may be expressed as types and measures of **morbidity** (illnesses due to a specific disease or health condition) and **mortality** (causes of death). Accurate clinical assessments of outcomes are vitally important to the quality of epidemiologic research and the strength of inferences that can be made. Without such assessments, it would not be possible to replicate the findings of research.

Quantification

Epidemiology is a quantitative discipline; the term **quantification** refers to the counting of cases of illness or other health outcomes. Quantification means the use of statistical measures to describe the occurrence of health outcomes and to measure their association with exposures. The field of descriptive epidemiology quantifies variation of diseases and health outcomes according to subgroups of the population.

Control of Health Problems

Epidemiology aids with health promotion, alleviation of adverse health outcomes (e.g., infectious and chronic diseases), and prevention of disease. Epidemiologic methods are applicable to the development of needs assessments, the design of prevention programs, the formulation of public health policies, and the evaluation of the success of such programs. Epidemiology contributes to health policy development by providing quantitative information that can be used by policy makers.

THE EVOLVING CONCEPTION OF EPIDEMIOLOGY AS A LIBERAL ART

Epidemiology is often considered to be a biomedical science that relies on a specific methodology and high-level technical skills.[6] Nevertheless, epidemiology in many respects also is a "low-tech" science that can be appreciated by those who do not specialize in this field.[7] The following text box lists skills acquired through the study of epidemiology; these skills enlarge one's appreciation of many academic fields: laboratory sciences, mathematics, the social sciences, history, and literature.

The Interdisciplinary Approach

Epidemiology is an **interdisciplinary science**, meaning that it uses information from many fields. Here are a few examples

Skills acquired through training in epidemiology

1. Use of the interdisciplinary approach
2. Use of the scientific method
3. Enhancement of critical-thinking ability
   a. Reasoning by analogy and deduction
   b. Problem solving
4. Use of quantitative and computer methods
5. Communication skills
6. Inculcation of aesthetic values

of the specializations that contribute to epidemiology and the types of input that they make:

- Mathematics and biostatistics (for quantitative methods)
- History (for historical accounts of disease and early epidemiologic methods)
- Sociology (social determinants of disease)
- Demography and geography (population structures and location of disease outbreaks)
- Behavioral sciences (models of disease; design of health promotion programs)
- Law (examining evidence to establish causality; legal bases for health policy)

Many of the issues of importance to contemporary society do not have clearly delineated disciplinary boundaries. For example, prevention of school violence requires an interdisciplinary approach that draws on information from sociology, behavioral sciences, and the legal profession. In helping to develop solutions to the problem of school violence, epidemiology leverages information from mathematics (e.g., statistics on the occurrence of violence), medicine (e.g., treatment of victims of violence), behavioral and social sciences (e.g., behavioral and social aspects of violence), and law (legal basis for development of school-related antiviolence programs). Through the study of epidemiology, one acquires an appreciation of the interdisciplinary approach and a broader understanding of a range of disciplines.

Use of the Scientific Method

Epidemiology is a scientific discipline that makes use of a body of research methods similar to those used in the basic sciences and applied fields, including biostatistics. The work of the epidemiologist is driven by theories, hypotheses, and empirical data. The scientific method employs a systematic approach and objectivity in evaluating the results of research. Comparison groups are used to examine the effects of exposures. Epidemiology uses rigorous study designs, which include cross-sectional, ecologic, case-control, and cohort studies.

Enhancement of Critical-Thinking Ability

Critical-thinking skills include the following: reasoning by analogy, making deductions that follow from a set of evidence, and solving problems. We will learn that epidemiologists use analogical reasoning to infer disease causality. Suppose there are two similar diseases. The etiology of the first disease is known, but the etiology of the second disease is unknown. By analogy, one can reason that the etiology of the second disease must be similar to that of the first.

Also, epidemiologists gather descriptive information on the occurrence of diseases; they use this information to develop hypotheses regarding specific exposures that might have been associated with those diseases. Finally, epidemiologists are called into action to solve problems, for example, trying to control foodborne disease outbreaks caused by *Salmonella* and *E. coli*, slowing epidemic diseases such as Ebola virus disease, and determining whether microcephaly is a consequence of Zika virus infection.

Use of Quantitative and Computer Methods

Biostatistics is one of the core disciplines of epidemiology. Because of the close linkage between the two fields, epidemiology and biostatistics are housed in the same academic department in some universities. Through your training in epidemiology, you will acquire quantitative skills, such as tabulating numbers of cases, making subgroup comparisons, and mapping associations between exposures and health outcomes. In research and agency settings, epidemiologists use computers to store, retrieve, and process health-related information and to perform these types of analyses. An intriguing development is the field of "big data," which processes massive reservoirs of data from sources that include social media and commercial transactions. Those who become tech savvy may be able to detect patterns that help to discern the presence and determinants of epidemics as well as risk factors for infectious and chronic diseases.

Communication Skills

As a core discipline of public health, epidemiology is an applied field. Information from epidemiologic analyses can be used to control diseases, improve the health of the community, evaluate intervention programs, and inform public policy. One of the skills needed by applied epidemiologists is the ability to disseminate information that could be useful for controlling health problems and improving the health status of the population.

Inculcation of Aesthetic Values

Aesthetic values are concerned with the appreciation of beauty, which would seem to have no relevance to epidemiology. Nevertheless, you can hone your aesthetic values by reading about the history of epidemiology and descriptions of epidemics and health problems found in literature. The writings of the great thinkers such as Hippocrates and John Snow, who contributed so greatly to epidemiology, are compelling as works of literature. Many other writings relevant to epidemiology are extant. Two are *The Jungle* (by Upton Sinclair), which describes deplorable sanitary conditions in Chicago slaughterhouses in 1906, and Camus' *The Plague*, an account of the ravages of disease.

APPLICATION OF DESCRIPTIVE AND ANALYTIC METHODS TO AN OBSERVATIONAL SCIENCE

In examining the occurrence of health and disease in human populations, researchers almost always are prohibited from using experimental methods because of ethical issues, such as potential harm to subjects. Studies of the population's health present a challenge to epidemiologic methods. First and foremost, epidemiology is an **observational science** that capitalizes on naturally occurring situations in order to study the occurrence of disease. Thus, in order to study the association of cigarette smoking with lung diseases, epidemiologists might examine and compare the frequency of lung cancer and other lung diseases among smokers and nonsmokers.

Descriptive Epidemiology

From past history until the present era, epidemiologists have implemented descriptive epidemiology (and descriptive epidemiologic studies) as one of the fundamental applications of the field.[8] The term **descriptive epidemiology** refers to epidemiologic studies that are concerned with characterizing the amount and distribution of health and disease within a population. Health outcomes are classified according to the variables of person, place, and time. Examples of person variables are demographic characteristics such as sex, age, and race/ethnicity. Place variables denote geographic locations, including a specific country or countries, areas within countries, and places where localized patterns of disease may occur. Illustrations of time variables are a decade, a year, a month, a week, or a day. These studies, which aid in

the development of hypotheses, set the stage for subsequent research that examines the etiology of disease.

Analytic Epidemiology

Analytic epidemiology examines causal (etiologic) hypotheses regarding the association between exposures and health conditions. The field of analytic epidemiology proposes and evaluates causal models for etiologic associations and studies them empirically. "Etiologic studies are planned examinations of causality and the natural history of disease. These studies have required increasingly sophisticated analytic methods as the importance of low-level exposures is explored and greater refinement in exposure–effect relationships is sought."[9(p945)] Note that the natural history of disease refers to the time course of disease from its beginning to its final clinical endpoints. For more information see the chapter on epidemiology and screening for disease.

One approach of analytic epidemiology is to take advantage of naturally occurring situations or events in order to test causal hypotheses. These naturally occurring events are referred to as **natural experiments**, defined as "[n]aturally occurring circumstances in which subsets of the population have different levels of exposure to a hypothesized causal factor in a situation resembling an actual experiment. The presence of people in a particular group is typically nonrandom."[4] An example of a natural experiment is the work of John Snow, discussed later in this chapter. Many past and ongoing natural experiments are relevant to environmental epidemiology. When new public health–related laws and regulations are introduced, their implementation becomes similar to natural experiments that could be explored in epidemiologic research. For example, epidemiologists could study whether motor vehicle laws that limit texting while driving reduce the frequency of automobile crashes. Other examples of natural experiments that have evolved from laws are the addition of fluoride to the public water supply in order to prevent tooth decay and the requirement that children wear safety helmets while riding bicycles.

HISTORY OF EPIDEMIOLOGY AND DEVELOPMENT OF EPIDEMIOLOGIC PRINCIPLES

The history of epidemiology originated as early as classical antiquity (before about 500 CE), and later during the medieval period, which was marked by bubonic plague epidemics in Europe. The Renaissance was the era of Paracelsus, a toxicologist, and John Graunt, a pioneering compiler of vital statistics. During the eighteenth and nineteenth centuries, breakthroughs occurred in the development of a vaccination against smallpox and the formulation of epidemiologic methods. The period from the beginning of the twentieth century to the present has seen a rapid growth in epidemiology; two of the achievements of this period were identification of smoking as a cause of cancer and eradication of smallpox. (Refer to **Figure 1-5** for a brief epidemiology history time line.)

The Period of Classical Antiquity (before 500 CE)

Hippocrates (460 BCE–370 BCE)

The ancient Greek authority Hippocrates contributed to epidemiology by departing from superstitious reasons for disease outbreaks. Until Hippocrates' time, supernatural explanations were used to account for the diseases that ravaged human populations. In about 400 BCE, Hippocrates suggested that environmental factors such as water quality and the air were implicated in the causation of diseases. He authored the historically important book *On Airs, Waters, and Places*. Hippocrates' work and the writings of many of the ancients did not delineate specific known agents involved in the causality of health problems but referred more generically to air, water, and food. In this respect, early epidemiology shares with contemporary epidemiology the frequent lack of complete knowledge of the specific agents of disease, especially those associated with chronic diseases.

FIGURE 1-5 History of epidemiology.

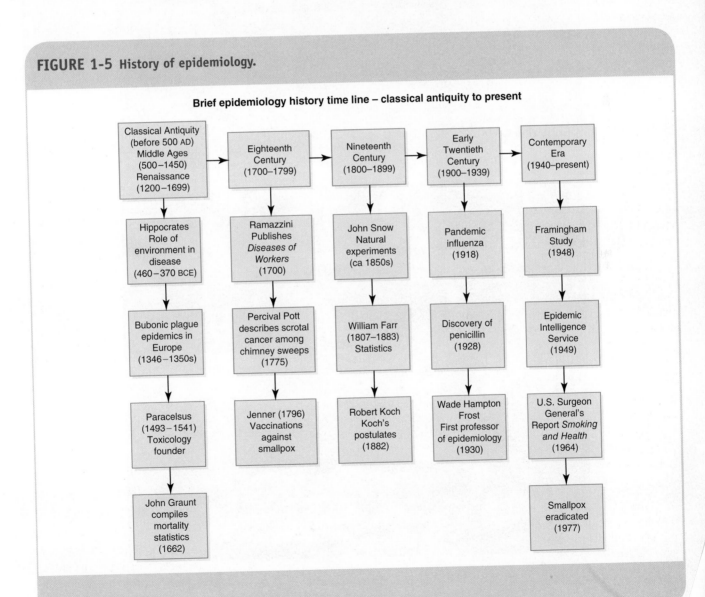

Brief epidemiology history time line – classical antiquity to present

Middle Ages (approximately 500–1450)

Black Death

Of great significance for epidemiology is the Black Death, which occurred between 1346 and 1352 and claimed up to one-third of the population of Europe at the time (20 to 30 million out of 100 million people). The Black Death was thought to be an epidemic of bubonic plague, a bacterial disease caused by *Yersinia pestis*. (Refer to **Figure 1-6** for a drawing of plague victims.) Bubonic plague is characterized by painful swellings of the lymph nodes (buboes) in the groin and elsewhere in the body. Other symptoms often

FIGURE 1-6 Black Death.

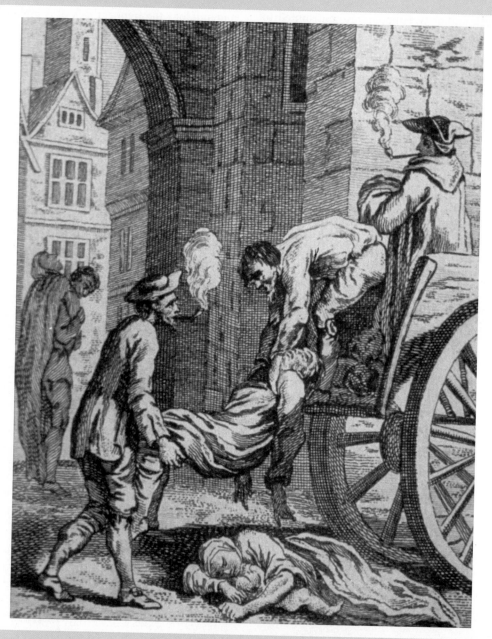

FIGURE 1-7 This patient presented with symptoms of plague that included gangrene of the right foot causing necrosis (tissue death) of the toes.

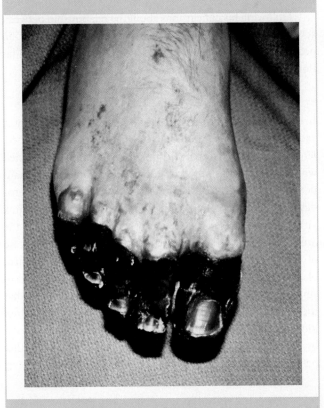

Reprinted from Centers for Disease Control and Prevention. Public Health Image Library, ID# 4139. Available at: http://phil.cdc.gov/phil/home.asp. Accessed February 6, 2016.

include fever and the appearance of black splotches on the skin. (Refer to **Figure 1-7**.) Untreated, bubonic plague kills up to 60% of its victims. The bites of fleas harbored by rats and some other types of rodents can transmit plague.

Renaissance (approximately 1200–1699)

Paracelsus (1493–1541)

Paracelsus was one of the founders of the field of toxicology, a discipline that is used to examine the toxic effects of chemicals found in environmental venues such as the workplace. Active during the time of da Vinci and Copernicus, Paracelsus advanced toxicology during the early sixteenth century. Among his contributions were several important concepts: the dose-response relationship, which refers to the observation that the effects of a poison are related to the strength of its dose, and the notion of target organ specificity of chemicals.

John Graunt (1620–1674)

In 1662, John Graunt published *Natural and Political Observations Mentioned in a Following Index, and Made Upon the Bills of Mortality*. This work recorded descriptive characteristics of birth and death data, including seasonal variations, infant mortality, and excess male over female mortality. Graunt is said to be the first to employ quantitative methods to describe population vital statistics by organizing mortality data in a mortality table. Because of his contributions to vital statistics, Graunt has been called the Columbus of statistics.

Eighteenth Century (1700–1799)

Ramazzini (1633–1714)

Bernardino Ramazzini is regarded as the founder of the field of occupational medicine.[10] He created elaborate descriptions of the manifestations of occupational diseases among many different types of workers.[11] His descriptions covered a plethora of occupations, from miners to cleaners of privies to fabric workers. The father of occupational medicine is also considered to be a pioneer in the field of ergonomics, by pointing out the hazards associated with postures assumed in various occupations. Ramazzini authored *De Morbis Artificum Diatriba* (Diseases of Workers), published in 1700. His book highlighted the risks posed by hazardous chemicals, dusts, and metals used in the workplace.

Sir Percival Pott (1714–1788)

Sir Percival Pott, a London surgeon, is thought to be the first individual to describe an environmental cause of cancer. In 1775, Pott made the astute observation that chimney sweeps had a high incidence of scrotal cancer (in comparison with male workers in other occupations.)[12] He argued that chimney sweeps were prone to this malady as a consequence of their contact with soot.

In a book titled *Chirurgical Observations Relative to the Cataract, the Polypus of the Nose, the Cancer of the Scrotum, the Different Kinds of Ruptures, and the Mortification of the Toes and Feet*, Pott developed a chapter called "A Short Treatise of the Chimney Sweeper's Cancer." This brief work of only 725 words is noteworthy because "... it provided the first clear description of an environmental cause of cancer, suggested a way to prevent the disease, and led indirectly to the synthesis of the first known pure carcinogen and the isolation of the first carcinogenic chemical to be obtained from a natural product. No wonder therefore that Pott's observation has come to be regarded as the foundation stone on w[h]ich the knowledge of cancer prevention has been built!"[13(p521)] In Pott's own words,

> ... every body... is acquainted with the disorders to which painters, plummers, glaziers, and the workers in white lead are liable; but there is a disease as peculiar to a certain set of people which has not, at least to my knowledge, been publickly noteced; I mean the chimney-sweepers' cancer.... The fate of these people seems singularly hard; in their early infancy, they are most frequently treated with great brutality, and almost starved with cold and hunger; they are thrust up narrow, and sometimes hot chimnies, where they are bruised, burned, and almost suffocated; and when they get to puberty, become peculiary [sic] liable to a noisome, painful and fatal disease. Of this last circumstance there is not the least doubt though perhaps it may not have been sufficiently attended to, to make it generally known. Other people have cancers of the same part; and so have others besides lead-workers, the Poictou colic, and the consequent paralysis; but it is nevertheless a disease to which they are particularly liable; and so

are chimney-sweepers to the cancer of the scrotum and testicles. The disease, in these people... seems to derive its origin from a lodgment of soot in the rugae of the scrotum.[13(pp521–522)]

Following his conclusions about the relationship between scrotal cancer and chimney sweeping, Pott established an occupational hygiene control measure—the recommendation that chimney sweeps bathe once a week.

Edward Jenner (1749–1823)

In 1798, Jenner's findings regarding his development of a vaccine that provided immunity to smallpox were published. Jenner had observed that dairymaids who had been infected with cowpox (transmitted by cattle) were immune to smallpox. The cowpox virus, known as the vaccinia virus, produces a milder infection in humans than does the smallpox virus. Jenner created a vaccine by using material from the arm of a dairymaid, Sarah Nelmes, who had an active case of cowpox. In 1796, the vaccine was injected into the arm of an 8-year-old boy, James Fipps, who was later exposed to smallpox and did not develop the disease. Concluding that the procedure was effective, Jenner vaccinated other children including his own son. **Figure 1-8** displays an 1802 cartoon by British satirist James Gillray. The cartoon implied that people who were vaccinated would become part cow.

FIGURE 1-8 The Cow Pock—or—the Wonderful Effects of the New Inoculation.

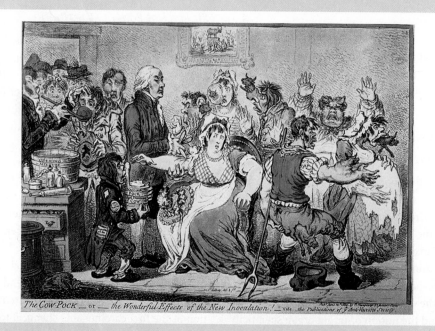

The Cow-Pock — or — the Wonderful Effects of the New Inoculation! — Vide. the Publications of ye Anti-Vaccine Society.

Drawing by James Gillray, 1802. Reprinted from National Institutes of Health, National Library of Medicine. Smallpox: A Great and Terrible Scourge. Available at: http://www.nlm.nih.gov/exhibition/smallpox/sp_vaccination.html. Accessed February 6, 2016.

Nineteenth Century (1800–1899)

John Snow and Cholera in London during the Mid-Nineteenth Century

Over the centuries, cholera has inspired great fear because of the dramatic symptoms and mortality that it causes. Cholera is a potentially highly fatal disease marked by profuse watery stools, called rice water stools. The onset of cholera is sudden and marked by painless diarrhea that can progress to dehydration and circulatory collapse; severe, untreated cholera outbreaks can kill more than one-half of affected cases. At present, the cause of cholera is known (the bacterium *Vibrio cholerae*); the level of fatality is often less than 1% when the disease is treated. One of the methods for transmission of cholera is through ingestion of contaminated water (see **Figure 1-9**).

John Snow (1813–1858), an English anesthesiologist, innovated several of the key epidemiologic methods that remain valid and in use today. In recognition of his groundbreaking contributions, many epidemiologists consider Snow to be the father of the field. For example, Snow believed that the disease cholera was transmitted by contaminated water and was able to demonstrate this association. In Snow's time, the mechanism for the causation of infectious diseases such as cholera was largely unknown. The Dutchman Anton van Leeuwenhoek had used the microscope to observe microorganisms (bacteria and yeast). However, the connection between microorganisms and disease had not yet been ascertained. One of the explanations for infectious diseases was the **miasmatic theory of disease**, which held that "… disease was transmitted by a miasm, or cloud, that clung low on the surface of the earth."[14(p11)] This theory was applied to malaria, among other diseases.

Snow noted that an outbreak of "Asiatic" cholera had occurred in India during the early 1800s. Snow wrote, "The first case of decided Asiatic cholera in London, in the autumn of 1848, was that of a seaman named John Harnold, who had newly arrived by the Elbe steamer from Hamburgh, where the disease was prevailing."[15(p3)] Cholera then began to appear in London.

During the mid-1800s, Snow conducted an investigation of a cholera outbreak in London. A section of London, designated the Broad Street neighborhood (now part of the Soho district), became the focus of Snow's detective work (refer to the map shown in **Figure 1-10**). His procedures for investigating the cholera outbreak demonstrated several important innovations (summarized in the text box titled "John Snow, MD, the forerunner of modern epidemiologists").

Here is Snow's graphic description of the cholera outbreak that occurred in 1849. "The most terrible outbreak of cholera which ever occurred in this kingdom, is probably that which took place in Broad Street, Golden Square, and the adjoining streets, a few weeks ago…. The mortality in this limited area probably equals any that was ever caused in this country, even by the plague; and it was much more sudden, as the greater number of cases terminated in a few hours…. Many houses were closed altogether, owing to the death of the proprietors; and, in a great number of instances, the tradesmen who remained had sent away their families: so that in less than six days from the commencement of the outbreak, the most afflicted streets were deserted by more than three-quarters of their inhabitants."[15(p38)]

Snow's pioneering approach illustrated the use of both descriptive and analytic epidemiology. One of his first activities was to plot the cholera deaths in relation to a pump that he hypothesized was the cause of the cholera outbreak. Each death was shown on the map (Figure 1-10) as a short line. An arrow in the figure points to the location of the Broad Street

---

FIGURE 1-9 Typical water supply that is contaminated with *Vibrio cholerae*, the infectious disease agent for cholera.

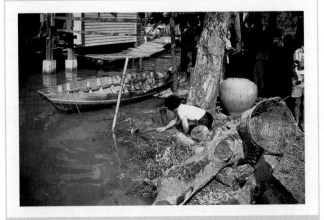

Reprinted from Centers for Disease Control and Prevention. Public Health Image Library, ID# 1940. Available at: http://phil.cdc.gov/phil/home.asp. Accessed February 6, 2016.

John Snow, MD, the forerunner of modern epidemiologists

Snow's contributions to epidemiology included:

- Powers of observation and written expression
- Application of epidemiologic methods
  - Mapping (spot maps)
  - Use of data tables to describe infectious disease outbreaks
- Participation in a natural experiment
- Recommendation of a public health measure to prevent disease (removal of the pump handle; see text)

FIGURE 1-10 Map of cholera cases in the Broad Street, London area. Each case is indicated by a short line.

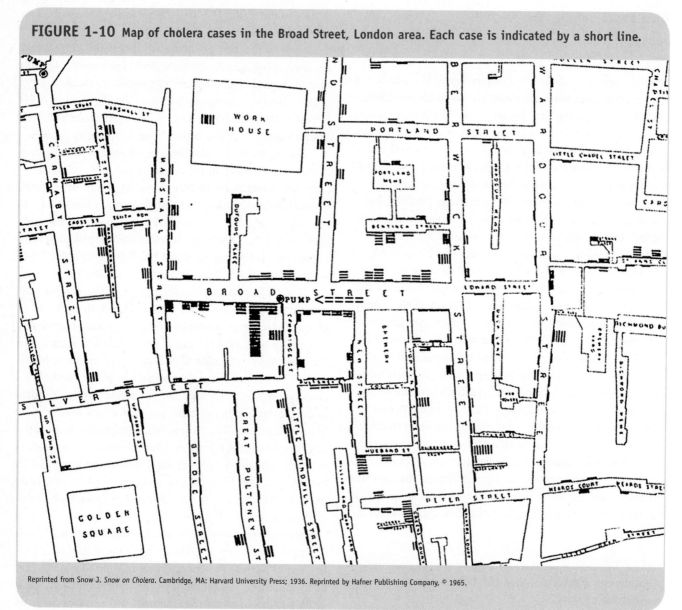

Reprinted from Snow J. *Snow on Cholera*. Cambridge, MA: Harvard University Press; 1936. Reprinted by Hafner Publishing Company, © 1965.

pump. "As soon as I became acquainted with the situation and the extent of this irruption of cholera, I suspected some contamination of the water of the much-frequented street-pump in Broad Street, near the end of Cambridge Street;... On proceeding to the spot, I found that nearly all the deaths had taken place within a short distance of the pump."[15(pp38–39)] The handle of the pump was later removed—a public health measure to control the outbreak. In Snow's time, many European cities took water for domestic use directly from rivers, which often were contaminated with microorganisms. (Refer to **Figure 1-11**, which suggests that pumps that dispensed river water were sources of deadly contamination.)

The natural experiment: Two water companies, the Lambeth Company and the Southwark and Vauxhall Company,

provided water in such a manner that adjacent houses could receive water from two different sources. In 1852, one of the companies, the Lambeth Company, relocated its water sources to a section of the Thames River that was less contaminated. During a later cholera outbreak in 1854, Snow observed that a higher proportion of residents who used the water from the Southwark and Vauxhall Company developed cholera than did residents who used water from the Lambeth Company. The correspondence between changes in the quality of the water supply and changes in the occurrence of cholera became known as a natural experiment.

Data from the outbreak of 1854 are presented in **Table 1-3**. The Lambeth Company provided cleaner water than the Southwark and Vauxhall Company. "The mortality

FIGURE 1-11 Death lurks at the pump.

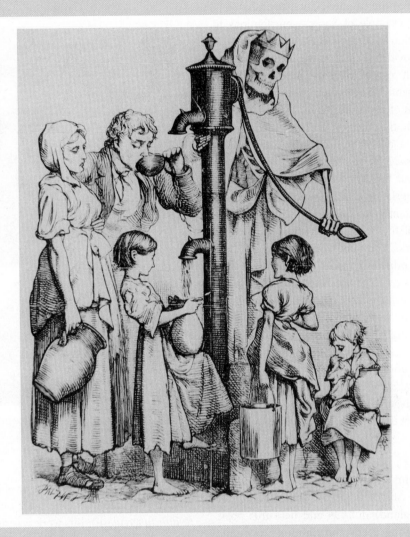

© SPL/Science Source.

TABLE 1-3 The Proportion of Deaths per 10,000 Houses—Cholera Epidemic of 1854

	Number of Houses	Deaths from Cholera	Deaths in Each 10,000 Houses
Southwark and Vauxhaul Company	40,046	1,263	315
Lambeth Company	26,107	98	37
Rest of London	256,423	1,422	59

Reprinted from Snow J. *Snow on Cholera*. Cambridge, MA: Harvard University Press; 1936; reprinted by Hafner Publishing Company © 1965:86.

in the houses supplied by the Southwark and Vauxhall Company was therefore between eight and nine times as great as in the houses supplied by the Lambeth Company….”[15(p86)]

Here is a second example of Snow's contributions to epidemiology. In addition to utilizing the method of natural experiment, Snow provided expert witness testimony on behalf of industry with respect to environmental exposures to potential disease agents.[16] Snow attempted to extrapolate from the health effects of exposures to high doses of environmental substances to the effects of exposure to low doses. On January 23, 1855, a bill was introduced in the British Parliament called the Nuisances Removal and Diseases Prevention Amendments bill. This bill was a reform of Victorian public health legislation that followed the 1854 cholera epidemic.[16] The intent of the bill was to control release into the atmosphere of fumes from operations such as gas works, silk-boiling works, and bone-boiling factories. Snow contended that these odiferous fumes were not a disease hazard in the community.[17] The thesis of Snow's argument was that deleterious health effects from the low levels of exposure experienced in the community were unlikely, given the knowledge about higher-level exposures among those who worked in the factories. Snow argued that the workers in the factories were not suffering any ill health effects or dying from the exposures. Therefore, it was unlikely that the much lower exposures experienced by the members of the larger community would affect their health.

William Farr (1807–1883)

A contemporary of John Snow, William Farr assumed the post of "Compiler of Abstracts" at the General Register Office (located in England) in 1839 and held this position for 40 years. Among Farr's contributions to public health and epidemiology was the development of a more sophisticated system for codifying medical conditions than that which was previously in use. Also noteworthy is the fact that Farr used data such as census reports to study occupational mortality in England. In addition, he explored the possible linkage between mortality rates and population density, showing that both the average number of deaths and births per 1,000 living persons increased with population density (defined as number of persons per square mile).

Robert Koch (1843–1910)

The German physician Robert Koch (**Figure 1-12**) verified that a human disease was caused by a specific living organism. He isolated the bacteria that cause anthrax (*Bacillus anthracis*)

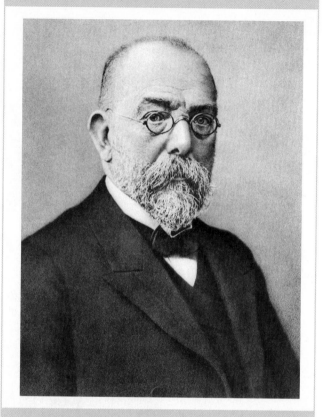

FIGURE 1-12 Robert Koch.

© National Library of Medicine.

and cholera (*Vibrio cholerae*). One of his most famous contributions was identifying the cause of tuberculosis (*Mycobacterium tuberculosis*); this work was described in 1882 in *Die Aetiologie der Tuberkulose*. Koch's four postulates to demonstrate the association between a microorganism and a disease were formatted as follows:

1. The organism must be observed in every case of the disease.
2. It must be isolated and grown in pure culture.
3. The pure culture must, when inoculated into a susceptible animal, reproduce the disease.
4. The organism must be observed in, and recovered from, the experimental animal.[18]

Early Twentieth Century (1900–1940)
Pandemic Influenza

Also known as the Spanish Flu, this pandemic raged from 1918 to 1919 and killed 50 to 100 million people globally.

Estimates suggest that one-third of the world's population, which then was 1.5 billion, became infected and developed clinically observable illness. Instead of primarily attacking the young and the elderly as is usually the situation with influenza, the Spanish Flu took a heavy toll on healthy young adults. One hypothesis is that the influenza virus interacted with respiratory bacteria, causing numerous deaths from bacterial pneumonias. The death rate was so high that morgues were overflowing with bodies awaiting burial; adequate supplies of coffins and the services of morticians were unavailable. To handle the influx of patients, special field hospitals were set up. (See **Figure 1-13**.)

Discovery of Penicillin

Scottish researcher Alexander Fleming (1881–1955) discovered the antimicrobial properties of the mold *Penicillium notatum* in 1928. This breakthrough led to development of the antibiotic penicillin, which became available toward the end of World War II.

The Contemporary Era (1940 to the present)

From the mid-twentieth century to the present (first quarter of the twenty-first century), epidemiology has made numerous contributions to society. These innovations include:

- Framingham Study. Begun in 1948, this pioneering research project is named for Framingham, Massachusetts, where initially, a random sample of 6,500 persons age 30 to 59 years participated. This project has been responsible for gathering basic information about aspects of health such as the etiology of coronary heart disease.
- Epidemic Intelligence Service. Alexander Langmuir was hired by the Centers for Disease Control and Prevention as the first chief epidemiologist. One of Langmuir's contributions was the establishment in 1949 of the Epidemic Intelligence Service (EIS). In the beginning, the mission of EIS was to combat bioterrorism. Presently, EIS officers aid in the rapid response to public health needs both domestically and internationally.

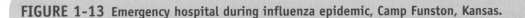

FIGURE 1-13 Emergency hospital during influenza epidemic, Camp Funston, Kansas.

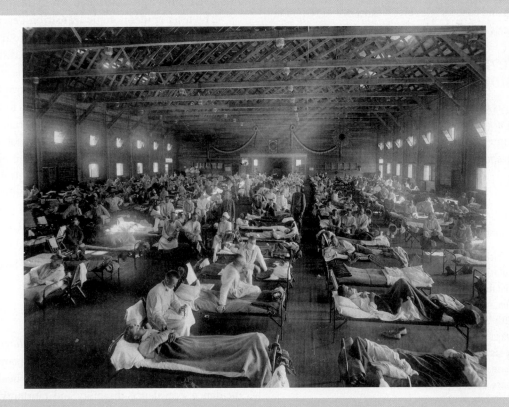

© National Museum of Health and Medicine, Armed Forces Institute of Pathology, (NCP 1603).

- Smoking and health. By the mid-twentieth century, a growing body of evidence suggested that cigarette smoking contributed to early mortality from lung cancer as well as other forms of morbidity and mortality. In 1964, the U.S. Surgeon General released *Smoking and Health*,[19] which asserted that cigarette smoking is a cause of lung cancer in men and is linked to other disabling or fatal diseases.
- Smallpox eradication. As noted previously, Jenner pioneered development of a smallpox vaccine during the 1800s. Smallpox is an incurable disease caused by a virus. One form of the virus, variola major, produces a highly fatal infection in unvaccinated populations. Because of a highly effective surveillance and vaccination program that was intensified during the late 1960s, the ancient scourge of smallpox was brought under control. The last known naturally acquired case was reported in Somalia in 1977.
- Some newer developments. More recent contributions of epidemiology include helping to discover the association between the human papillomavirus and cervical cancer, the correspondence between a bacterium (*Helicobacter pylori*) and peptic ulcers, the correlation between genetic factors and cancers (e.g., breast cancer), and responding to threats from emerging infectious diseases.

BRIEF OVERVIEW OF CURRENT USES OF EPIDEMIOLOGY

Epidemiologists are indebted to J.N. Morris,[20] who published a list of seven uses of epidemiology; Morris' original formulation has continued to be relevant to the modern era. Five of these uses are shown in the following text box.

Among the principal uses of epidemiology are the following:

- Historical use: Study the history of the health of populations.
- Community health use: Diagnose the health of the community.
- Health services use: Study the working of health services.
- Risk assessment use: Estimate individuals' risks of disease, accident, or defect.
- Disease causality use: Search for the causes of health and disease.

Adapted from Morris JN. *Uses of Epidemiology*. 3rd ed. Edinburgh, UK: Churchill Livingstone; 1975:262–263.

Historical Use

The historical use of epidemiology documents the patterns, types, and causes of morbidity and mortality over time. Since the early 1900s, in developed countries the causes of mortality have shifted from those related primarily to infectious and communicable diseases to chronic conditions. This use is illustrated by changes over time in the causes of mortality in the United States. For example, **Figure 1-14** shows the decline in the rate of influenza and pneumonia mortality between 1900 and 2013. Mortality from infectious diseases rose sharply during the influenza pandemic of 1918 and then resumed its downward trend. In the early 1980s, mortality from infectious diseases increased again because of the impact of human immunodeficiency virus (HIV) disease. Mortality from HIV disease subsequently declined and caused 12,543 deaths in 2005; during that year, the leading causes of death in the United States were heart disease, cancer, and stroke. In 2013, heart disease and cancer remained as the top two leading causes of mortality, but the category chronic lower respiratory diseases (chronic bronchitis, emphysema, and asthma) replaced stroke as the third leading cause of death; a total of 6,955 deaths were associated with HIV.[21]

The term **epidemiologic transition** describes a shift in the patterns of morbidity and mortality from causes related primarily to infectious and communicable diseases to causes associated with chronic, degenerative diseases. The epidemiologic transition coincides with the **demographic transition**, a shift from high birth rates and death rates found in agrarian societies to much lower birth and death rates in developed countries. **Figure 1-15** shows the stage of epidemiologic transition across the top and the stage of demographic transition across the bottom. These two kinds of transition parallel one another over time. The figure is subdivided into four segments: pre, early, late, and post. Refer to the figure for the definitions of these stages. At present, the United States is in the posttransition stage, which is dominated by diseases associated with personal behavior, adverse lifestyle, and emerging infections.

Community Health Use

Morris described this use as follows: "To *diagnose the health of the community* and the condition of the people, to measure the true dimensions and distribution of ill-health in terms of incidence, prevalence, disability and mortality; to set health problems in perspective and define their relative importance; to identify groups needing special attention."[20(p262)]

Examples of characteristics that affect the health of the community are age and sex distributions, racial/ethnic

FIGURE 1-14 Rate* of influenza and pneumonia mortality, by year—United States, 1900–2013.

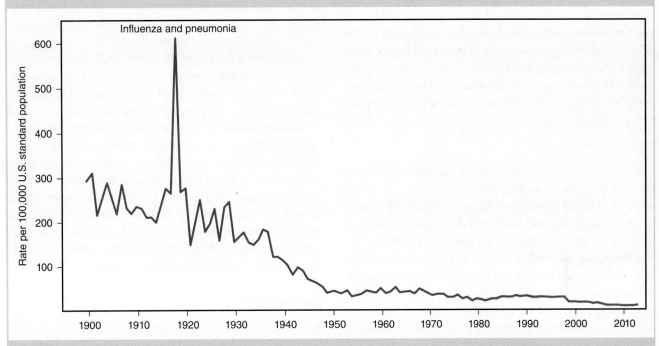

*Age-adjusted
Reproduced from Chong Y, Tejada Vera B, Lu L, Anderson RN, Arias E, Sutton PD: Deaths in the United States, 1900–2013. Hyattsville, MD: National Center for Health Statistics. 2015. Available at: https://blogs.cdc.gov/nchs-data-visualization/deaths-in-the-us/. Accessed November 17, 2016.

FIGURE 1-15 Demographic/epidemiologic transition framework.

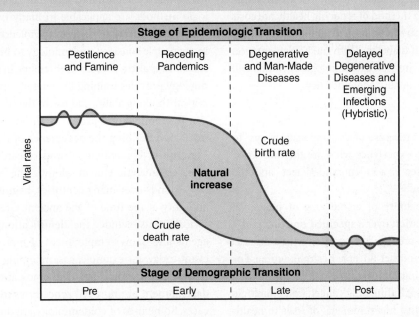

Reprinted from Rockett IRH. Population and health: an introduction to epidemiology, 2nd ed. *Population Bulletin,* December 1999;54(4):9. Reprinted with permission of Population Reference Bureau.

makeup, socioeconomic status, employment and unemployment rates, access to healthcare services, population density, and residential mobility. These variables are reflected in a wide range of outcomes: life expectancy, social conditions, and patterns of morbidity and mortality. Concerning for the field of epidemiology and public health professionals is the impact of demographic and socioeconomic factors on health disparities observed in many communities. The communities where people live are very salient for adverse health outcomes and, conversely, a healthy life.

Health Services Use

Morris also proposed that epidemiology could be used "to study the *working of health services* with a view to their improvement. Operational (operations) research translates knowledge of (changing) community health and expectations in terms of needs for services and measure [sic] how these are met."[20(p262)]

Operations research is defined as a type of study of the placement of health services in a community and the optimum utilization of such services. Epidemiology helps to provide quantitative information regarding the availability and cost of healthcare services. Epidemiologic studies aid planners in determining what services are needed in the community and what services are duplicated unnecessarily. Provision of healthcare services is exceedingly costly for society; epidemiologic methods can provide inputs into cost-benefit analyses, which balance cost issues against quality of services in order to maximize cost effectiveness. Epidemiologic findings are relevant to the current era of managed care through **disease management**; this term refers to a method of reducing healthcare costs by providing integrated care for chronic conditions (e.g., heart disease, hypertension, and diabetes). With the implementation of the 2010 Affordable Care Act, epidemiologic methods will be germane to healthcare quality and efficiency.

Risk Assessment Use

According to Morris, the purpose of this application was "to estimate from the group experience what are the *individual* risks on average of disease, accident and defect, and the *chances* of avoiding them."[20(p262)]

Risk is "[t]he probability of an adverse or beneficial event in a defined population over a specified time interval."[4] A **risk factor** is an exposure that is associated with a disease, morbidity, mortality, or another adverse health outcome. For example, cigarette smoking increases the risk of contracting certain forms of cancer, including lung cancer. Epidemiologic studies provide quantitative measurements of risks to health through a methodology known as risk assessment, which is one of the major cornerstones of health policy development.

Disease Causality Use

With respect to this use, Morris wrote, "To *search for causes* of health and disease by computing the experience of groups defined by their composition, inheritance and experience, their behaviour [sic] and environments."[20(p262)]

The search for causes of disease and other health outcomes is one of the most important uses of epidemiology. In order to assess potential causal associations, epidemiologists need to consider a set of causal criteria, such as the strength of association between exposure and health outcome. Descriptive epidemiologic studies can suggest hypotheses to be studied by employing analytic study designs. Possible associations can be evaluated by analytic study designs; these designs include case-control and cohort studies. Other analytic studies involve natural experiments, clinical trials, and community trials. We will learn that study designs, whether observational or analytic, can be arranged in a hierarchy according to our confidence in the validity of the information that they provide.

CONCLUSION

Epidemiologists study the occurrence of diseases and health outcomes in populations. Findings from epidemiologic research are reported frequently in the popular media. For example, disease outbreaks such as those caused by foodborne illnesses often command public attention. Chapter 1 defined some of the terms that are used to describe disease outbreaks, discussed the scope and applications of epidemiology, and presented information on its interdisciplinary composition. Epidemiologic methods are applicable to many types of health-related issues, from infectious diseases to violence in schools. Although many people consider epidemiology to be essentially a medical subject, it is also a liberal arts discipline in many respects; epidemiology provides training in generally applicable skills such as critical-thinking ability and use of the scientific method.

Epidemiology is primarily an observational science that involves describing the occurrence of disease in populations (descriptive epidemiology) and researching the etiology of diseases (analytic epidemiology). The history of epidemiology extends over many centuries, beginning during classical antiquity at the time of the ancient Greeks. Subsequent historical events included the identification of infectious disease agents and Snow's employment of methods that remain relevant today, for example, case mapping and data tabulation. Recent history has included eradication of smallpox and development of improved procedures to control chronic diseases. Some uses of epidemiology are documenting trends in health and disease, diagnosing the health of the community, and identifying needed health services.

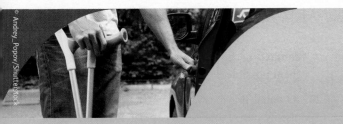

Study Questions and Exercises

1. Define the following terms:
   a. Epidemic
   b. Pandemic
   c. Epidemiology

2. Name and discuss three of the key characteristics of epidemiology.

3. In what respects does epidemiology differ from clinical medicine?

4. What are some examples of risk factors for disease that you experience in your life? Be sure to define what is meant by a risk factor.

5. Check your local library or go online to find works of literature that describe epidemics and epidemic detective work. A recommended title is Berton Roueché's classic, *The Medical Detectives* (New York, NY: Penguin Books; 1991). This work describes "Eleven Blue Men" and other fascinating episodes of medical investigations.

6. Distinguish between the descriptive and analytic approaches to epidemiology.

7. The following list shows individuals who contributed to the history of epidemiology. Describe each of their contributions.
   a. Hippocrates
   b. John Graunt
   c. Sir Percival Pott
   d. Robert Koch
   e. Alexander Fleming

8. Discuss four uses of epidemiology. For each use, give examples that were not mentioned in the textbook. Rank the uses according to their importance for public health.

9. Find an article in the popular media (either in the print media or online) that illustrates one or more uses of epidemiology. Write a one-page summary of the article and highlight the uses of epidemiology that are relevant to the topic presented. If you are enrolled in a class, be prepared to discuss the article in the class.

10. How could epidemiology be used to research and develop solutions to the problems of electronic bullying and bullying on school campuses? In what sense are the events an appropriate topic for epidemiologic investigation? Why do you think a greater percentage of females than males report electronic bullying?

11. New outbreaks of disease erupt periodically in the United States and elsewhere around the globe. Some of these conditions are familiar, whereas others are entirely new. List at least three outbreaks of disease that have happened in the last 6 months. If you are enrolled in a class, create an online forum in which you catalog recent and current epidemics.

12. What are your objectives for studying epidemiology? What skills do you hope to acquire? How will this information help you to advance your career in public health? Demonstrate ways in which this course can help you with your present position, regardless of whether it is connected with the health field.

13. The Ebola virus scare, the Zika virus infection, and foodborne illnesses associated with a restaurant chain are examples of challenges to epidemiology. Compare the similarities and differences among these events. State at least one general principle that you can distill from these episodes.

14. What would be the response of epidemiologists to a single case of a long absent infectious disease, e.g., polio, should it happen in New York City? Describe the circumstances under which a single case of a disease is considered to be an epidemic.

15. Illustrate four ways in which epidemiology contributes as the basic science of public health.

16. Often, programs in epidemiology and biostatistics are housed in the same department. Why do you think this would be the case?

17. John Snow removed the handle from the pump featured in the Broad Street cholera epidemic. Using your own ideas, state why or why not this was an effective public health intervention.

18. Describe John Snow's natural experiment. Based on your own knowledge, discuss at least two contemporary examples of natural experiments that have been implemented within the past decade.

19. In your own opinion, why do you think many public health professionals regard John Snow as the father of epidemiology? Provide three reasons to support your position.

20. Using your own ideas, define the terms Black Death and Spanish flu and state why these events were historically significant for epidemiology.

21. In your opinion, under what present-day circumstances could Edward Jenner conduct his experiments with smallpox vaccinations? Do you think that any of his procedures would be prohibited in a modern research study?

22. Name three contemporary achievements of epidemiology. Discuss how the historical context of epidemiology helped to make them possible.

23. As noted previously, epidemiology studies the distribution of diseases in populations. Conduct a discussion in your class or an online forum in which you cite examples of the differential distributions of adverse health outcomes among various subgroups of the American population and explanations for their occurrence.

Young Epidemiology Scholars (YES) Exercises

The Young Epidemiology Scholars: Competitions website provides links to teaching units and exercises that support instruction in epidemiology. The YES program, discontinued in 2011, was administered by the College Board and supported by the Robert Wood Johnson Foundation. The exercises continue to be available at the following website: http://yes-competition.org/yes/teaching-units/title.html. The following exercises relate to topics discussed in this chapter and can be found on the YES competitions website.

History of epidemiology

1. McCrary F, Stolley P. Examining the Plague: An Investigation of Epidemics Past and Present.

2. McCrary F, St. George DMM. Mortality and the Trans-Atlantic Slave Trade.

3. McCrary F, Baumgarten M. Casualties of War: The Short- and Long-Term Effects of the 1945 Atomic Bomb Attacks on Japan.

Uses of epidemiology

1. Huang FI, Bayona M. Disease Outbreak Investigation.

REFERENCES

1. Centers for Disease Control and Prevention. Possible Zika virus infection among pregnant women—United States and territories, May 2016. *MMWR*. 2016;65(20):514–519.

2. Centers for Disease Control and Prevention. *Escherichia coli* O26 infections linked to Chipotle Mexican Grill restaurants (Final Update). November 2015. Available at: http://www.cdc.gov/ecoli/2015/o26-11-15/index.html. Accessed August 9, 2016.

3. Centers for Disease Control and Prevention. Multistate outbreak of *Salmonella* Saintpaul infections linked to raw produce. Available at: http://www.cdc.gov/salmonella/2008/raw-produce-8-28-2008.html. Accessed June 10, 2016.

4. Porta M, ed. *A Dictionary of Epidemiology*. 6th ed. New York, NY: Oxford University Press; 2014.

5. Friis RH, Sellers TA. *Epidemiology for Public Health Practice*. 5th ed. Burlington, MA: Jones & Bartlett Learning; 2014.

6. Oppenheimer GM. Comment: epidemiology and the liberal arts—toward a new paradigm? *Am J Public Health*. 1995;85:918–920.

7. Fraser DW. Epidemiology as a liberal art. *N Engl J Med*. 1987;316:309–314.

8. Grufferman S. Methodological approaches to studying environmental factors in childhood cancer. *Environ Health Perspect*. 1998;106 (Suppl 3):881–886.

9. Wegman DH. The potential impact of epidemiology on the prevention of occupational disease. *Am J Public Health*. 1992;82:944–954.

10. Franco G. Ramazzini and workers' health. *Lancet*. 1999;354:858–861.

11. Gochfeld M. Chronologic history of occupational medicine. *J Occup Environ Med*. 2005;47:96–114.

12. National Institutes of Health, The clinical center. Medicine for the layman environment and disease. Available at: http://www.mindfully.org/Health/Layman-Medicine.htm. Accessed December 27, 2015.

13. Doll R. Pott and the path to prevention. *Arch Geschwulstforsch*. 1975;45:521–531.

14. Gordis L. *Epidemiology*. 5th ed. Philadelphia, PA: Elsevier Saunders; 2014.

15. Snow J. *Snow on Cholera*. New York, NY: Hafner Publishing Company, by arrangement with Harvard University Press; 1965.

16. Lilienfeld DE. John Snow: the first hired gun? *Am J Epidemiol*. 2000;152:4–9.

17. Sandler DP. John Snow and modern-day environmental epidemiology. *Am J Epidemiol*. 2000;152:1–3.

18. King LS. Dr. Koch's postulates. *J Hist Med*. Autumn 1952;350–361.

19. U.S. Department of Health, Education and Welfare, Public Health Service. *Smoking and Health, Report of the Advisory Committee to the Surgeon General of the Public Health Service*. Public Health Service publication 1103, Washington, DC: Government Printing Office; 1964.

20. Morris JN. *Uses of Epidemiology*. 3rd ed. Edinburgh, UK: Churchill Livingstone; 1975.

21. Xu JQ, Murphy SL, Kochanek KD, Bastian BA. Deaths: final data for 2013. *National Vital Statistics Reports*, 64(2). Hyattsville, MD: National Center for Health Statistics; 2016.

CHAPTER 2

Epidemiology and Data Presentation

With Practice Questions for the MCAT® Examination

LEARNING OBJECTIVES

By the end of this chapter you will be able to:

- Create graphs and tables from a data set.
- Interpret data presented as figures, graphs, and tables.
- Calculate and make inferences from measures of central tendency and measures of dispersion.
- Explain how measures of association are used in epidemiology.
- Calculate a point estimate and an interval estimate of a parameter.

CHAPTER OUTLINE

INTRODUCTION

In this chapter you will learn how epidemiologists acquire, organize, and present health-related data. First, we will cover alternative sampling methods for selecting epidemiologic data. Then we will explore procedures for organizing the data contained in a chosen data set. These procedures include describing the central tendency and variability of the data and displaying how the data are distributed. Additional topics will be the definition of the term *variable* and measures of bivariate association between variables. This chapter will disclose how summary information about a data set helps to reveal important characteristics about a population. The methods for developing summary information about data sets and assessing relationships between variables are essential for formulating hypotheses in descriptive studies and for establishing the foundation for more complex statistical analyses. Refer to **Table 2-1** for a list of important terms discussed in this chapter.

TERMINOLOGY OF SAMPLES

The terms covered in this section are *populations, samples, simple random sampling, convenience sampling, systematic sampling*, and *stratified random sampling*. An appreciation of these fundamental concepts will aid in applying epidemiologic methods to the study of the health of populations.

Distinguishing Between Populations and Samples

Epidemiology and public health, for that matter, are concerned with health outcomes in the population. Very precise definitions apply to the designation of populations and the variables used to describe them. The term **population** refers to a collection of people who share common observable characteristics.[1] Human populations can be demarcated in several ways, such as all of the residents of a particular geographic

TABLE 2-1 Selected List of Important Mathematical and Epidemiologic Terms Used in This Chapter

Bar chart	Mean deviation	Quartile
Bivariate association	Measure of central tendency	Range, midrange, and interquartile range
Central tendency (location)	Measures of variation	Representativeness
Cluster sampling	Median	Sample (simple random, systematic)
Contingency table	Mode	Sampling bias
Convenience sampling	Multimodal curve	Scatter plots (scatter diagrams)
Dichotomous data	Normal distribution	Skewed distribution
Discrete versus continuous data	Outlier	Standard deviation
Distribution curve	Parameter	Standard normal distribution
Dose-response curve	Pearson correlation coefficient	Statistic
Estimation	Percentiles	Stevens' measurement scales
Epidemic curve	Pie chart	Stratum
Histogram	Point versus interval estimate	Unbiased
Line graph	Population (universe)	Variable (continuous, discrete)
Mean	Quantitative and qualitative data and variables	Variance

area,[2] or delimited by some other characteristic. See the following examples:

- All of the inhabitants of a country (e.g., China)
- All of the people who live in a city (e.g., New York)
- All students currently enrolled in a particular university
- All of the people diagnosed with a disease such as type 2 diabetes or lung cancer

A variable for describing a characteristic of a population is a **parameter**, which is defined as a measureable attribute of a population. An example of a parameter is the average age of the population, designated by the symbol μ.

A goal of statistical inference is to characterize a population by using information from samples. Thus samples must be representative of their parent population. **Representativeness** means that the characteristics of the sample correspond to the characteristics of the population from which the sample was chosen.

In order to infer the characteristics of samples, biostatisticians use sample-based data. A **sample** is a subgroup that has been selected, by using one of several methods, from the population (universe). In the terminology of sampling, the **universe** describes the total set of elements from which a sample is selected.

Numbers that describe a sample are called **statistics**. Returning to the average age of a population (μ), the sample estimate of μ is denoted by $\bar{X}$ (the sample mean). Inferential statistics use sample-based data to make conclusions about the population from which a sample has been selected; this process is known as **estimation**. Thus, $\bar{X}$ can be used as an estimate for μ, the population mean (a parameter).

Rationale for Using Samples

The rationale for using samples includes improved parameter estimates and possible cost savings. Four illustrations of using sampling techniques are reviewing income tax returns, verifying signatures on ballot initiatives, enumerating the U.S. population, and assuring the quality of manufactured goods. (Refer to the bullets in the next paragraph.) Sometimes economic and personnel constraints limit the ability of many organizations to assess each individual member of a population. Government agencies, manufacturers, and firms that poll public opinion achieve cost savings by using random sampling.

- *The Internal Revenue Service (IRS)*, instead of auditing every single income tax return, selects a sample of returns for audit by using statistical criteria developed by the agency. The statistical methods enable the IRS to detect returns with mistakes or incorrect information. Accordingly, the IRS is able to reduce personnel costs.
- *The U.S. Census Bureau,* which conducts the U.S. decennial census, is mandated to enumerate the nation's entire population. However, the Census Bureau applies sampling techniques to improve estimates for important subpopulations (e.g., states, counties, cities, or precincts).
- Some *boards of election* use random sampling to verify the authenticity of signatures on petitions to place initiatives on a ballot. This procedure cuts the workload of election officials.
- *Pharmaceutical and other manufacturers* employ sampling to ensure product quality when testing the product requires that it be damaged or destroyed. For example, testing might require compromising hygienic sealing; loss of product can be very costly. Instead of testing a large percentage of their output, a manufacturer could obtain a small random sample of the output from the production line in order to reduce waste.

Methods for Selecting a Sample

The two methods for selecting a sample are random sampling (simple random sampling and stratified random sampling) and nonrandom sampling (convenience sampling, systematic sampling, and cluster sampling). Regardless of which of these two methods is applied, researchers need to be able to obtain a sample efficiently and in a manner that permits an accurate estimate of a parameter. Improperly chosen samples can produce misleading and erroneous findings.

Limitations of Nonrandom Samples

A limitation of nonrandom samples is that they are prone to sampling bias. In this instance, **sampling bias** means that the individuals who have been selected are not representative of the population to which the epidemiologist would like to generalize the results of the research.

Two examples of nonrandom samples are data from surveys conducted on the Internet and media-based polling. These two methods are likely to produce nonrepresentative samples. Increasingly, the Internet has been used for conducting surveys; the resulting sample of respondents is likely to be a biased sample because of self-selection—only people who are interested in the survey topic respond to the survey. We do not know about the nonrespondents and consequently have very little information about the target population (the population denominator, as it is called in epidemiology).

Television and radio shows, when polling audience members, also generate self-selected samples, which can be biased. Hypothetically, the show's moderator might request that the audience voice their opinions regarding a political issue or other matter by accessing a call-in line. Other potentially biased samples arise from the use of membership lists of organizations or magazine subscription lists. Not only are the respondents self-selected, but also the universe of members or subscribers may differ from the general population in important ways.

Simple Random Sampling

Simple random sampling (SRS) refers to the use of a random process to select a sample. A simplistic example of SRS is drawing names from a hat. Random digit dialed (RDD) telephone surveys are a more elaborate method for selecting random samples. At one time, RDD surveys obtained high response rates from the large proportion of the U.S. homes with telephones. However, as more people transition from land lines to cellular phones, RDD surveys of land-based telephones have had declining population coverage and reduced response rates. Another method of SRS is to draw respondents randomly from lists that contain large and diverse populations (e.g., licensed drivers).

In simple random sampling, one chooses a sample of size n from a population of size N. Each member of a population has an equal chance of being chosen for the sample. In addition, all samples of size n out of a population of size N are equally possible. Considerable effort surrounds the determination of the size of n.

According to statistical theory, random sampling produces unbiased estimates of parameters. In addition, random sampling permits the use of statistical methods to make inferences about population characteristics. In the context of sampling theory, the term **unbiased** means that the average of the sample estimates over all possible samples of a fixed size is equal to the population parameter. For example, if we select all possible samples of size n from N and compute $\overline{X}$ for each sample, the mean of all of the $\overline{X}$s (symbol, $\mu_{\overline{x}}$) will be equal to μ ($\mu_{\overline{x}} = \mu$). However, any individual sample mean ($\overline{X}$) is likely to be slightly different from μ. This difference is from random error, which is defined as error due to chance.[2] Beware, therefore, that the unbiasedness property of random samples does not guarantee that any particular sample estimate will be close to the parameter value; also, a sample is not guaranteed to be representative of the population.

Stratified Random Sampling

Most large populations in the United States and other countries comprise numerous subgroups. An epidemiologist may want to investigate the characteristics of these subgroups. Unfortunately, when a simple random sample of a large population is selected, members of subgroups of interest may not appear in sufficient numbers in the chosen sample to permit statistical analyses of them. The underrepresentation of interesting subgroups in random samples is a conundrum for epidemiologists. Stratified random sampling offers a work-around for this problem.

Returning to statistical terminology, we will designate N as the number in the population and n as the number in the sample. Suppose an epidemiologist wants to study the health characteristics of racial or ethnic subgroups that are uncommon in the general population. The size of n is limited by our available budget. If n is small (which is often the case) in comparison to N, then only a few individuals from the minority group will enter the sample.

We will define a **stratum** as a subgroup of the population. For example, a population can be stratified by racial or ethnic group, age category, or socioeconomic status. Stratified random sampling uses oversampling of strata in order to ensure that a sufficient number of individuals from a particular stratum are included in the final sample. Statisticians have demonstrated that stratified random sampling can improve parameter estimates for large, complex populations, especially when there is substantial variability among subgroups.

Let's address how stratified random sampling helps to increase the numbers of respondents from underrepresented groups. As an illustration, the author used stratified random sampling in order to study tobacco use among a minority Asian group (Cambodian Americans). In the city where the research was conducted, individuals from this stratum were oversampled for inclusion in the research sample. As a result, the investigators obtained sufficient information from this stratum for a descriptive epidemiologic analysis.

Convenience Sampling

Convenience sampling uses available groups selected by an arbitrary and easily performed method. Samples generated by convenience sampling sometimes are called "grab bag" samples. An example of a convenience sample is a group of patients who receive medical service from a physician who is treating them for a chronic disease. Convenience samples are highly likely to be biased and are not appropriate for application of inferential statistics. However they can be helpful in descriptive studies and for suggesting additional research.

Systematic Sampling

Systematic sampling uses a systematic procedure to select a sample of a fixed size from a sampling frame (a complete list of people who constitute the population). Systematic sampling is feasible when a sampling frame such as a list of names is available. As a hypothetical example of systematic sampling, an epidemiologist wants to select a sample of 100 individuals from an alphabetical list that contains 2,000 names. A way to determine the sample size is to select a desired percentage of cases (e.g., 5%). After specifying a sample size, a sampling interval must be created, say, every tenth name. An arbitrary starting point on the list is identified (e.g., the top of the list or a randomly selected name in the list); then from that point every tenth name is chosen until the quota of 100 is reached.

A systematic sample may not be representative of the sampling frame for various reasons, especially when samples are not taken from the entire list. As an example, if the sampling quota is reached by the first third of an alphabetized list, people in the remainder of the list will not be chosen. Perhaps these individuals are from a particular ethnic group with names concentrated at the end of the list. Consequently, exclusion of these names may result in a biased sample.

Cluster Sampling

Cluster sampling is another common method for sample selection. **Cluster sampling** refers to a method of sampling in which the element selected is a group (as distinguished from an individual) called a cluster. An example of a selected element is a city block (block cluster). The U.S. Census Bureau employs cluster sampling procedures to conduct surveys in the decennial census. Because it is a more parsimonious design than random sampling, cluster sampling can produce cost savings; also, statistical theory demonstrates that cluster sampling is able to create unbiased estimates of parameters.

DATA AND MEASUREMENT SCALES

Two types of data for use in epidemiology are qualitative and quantitative data, both of which comprise variables. The term *variable* encompasses discrete and continuous variables. Noteworthy is the contribution of psychologist Stanley Stevens, who formalized scales of measurement. Scales of measurement delimit analyses that are permissible with different kinds of data.

Types of Data Used in Epidemiology

As noted, epidemiology uses qualitative and quantitative data, terms that are straightforward but can be confusing. Another way to classify data is as discrete or continuous.

Qualitative data employ categories that do not have numerical values or rankings. Qualitative data are measured on a categorical scale.[2] Occupation, marital status, and sex are examples of qualitative data that have no natural ordering.[1]

Quantitative data are data reported as numerical quantities.[2] "Quantitative data [are] data expressing a certain quantity, amount or range."[3] Such data are obtained by counting or taking measurements, for example, measuring a patient's height.

Discrete data are data that have a finite or countable number of values. Discrete data can take on the values of integers (whole numbers). Examples of discrete data are: number of children in a family (there cannot be fractional numbers of children such as half a child); a patient's number of missing teeth; and the number of spots on a die (one to six spots). If discrete data have only two values, they are **dichotomous data** (binary data). Examples are dead or alive, present or absent, male or female.

Continuous data have an infinite number of possible values along a continuum.[2] Weight, for example, is measured on a continuous scale. A scientific weight scale in a school chemistry lab might report the weight of a substance to the nearest 100th of a gram. A research laboratory might have a scale that can report the weight of the same material to the nearest 1,000th of a gram or even more precisely.

Classification of Variables

The term **variable** is used to describe a quantity that can vary (that is, take on different values), such as age, height, weight, or sex. In epidemiology, it is common practice to refer to exposure variables (for example, contact with a microbe or toxic chemical) and outcome variables (for example, a health outcome such as a disease).

Variables can be discrete or continuous. A **discrete variable** is made up of discrete data. Examples of discrete variables are ones that use data such as household size (number of people who reside in a household) or number of doctor visits.

A **continuous variable** is a variable composed of continuous data; examples of continuous variables are age, height, weight, heart rate, blood cholesterol, and blood sugar levels. However, as soon as one takes a measurement, for example, someone's blood pressure, the result becomes a discrete value.

Stevens' Measurement Scales

In 1946, Stanley Smith Stevens, a psychologist at Harvard University, published a seminal work titled "On the Theory of Scales of Measurement." Stevens wrote "… that scales of measurement fall into certain definite classes. These classes are determined both by the empirical operations invoked in the process of 'measuring' and by formal (mathematical) properties of the scales. Furthermore—and this is of great concern to several of the sciences—the statistical manipulations that can be legitimately applied to empirical data depend on the type of scale against which the data are ordered."[4(p677)] The implication of Stevens' statement is that before conducting a data analysis, one should choose an analysis that is appropriate to the scale of measurement being used. **Table 2-2** illustrates **Stevens' measurement scales**, which encompass four categories: nominal, ordinal, interval, and ratio. The following section further defines the terms used in scales of measurement.

Nominal scales are a type of qualitative scale that consists of categories that are not ordered. (Ordered data have categories such as worst to best.) Examples of nominal scales are race (e.g., black, white, Asian) and religion (e.g., Christian, Jewish, Muslim). Note that nominal scales include dichotomous scales.

Ordinal scales comprise categorical data that can be ordered (ranked data) but are still considered qualitative data.[1] The intervals between each point on the scale are not equal intervals. Permissible data presentations with ordinal data include the use of bar graphs. An example of an ordinal scale with qualitative data that can be ordered is a scale that measures self-perception of health (e.g., strongly agree, agree, disagree, and strongly disagree). Other ordinal scales measure the following characteristics (all in gradations from low to high):

- Levels of educational attainment
- Socioeconomic status
- Occupational prestige

TABLE 2-2 Scales of Measurement

Scale	Basic Empirical Operations	Permissible Statistics
Nominal	Determination of equality	Number of cases (e.g., counts of the number of cases of a category in a nominal scale)
Ordinal	Determination of greater or less	Median Percentiles
Interval	Determination of equality of intervals or differences	Mean Standard deviation Correlation (e.g., Pearson product-moment)
Ratio	Determination of equality of ratios	Coefficient of variation*

*The coefficient of variation for a sample is the ratio of the sample standard deviation to the sample mean. It can be used to make comparisons among different distributions. This term is not discussed further in this chapter.

Adapted and reprinted from Stevens SS. On the theory of scales of measurement. *Science*. 1946;103(2648):678.

An **interval scale** consists of continuous data with equal intervals between points on the measurement scale and without a true zero point. Interval scales do not permit the calculation of ratios. (Ratios are numbers obtained by dividing one number by another number.) An example of an interval scale is the Fahrenheit temperature scale, which does not have a true zero point. Therefore, it is not possible to say that 100°F is twice as hot as 50°F. The intelligence quotient (IQ) is measured on an interval scale. We cannot state that a person with an IQ of 120 is twice as smart as a person with an IQ of 60.

A **ratio scale** retains the properties of an interval level scale. In addition, it has a true zero point. The fact that ratio scales have a zero point permits one to form ratios with the data. To illustrate, the Kelvin temperature scale is a ratio scale because it has a meaningful zero point, which permits the calculation of ratios. A temperature of 0°K signifies the absence of all heat; also, one can say that 200°K is twice as hot as 100°K.

PRESENTATION OF EPIDEMIOLOGIC DATA

When you have acquired a data set, you need to know the basic methods for displaying and analyzing data. This information comes in handy for interpreting epidemiologic reports and performing simple, but powerful, data analyses. The methods for displaying and analyzing data depend on the type of data being used. This section covers frequency tables and graphical presentations of data, for example, bar charts, line graphs, and pie charts.

Creating Frequency Tables

A frequency table provides one of the most convenient ways to summarize or display data in a grouped format. A prior step to creating the table is counting and tabulating cases; this process must take place after the data have been reviewed for accuracy and completeness (a process called data cleaning). A clean data set contains a group of related data that are ready for coding and data analysis. Frequency tables are helpful in identifying **outliers**, extreme values that differ greatly from other values in the data set. These cases may be actual extreme cases or originate from data entry errors. For example, in a frequency table of ages, an age of 149 years would be an outlier.

Table 2-3 presents a data set for 20 patients with hepatitis C virus infection. As shown in the table, the variables "interviewed, sex, race, reason for test, injection-drug use (IDU), shared needles, and noninjection drug use" are all nominal, discrete data. Statistical analysts often refer to the type of formatting of the information shown in the table as a *line listing* of data.

Across the top row are shown the column headings that designate the study variables (e.g., case number, interview status, age, sex, and race). Each subsequent row contains the data for a single case (a record). What can be done with the data at this stage? One possibility is to tabulate the data. For large data sets, computers simplify this task; here is what is involved. The process of tabulation creates frequencies of the study variables, for example, "Interviewed." This is a nominal,

TABLE 2-3 [Data Set] Demographic Characteristics, Risk Factors, Surveillance Status, and Clinical Information for 20 Patients with Hepatitis C Virus (HCV) Infection—Postal Code A, Buffalo, New York, November 2004–April 2007*

Case	Interviewed	Age (yrs)	Sex	Race	Date of Diagnosis	Reason for Test	IDU[†]	Shared Needles	Noninjection Drug Use
1	Yes	17	Male	White	11/3/04	Risk factors	Yes	Yes[††]	Yes
2	No	23	Female	White	1/25/05	Symptomatic	Yes	—	Yes
3	No	26	Male	White	3/9/05	Risk factors	Yes	—	—
4	Yes	28	Male	White	12/6/05	Symptomatic	Yes	Yes	Yes
5	Yes	17	Male	White	12/29/05	Risk factors	Yes	Yes[††]	Yes
6	No	19	Male	White	1/20/06	Symptomatic	Yes	Yes[††]	Yes
7	Yes	17	Male	White	1/24/06	Risk factors	Yes	Yes[††]	Yes
8	Yes	16	Female	White	2/17/06	Risk factors	Yes	Yes[††]	Yes
9	Yes	21	Male	White	2/23/06	Risk factors	Yes	Yes[††]	Yes
10	No	22	Male	White	3/2/06	Risk factors	Yes	—	—
11	Yes	18	Female	White	5/17/06	Risk factors	Yes	Yes	Yes
12	Yes	19	Male	White	5/24/06	Risk factors	Yes	Yes	Yes
13	No	19	Male	White	5/24/06	Risk factors	Yes	—	—
14	No	20	Male	White	5/26/06	Symptomatic	Yes	Yes[††]	Yes
15	Yes	17	Female	White	8/14/06	Risk factors	No	No	No
16	Yes	23	Male	White	10/10/06	Risk factors	Yes	Yes[††]	Yes
17	No	19	Male	White	12/19/06	Risk factors	Yes	Yes[††]	Yes
18	No	26	Female	White	1/6/07	Risk factors	Yes	Yes	Yes
19	No	17	Female	White	3/13/07	Risk factors	Yes	Yes[††]	Yes
20	Yes	19	Male	White	4/26/07	Risk factors	Yes	Yes[††]	Yes

*Data were compiled from standard surveillance forms and patient interviews.

[†]Injection-drug use.

[††]Shared needles with a person known or believed to be HCV positive.

Adapted and reprinted from Centers for Disease Control and Prevention. Use of enhanced surveillance for hepatitis C virus infection to detect a cluster among young injection-drug users—New York, November 2004–April 2007. *MMWR*. 2008;57:518.

discrete variable that has the response categories "yes" and "no." The tabulated responses to the variable "Interviewed" are:

Yes: ||||| ||||| |

Total number of "yes" responses: 11

No: ||||| ||||

Total number of "no" responses: 9
Total number of cases = 11 + 9 = 20

Similar tabulations could be performed for the other study variables in Table 2-3. The results can then be presented in a frequency table (frequency distribution). Refer to **Table 2-4** for an example of a frequency table based on the tabulated data.

Graphical Presentations

After tabulating the data, an epidemiologist might plot the data graphically as a bar chart, histogram, line graph, or pie chart. Such graphical displays summarize the key aspects of the data set. Although visual displays facilitate an intuitive understanding of the data, they omit some of the detail contained in the data set. The following sections cover three methods for data presentation.

TABLE 2-4 Tabulations of Discrete Variables by Using Data in Table 2-3

Variable	Frequency	Variable	Frequency
Interviewed	—	Injection drug use	—
Yes	11	Yes	19
No	9	No	1
Unknown	0	Unknown	0
Total	20	Total	20
Sex	—	Shared needle	—
Male	14	Yes	15
Female	6	No	1
Unknown	0	Unknown	4
Total	20	Total	20
Race	—	Noninjection drug use	—
White	20	Yes	16
Other	0	No	1
Unknown	0	Unknown	3
Total	20	Total	20

Bar Charts and Histograms

The first presentation method described here is the use of two similar charts, bar charts and histograms. Although similar, there are crucial distinctions between the two kinds of charts—whether they are used to present qualitative or quantitative data.

A **bar chart** is a type of graph that shows the frequency of cases for categories of a discrete variable. An example is a qualitative, discrete variable such as the Yes/No variable described in the foregoing example of data for hepatitis C patients. Along the base of the bar chart are categories of the variable; the height of the bars represents the frequency of cases for each category. Selected data from Table 2-4 are graphed in **Figure 2-1**, which shows a bar chart.

Figure 2-2 presents another example of a bar chart—the percentage of nutrient-fortified wheat flour processed in roller mills in seven World Health Organization (WHO) regions for 2004 and 2007. Fortification of wheat increases its nutritional value. The chart demonstrates that the highest percentage of fortified wheat was produced in the Americas and that the percentage showed an increasing trend in all regions between 2004 and 2007.

Similar to bar charts, **histograms** are charts that are used to display the frequency distributions for grouped categories of a continuous variable. See the example shown in **Figure 2-3**. When continuous variables are plotted as histograms, coding procedures have been applied to convert them into categories, as indicated on the X-axis.

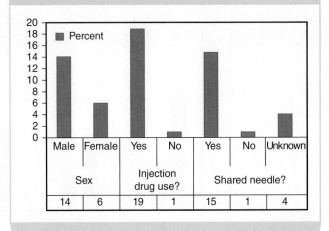

FIGURE 2-1 Bar chart of selected information from Table 2-4.

Line Graphs

A second type of graphical display is a line graph, which enables the reader to detect trends, for example, time trends in the data. A **line graph** is a type of graph in which the points in the graph have been joined by a line. A single point represents the frequency of cases for each category of a variable. When using more than one line, the epidemiologist is able to demonstrate comparisons among subgroups. **Figure 2-4**

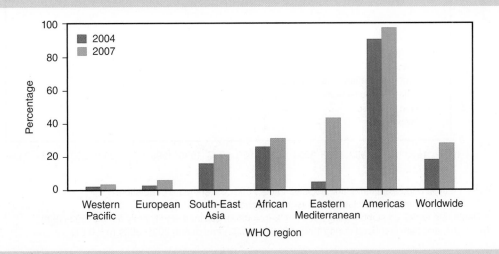

FIGURE 2-2 Percentage of wheat flour processed in roller mills that was fortified—worldwide and by World Health Organization (WHO) region, 2004 and 2007.

Reprinted from Centers for Disease Control and Prevention. Trends in wheat-flour fortification with folic acid and iron—worldwide, 2004 and 2007. *MMWR.* 2008;57:9.

FIGURE 2-3 Average number of annual visits to physicians' offices by males age 15–39 years, by age group and race/ethnicity—National Ambulatory Medical Care Survey, United States, 2009–2012.

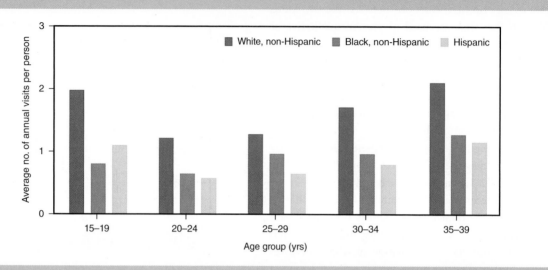

Reprinted from Centers for Disease Control and Prevention. Health care use and HIV testing of males aged 15–39 years in physicians' offices--United States, 2009-2012. *MMWR.* 2016;65(24):620.

FIGURE 2-4 Rates* of childhood cancer deaths, by race and ethnicity†—United States, 1990–2004.

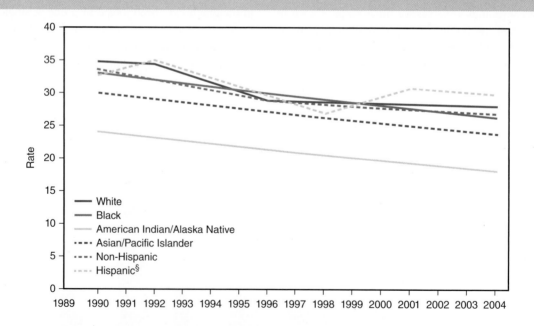

* Per 1 million population; rates age adjusted to the 2000 U.S. standard population.
† Ethnicity is not mutually exclusive from race categories.
§ Death rate remained stable during 1990–1992 (p = 0.53), declined significantly during 1992–1998 (p = 0.01), and then stabilized during 1998–2001 (p = 0.32) and during 2001–2004 (p = 0.57).

Reprinted from Centers for Disease Control and Prevention. Trends in childhood cancer mortality—United States, 1990–2004. *MMWR.* 2007;56:1260.

shows a line graph of childhood cancer deaths by race and ethnicity between 1990 and 2004. In almost all subgroups, the lines show a declining trend.

Pie Chart

A third method for the graphical presentation of data is to construct a **pie chart**, which is a circle that shows the proportion of cases according to several categories. The size of each piece of "pie" is proportional to the frequency of cases. The pie chart demonstrates the relative importance of each subcategory. For example, the pie chart in **Figure 2-5** represents the percentage of childhood cancer deaths by primary site/leading diagnosis for the United States in 2004. The data reveal that leukemias and brain/nervous system cancers accounted for the most frequent percentages of childhood cancer deaths.

MEASURES OF CENTRAL TENDENCY

A **measure of central tendency** (also called a measure of location) is a number that signifies a typical value of a group of numbers or of a distribution of numbers. The number gives the center of the distribution or can refer to certain numerical values in the distribution where the numbers tend to cluster. The measures of central tendency covered in this section are the *mode, median*, and *arithmetic mean*.

Mode

The **mode** is defined as the number occurring most frequently in a set or distribution of numbers.[2] An example of a mode is given in **Table 2-5**. The mode is 2.

TABLE 2-5 Example of a Mode

Number	Frequency	Mode
1,1,1,1	4	
2,2,2,2,2	5	Mode = 2
3,3	2	
4,4,4	3	

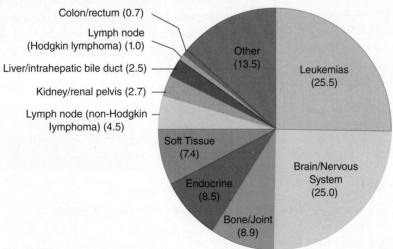

FIGURE 2-5 Percentage of childhood cancer deaths,* by primary cancer site/leading diagnosis†—United States, 2004.

*N = 2,223.

†Based on *International Classification of Diseases, Tenth Revision* codes for leukemias (C91.0 – C91.4, C91.7, C91.9, C92.0–C92.5, C92.7, C92.9, C93.0 – C93.2, C93.7, C93.9, C94.0, C94.2, C94.4, C94.5, and C95.0) and brain and other nervous system neoplasms (C70–C72).

Reprinted from Centers for Disease Control and Prevention. Trends in childhood cancer mortality—United States, 1990–2004. *MMWR.* 2007;56:1258.

Median

The **median** is the middle point of a set of numbers. If a group of numbers is ranked from the smallest value to the highest value, the median is the point that demarcates the lower and upper half of the numbers. Let's compute the median for a small data set (n). The median is computed differently for an odd group of numbers than for an even group of numbers. The first step in computing the median is to rank order the numbers from the lowest to the highest values as described in the following section:

- *Median (m)* = the middle number of an array when n is odd.
  Data set ($n = 9$): [8,1,2,9,3,2,8,1,2]
  a. Rank order the numbers from the lowest to the highest.
  b. The result is [1,1,2,2,2,3,8,8,9]; m = 2

- *Median* = the average of two middle numbers when n is even.
  Data set ($n = 8$): [8,1,7,9,3,2,8,1]
  a. As above, rearrange the numbers in an array and then calculate the median.
  b. The result is [1,1,2,3,7,8,8,9]. The two middle numbers are 3 and 7; m = (7 + 3)/2 = 5.

Mean

The **mean** is also called the arithmetic mean or average. It is a common measure of central tendency with many uses in epidemiology. For example, the mean could be used to describe the average systolic blood pressure of patients enrolled in a primary care clinic. The formula for the mean is presented in **Formula 2-1**. The symbol sigma (Σ) refers to summing or adding numbers as shown in the calculation example.

FORMULA 2-1 Arithmetic Mean of a Sample ($\bar{X}$)

$$\bar{X} = \frac{\sum X}{n}$$

$$\bar{X} = \frac{X_1 + X_2 + X_3 + \ldots + X_n}{n}$$

Calculation example:
We have the following cholesterol values from a heart disease study: 201, 223, 194, 122, 241. Calculate the mean cholesterol level. Answer:

$$\sum X = 201 + 223 + 194 + 122 + 241$$

$$\bar{X} = \frac{201 + 223 + 194 + 122 + 241}{5} = \frac{981}{5} = 196.2$$

MEASURES OF VARIATION

Synonyms for variation are *dispersion* and *spread*. **Measures of variation** are range, midrange, mean deviation, and standard deviation.

Range and Midrange

- The **range** is the difference between the highest (H) and lowest (L) value in a group of numbers. Calculation example:

The respective ages of residents of a board and care facility are 67, 71, 75, 80, and 98 years. Use the formula:

$$[\text{Range} = H - L]$$

Range is 98 years − 67 years = 31 years

- The **midrange** is the arithmetic mean of the highest and lowest values. Calculation example (using the previous data):

Use the formula:

$$\text{Midrange} = \frac{(H - L)}{2} = \frac{31}{2} = 15.5$$

Variance and Standard Deviation, Mean Deviation

The term **variance** refers to the degree of variability in a set of numbers. The variance reflects how different the numbers are from one another. The variance of sample denoted by s^2 indicates how variable the numbers in a sample are. The **standard deviation** of a sample (s) is the square root of the variance. Refer to **Formula 2-2** for the formulas for these terms. The formulas shown are for the deviation score method for the computations. The standard deviation can be used the quantify degree of spread of a group of numbers. We will return to the standard deviation when we cover the spread of distributions of variables.

FORMULA 2-2 Variance and Standard Deviation of a Sample

s^2 = variance of a sample
s = standard deviation of a sample

$$s^2 = \frac{\sum (X - \bar{X})^2}{n - 1}$$

(variance of a sample, deviation score method)

$$s = \sqrt{\frac{\sum (X - \bar{X})^2}{n - 1}}$$

(standard deviation of a sample, deviation score method)

TABLE 2-6 Calculation of a Standard Deviation of a Sample

Case Number	Age (years) X	Deviation about Mean $(X-\overline{X})$	Absolute Value of Deviation $|X-\overline{X}|$	Squared Deviation $(X-\overline{X})^2$
1	17	–3.6	3.6	13.0
2	23	2.4	2.4	5.8
3	26	5.4	5.4	29.2
4	28	7.4	7.4	54.8
5	17	Stratum 3.6	3.6	13.0
6	19	Stratum 1.6	1.6	2.6
7	17	Stratum 3.6	3.6	13.0
8	16	Stratum 4.6	4.6	21.2
9	21	0.4	0.4	0.2
10	22	1.4	1.4	2.0
Sum (Σ)	206	0.0	34.0	154.4
	$\dfrac{\sum X}{n}$ (Mean) = 20.6		Mean deviation = $\dfrac{\sum|X - \overline{X}|}{n} = 3.4$	

Standard deviation (s) $\longrightarrow$ $\sqrt{\dfrac{\sum(X - \overline{X})^2}{n-1}} = 4.1$

A calculation example of the variance and standard deviation of a small data set is shown in the following example using data extracted from Table 2-3. Our task is to compute the variance, standard deviation, and mean deviation of the first 10 cases in **Table 2-6**. Follow the steps shown in Table 2-6. The formula for the **mean deviation** (the average of the absolute values of the deviations of each observation about the mean) is:

$$\text{Mean deviation} = \frac{\sum|X-\overline{X}|}{n}$$

DISTRIBUTION CURVES

A **distribution curve** is a graph that is constructed from the frequencies of the values of a variable, for example, variable X. The values are a "... complete summary of the frequency of values of... a measurement..." for variable X collected on a group of people.[2] Such curves can take various forms, including symmetric and nonsymmetric (skewed) shapes.

Distribution curves can be described in terms of central tendency and dispersion. Defined previously, measures of central tendency (location)—the mean, median, and mode—can be applied to distribution curves. The mode of a distribution curve is the most frequently occurring value of the variable. Distributions can have one mode or more than one mode. Different distributions may exhibit different degrees of spread or dispersion, which is the tendency for observations to depart from central tendency. The standard deviation is a measure of the dispersion (spread) of a distribution curve, as are the range, percentile, and quartiles.

Measures of Variability

Synonyms for measures of the variability of a distribution curve are *dispersion* and *spread*. Distribution curves can exhibit different degrees of spread or dispersion, which is the tendency for observations to depart from central tendency. An application of measures of variability is for comparison of distributions with respect to their dispersion. These measures include the range, percentiles, quartiles, mean deviation, and standard deviation.

Percentiles and Quartiles

Percentiles are created by dividing a distribution into 100 parts. The pth percentile is the number for which p% of the data have values equal to or smaller than that number. Thus, a value at the 80th percentile includes 80% of the values in the distribution. **Quartiles** subdivide a distribution into units of 25% of the distribution. For example:

- 1st quartile (Q1) = 25%
- 2nd quartile (Q2) = 50%
- 3rd quartile (Q3) = 75%

The **interquartile range (IQR)**, which is a measure of the spread of a distribution, is the portion of a distribution between the 1st quartile and 3rd quartile. The formula is:

$$IQR = Q3 - Q1$$

Normal Distribution

Many human characteristics, such as intelligence, follow a normal pattern of distribution. A **normal distribution** (also called a Gaussian distribution) is a symmetrical distribution with several interesting properties that pertain to its central tendency and dispersion. **Figure 2-6** shows a normal distribution.

Measures of Central Tendency (Location) of a Normal Distribution

The mean, median, and mode of a normal distribution are identical and fall exactly in the middle of the distribution as shown in Figure 2-6.

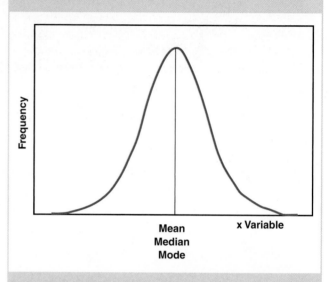

FIGURE 2-6 **A normal distribution and measures of location.**

Adapted from Centers for Disease Control and Prevention (CDC). Office of Workforce and Career Development. *Principles of Epidemiology in Public Health Practice.* 3rd ed. Atlanta, GA: CDC; May 2012:2-12.

The mean is a measure of location on the X-axis. **Figure 2-7** shows three identical normal curves with different means. You can see how the means have different locations on the X-axis.

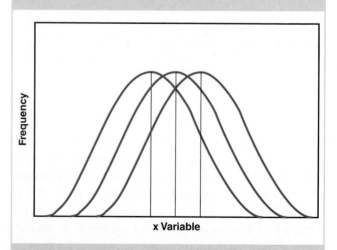

FIGURE 2-7 **Three curves with the same distributions and different means.**

Reprinted from Centers for Disease Control and Prevention (CDC). Office of Workforce and Career Development. *Principles of Epidemiology in Public Health Practice.* 3rd ed. Atlanta, GA: CDC; May 2012:2-12.

Standard Normal Distribution

The **standard normal distribution** is a type of normal distribution with a mean of zero and a standard deviation of one unit. The standard normal distribution has interesting properties (e.g., areas between standard deviation units) that are used for statistical analyses. Refer to **Figure 2-8**. The figure demonstrates the percentage of cases contained within ranges of standard deviation (SD) units. Note that the area between one standard deviation above and one standard deviation below the mean covers about 68% of the distribution.

Distributions with the Same Mean and Different Dispersions

Remember that dispersion is a measure that shows the degree of spread of the distribution. In **Figure 2-9**, the three distributions have the same mean (location on the X-axis) and different dispersions.

Skewed Distributions

Instead of being symmetric, a **skewed distribution** is one that is asymmetric; it has a concentration of values on either the left or right side of the X-axis. Skewness is defined by the direction in which the tail of the distribution points. **Figure 2-10** shows a symmetrical distribution (B) in comparison with a distribution that is skewed to the right (A; positively skewed; tail trails off to the right) and skewed to the left (C; negatively skewed; tail trails off to the left).

FIGURE 2-8 The standard normal distribution.

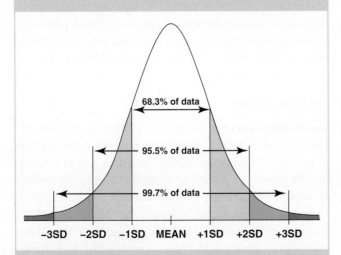

Reprinted from Centers for Disease Control and Prevention (CDC). Office of Workforce and Career Development. *Principles of Epidemiology in Public Health Practice*. 3rd ed. Atlanta, GA: CDC; May 2012:2-46.

FIGURE 2-9 Three distributions with the same mean and different dispersions.

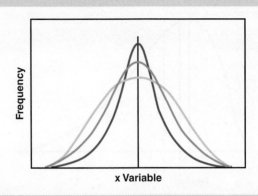

Reprinted from Centers for Disease Control and Prevention (CDC). Office of Workforce and Career Development. *Principles of Epidemiology in Public Health Practice*. 3rd ed. Atlanta, GA: CDC; May 2012:2-13.

FIGURE 2-10 Skewed distributions in comparison with a symmetrical distribution.

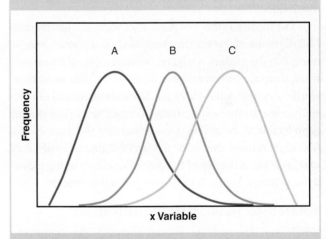

Reprinted from Centers for Disease Control and Prevention (CDC). Office of Workforce and Career Development. *Principles of Epidemiology in Public Health Practice*. 3rd ed. Atlanta, GA: CDC; May 2012:2-14.

Measures of Central Tendency (Location) of a Skewed Distribution

The mean, median, and mode have different values in a skewed distribution. (See **Figure 2-11**.) When a distribution is skewed, the median is a more appropriate measure of central tendency than the mean. This is because the median divides the distribution into halves. In comparison, the mean

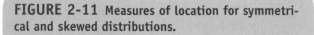

FIGURE 2-11 Measures of location for symmetrical and skewed distributions.

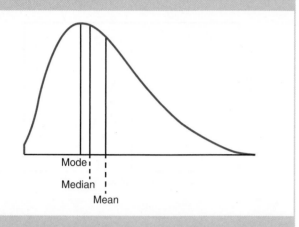

Adapted from Centers for Disease Control and Prevention (CDC). Office of Workforce and Career Development. *Principles of Epidemiology in Public Health Practice.* 3rd ed. Atlanta, GA: CDC; May 2012:2-53.

is a center of gravity (balancing point) of a distribution and does not indicate the central tendency of the skewed distribution.

The median is the 50% point of continuous distributions (distributions of continuous variables). You should bear in mind that the median is a better measure of central tendency when there are several extreme values in the data set. A noteworthy example is the use of median income instead of average income to represent central tendency. The median income is preferable to the average income because the incomes of a few high earners can raise the average disproportionately, making it not reflective of the central tendency of the majority of incomes. Figure 2-11 demonstrates this concept.

Symmetrical (Non-Skewed) Distributions

When the distributions are symmetrical, the mean and median are identical and can be used interchangeably. As a general rule, the arithmetic mean is generally preferred over the median as a measure of central tendency because it tends to be a more stable value; i.e., it varies less under sampling from one sample to the next.

Distributions with Multimodal Curves

As defined previously, the mode is the value in a frequency distribution that has the highest frequency of cases; there can be more than one mode in a frequency distribution. A **multimodal curve** is one that has several peaks in the frequency of a condition. **Figure 2-12** demonstrates a hypothetical multimodal plot

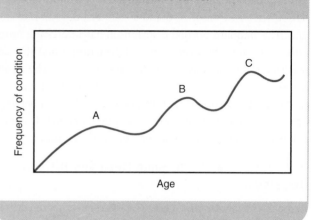

FIGURE 2-12 A multimodal curve.

of age on the horizontal axis and frequency of the condition on the vertical axis. When plotted as a line graph, a multimodal curve takes the form shown in Figure 2-12, a multimodal distribution with three modes: A, B, and C.

Among the reasons for multimodal distributions are age-related changes in the immune status or lifestyle of the host (the person who develops a disease). Another explanation might be the occurrence of conditions such as chronic diseases that have long latency periods and appear later in life. (The term latency refers to the time period between initial exposure and a measurable response.) Referring back to Figure 2-12: As a purely hypothetical example, the increase at point A (for children) might be due to their relatively low immune status; the spike at point B (for young adults) might be due to the effect of behavioral changes that bring potential hosts into contact with other people, resulting in person-to-person spread of disease; and the increase at point C (for the oldest people) might reflect the operation of latency effects of exposures to carcinogens.

Epidemic Curve

An **epidemic curve** is "[a] graphic plotting of the distribution of cases by time of onset."[2] An epidemic curve is a type of unimodal (having one mode) curve that aids in identifying the cause of a disease outbreak. Let's apply the concept of an epidemic curve to an outbreak of foodborne illness caused by *Salmonella* (associated illness: salmonellosis). An outbreak of *Salmonella* Heidelberg erupted in the United States from about mid-2012 to mid-2013.[5] The Pacific Northwest outbreak of 134 cases was linked with Foster Farms chickens. How did the epidemic curve support the investigation of the outbreak?

FIGURE 2-13 Number of clinical isolates matching the *Salmonella* Heidelberg outbreak strain and 5-year baseline mean number of cases with the same strain, by week of uploads—PulseNet,[*] United States, 2012–2013.

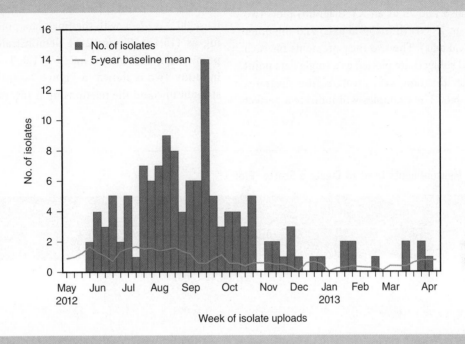

Reprinted from Disease Control and Prevention. Outbreak of *Salmonella* Heidelberg infections linked to a single poultry producer—13 states, 2012–2013. *MMWR*. 2013;62(27):555.

Salmonellosis is one of the leading forms of bacterially associated foodborne illnesses. Microbiologists classify the bacterium according to serotypes, which are subgroups of *Salmonella*. Heidelberg is a serotype of *Salmonella*.

Figure 2-13 provides the epidemic curve for the outbreak. The solid line shows baseline cases of *Salmonella* Heidelberg. These are sporadic cases (four to eight per month) that typically occur. During the outbreak, the number of cases spiked and exceeded the 5-year baseline mean. All of the cases in the outbreak matched on the same serotype of *Salmonella* (*Salmonella* Heidelberg). A large percentage of the people who were sickened revealed that they had purchased Foster Farms chickens. The figure indicates that the outbreak peaked during September 2012. The epidemic curve aided in verifying the waxing and waning of the outbreak.

ANALYSES OF BIVARIATE ASSOCIATION

Analyses of **bivariate association** examine relationships between two variables. Some of the types of bivariate analyses described in this section involve the use of scatter plots, correlation coefficients, and contingency tables. One should remember that an association between two variables signifies only that they are related and *not* that the association is causal. The matter of a causal association is complex and relies on a body of additional information beyond the observation of a relationship between two variables.

Pearson Correlation Coefficient

A measure of the strength of association (that you may have already encountered in a statistics course) is the **Pearson correlation coefficient** (*r*), used with continuous variables. Pearson's *r* is also called the Pearson product-moment correlation. Pearson correlation coefficients (*r*) range from –1 to 0 to +1. When *r* is negative, the relationship between two variables is said to be inverse, meaning that as the value of one variable increases, the value of the other variable decreases. A positive *r* denotes a positive association: when one variable increases, so does the other variable. The closer *r* is to either +1 or –1, the stronger the association is between the two variables. As *r* approaches 0, the association becomes weaker; the value 0 means that there is no association.

Scatter Plots

Let's explore the concept of association more generally by examining a **scatter plot** (scatter diagram), a method for graphically displaying relationships between variables. A scatter diagram (also known as an XY diagram) plots two variables, one on an X-axis (horizontal axis) and the other on a Y-axis (vertical axis). The two measurements for each case (or individual subject) are plotted as a single data point (dot) in the scatter diagram. Let's create scatter diagrams from simple data sets. The examples will indicate a perfect direct linear relationship ($r = +1.0$) and a perfect inverse linear relationship ($r = -1.0$); later we will examine other types of relationships. First examine the data for Study One shown in **Table 2-7** and then see how the graphs turn out. The first data point (case 001) is (1,1), and the second point (case 002) is (2,2), with the final data point (case 015) ending as (15,15). **Figure 2-14** demonstrates that all of the points fall on a straight line; $r = 1.0$. The plot of the data in Study Two is shown in **Figure 2-15**; the graph is also a straight line and the relationship is inverse ($r = -1.0$).

TABLE 2-7 Measurements Used to Create a Scatter Plot

Study One			Study Two		
Case Number	X Variable	Y Variable	Case Number	X Variable	Y Variable
001	1	1	001	1	15
002	2	2	002	2	14
003	3	3	003	3	13
004	4	4	004	4	12
005	5	5	005	5	11
006	6	6	006	6	10
007	7	7	007	7	9
008	8	8	008	8	8
009	9	9	009	9	7
010	10	10	010	10	6
011	11	11	011	11	5
012	12	12	012	12	4
013	13	13	013	13	3
014	14	14	014	14	2
015	15	15	015	15	1

FIGURE 2-14 The graph of a perfect direct linear association between two variables, *X* and *Y* (using data from Study One).

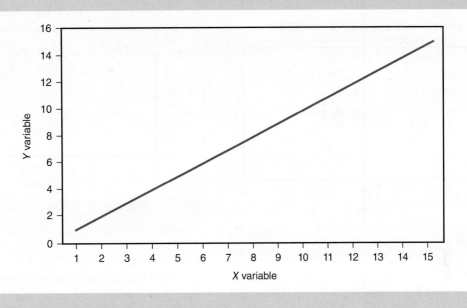

Next, we will plot the relationship between age and weight using data from a heart disease study (see **Figure 2-16**). The circular shape of this cloud reveals that there is no association between these two variables in the particular data set examined; the value of *r* is close to 0. When there is no association between two variables, they are *statistically independent*.

FIGURE 2-15 The graph of a perfect inverse linear association between two variables, *X* and *Y* (using data from Study Two).

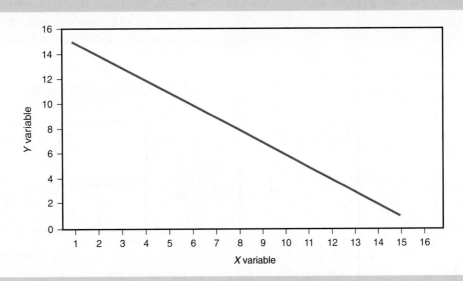

FIGURE 2-16 A scatter plot that demonstrates no relationship between age and weight.

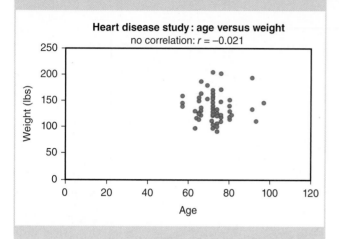

FIGURE 2-18 Inverted U-shaped curve.

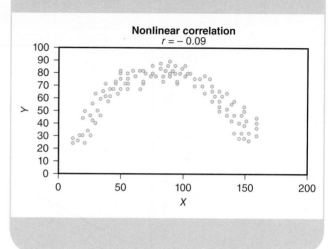

Figure 2-17 plots the relationship between systolic and diastolic blood pressure, which are positively related to one another ($r = 0.7$). Because this relationship is fairly strong, the points are close together and almost form a straight line. If we were to draw an oval around the points, the oval would be cigar shaped.

Some additional notes about scatter plots: The closer the points lie with respect to the straight "line of best fit" through them (called the regression line), the stronger the association

between variable X and variable Y. As noted, a perfect linear association between two variables is indicated by a straight line.

It is also possible for scatter plots to conform to nonlinear shapes, such as a curved line, which suggests a nonlinear or curvilinear relationship. **Figure 2-18** shows an inverted U-shaped relationship. The linear correlation between X and Y is essentially 0 (-0.09), indicating that there is no linear association. However, nonlinear curves do not imply that there is no relationship between two variables, only that their relationship is nonlinear.

Dose-Response Curves

A **dose-response curve** is the plot of a dose-response relationship, which is a type of correlative association between an exposure (e.g., dose of a toxic chemical) and effect (e.g., a biologic outcome). **Figure 2-19** illustrates a dose-response

FIGURE 2-17 A scatter plot that demonstrates a positive relationship between systolic and diastolic blood pressure.

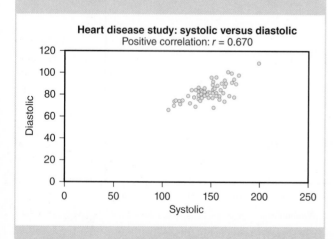

FIGURE 2-19 A dose-response curve.

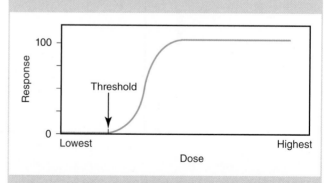

curve. The dose is indicated along the X-axis, with the response shown along the Y-axis. At the beginning of the curve, the flat portion suggests that at low levels of the dose, no or a minimal effect occurs. This is also known as the subthreshold phase. After the threshold is reached, the curve rises steeply and then progresses to a linear state in which an increase in response is proportional to an increase in dose. The threshold refers to the lowest dose at which a particular response occurs. When the maximal response is reached, the curve flattens out.

A dose-response relationship is one of the indicators used to assess a causal effect of a suspected exposure associated with an adverse health outcome. For example, there is a dose-response relationship between the number of cigarettes smoked daily and mortality from lung cancer.[6] As the number of cigarettes smoked per day increases, so do the rates of lung cancer mortality. This dose-response relationship was one of the considerations that led to the conclusion that smoking is a cause of lung cancer mortality.

Contingency Tables

Another method for demonstrating associations is to use a **contingency table**, which is a type of table that tabulates data according to two dimensions (refer to **Table 2-8**).

The type of contingency table illustrated by Table 2-8 is also called a 2 by 2 table or a fourfold table because it contains four cells, labeled A through D. The column and row totals are known as marginal totals. As noted previously, analytic epidemiology is concerned with the associations between exposures and health outcomes (disease status). Two study designs employ variations of a contingency table to present the results. One of these designs is a case-control study and the other is a cohort study. We will examine these study

designs further in Chapter 7. The definitions of the cells in Table 2-8 are as follows:

A = Exposure is present and disease is present.
B = Exposure is present and disease is absent.
C = Exposure is absent and disease is present.
D = Exposure is absent and disease is absent.

Here is an example of how a contingency table can be used to study associations. Consider the relationship between advertisements for alcoholic beverages and binge drinking. We can pose the question of whether teenagers who view television commercials that promote alcoholic beverages are more prone to engage in binge drinking than teenagers who do not view such advertisements. The contingency table would be labeled as shown in **Table 2-9**. In the example, the exposure status variable is viewing or not viewing alcoholic beverage commercials; the outcome variable is whether study subjects engage in binge drinking. The totals refer to the column totals, row totals, and grand total.

What information can we glean from this contingency table? If there is an association between binge drinking and viewing alcoholic beverage commercials, the proportions of binge drinkers in each cell would be different from one another. In fact, we would expect a higher proportion of teenage binge drinkers among those who view alcoholic beverage commercials in comparison with those who do not view such commercials. However, this statement is somewhat of an oversimplification. Later in the book, the author will present an in-depth discussion of measures for quantifying associations between exposure and outcome variables. The two measures that will be described are the odds ratio and relative risk. Suffice it to say that the choice of measures of association must be appropriate to the type of study design chosen.

PARAMETER ESTIMATION

Recall that epidemiologists use statistics to estimate parameters. Two types of estimates of parameters are a point estimate and a confidence interval estimate. A **point estimate** is a single value used to estimate a parameter. An example is the use of $\overline{X}$, the sample mean, to estimate μ, which is the corresponding population mean. An alternative to a point estimate is an **interval estimate**, defined as a range of values that with a certain level of confidence contains the parameter. One of the common levels of confidence is the 95% confidence level, although others are possible. This level of confidence means that one is 95% certain the confidence interval contains the parameter. Refer to **Formula 2-3**. In order to obtain a more precise or narrower estimate of the confidence interval for μ, one needs

TABLE 2-8 Generic Contingency Table

	Disease Status		
Exposure status	Yes	No	Total
Yes	A	B	A + B
No	C	D	C + D
Total	A + C	B + D	A + B + C + D

TABLE 2-9 The Association Between Viewing Alcohol Advertisements and Binge Drinking

	Binge Drinking		
Exposure Status	Binge Drinkers	Non-Binge Drinkers	Total
View alcoholic beverage commercials	(A) Binge drinkers who view alcoholic beverage commercials	(B) Non-binge drinkers who view alcoholic beverage commercials	(A + B) All viewers of alcoholic beverage commercials
Do not view alcoholic beverage commercials	(C) Binge drinkers who do not view alcoholic beverage commercials	(D) Non-binge drinkers who do not view alcoholic beverage commercials	(C + D) All nonviewers of alcoholic beverage commercials
Total	(A + C) All binge drinkers	(B + D) All non-binge drinkers	(A + B + C + D) All study subjects

FORMULA 2-3 The 95% confidence interval (CI)

$$95\% \text{ CI} = \bar{X} \pm \frac{1.96\sigma}{\sqrt{n}}$$

Calculation example: In Table 2-6, the mean ($\bar{X}$) was 20.6. The sample size (n) was 10. Assume that the population standard deviation (σ) is 3.1.

$$95\% \text{ CI} = 20.6 \pm \frac{(1.96)(3.1)}{\sqrt{10}} = 20.6 \pm 1.9$$

The 95% CI: 18.7 ↔ 22.5

The values 18.7 and 22.5 are the lower and upper confidence limits, respectively.

Alternative formula:

The term $\frac{\sigma}{\sqrt{n}}$ is called the standard error of the mean (SEM). The alternative formula for the 95% CI is:

$$95\% \text{ CI} = \bar{X} \pm 1.96 \times \text{SEM}$$

to increase the sample size, n. As shown in the formula: the denominator of the standard error of the mean:

$$\left(\frac{\sigma}{\sqrt{n}}\right) \text{ is } \sqrt{n}$$

As n increases, the standard error of the mean decreases; the result is a narrower confidence interval.

CONCLUSION

This chapter focused on acquisition, organization, and presentation of health-related data. Methods for sampling data include random and nonrandom sampling. Information from samples (statistics) is used to make inferences about the characteristics of populations (parameters). Among the types of data used in epidemiology are qualitative and quantitative data. Epidemiologic variables can be composed of discrete and continuous data (scales). Stevens' treatise classified measurement scales into nominal, ordinal, interval, and ratio levels of measurement.

The methods for display of data covered in this chapter were frequency tables, bar charts and histograms, line graphs, and pie charts. Statistical indices included measures of central tendency (e.g., mode, median, and mean) and measures of variation (e.g., range, variance, and standard deviation). Regarding distribution curves, the author defined the standard normal distribution, skewed distributions, and multimodal distributions. Measures of bivariate associations presented were correct coefficients, scatter plots, and contingency tables. Among the types of relationships between two variables discussed were linear direct, linear inverse, and nonlinear, e.g., curvilinear (as in an inverted U-shaped curve).

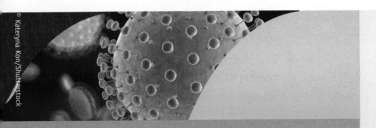

Study Questions and Exercises

1. Define the following terms used for populations and samples and give examples of each term:
   a. Population
   b. Sample
   c. Parameter
   d. Statistic
   e. Representativeness

2. Define the terms *qualitative* and *quantitative* data and indicate which of the two types the following data represent:
   a. Sex
   b. Race
   c. Weight

3. List Stevens' four scales of measurement. Indicate the permissible statistics that can be computed with each of the levels of measurement. What type of scale is the Fahrenheit temperature scale? What type of scale is the Kelvin temperature scale?

4. Distinguish between random and nonrandom samples, stating the advantages and disadvantages of each type of sample.

5. Define each of the following terms, citing their applications:
   a. Stratified random sample
   b. Systematic sample
   c. Convenience sample
   d. Cluster sampling

6. Why is a random sample unbiased?

7. Define and compare the terms *central tendency* and *variation*, giving examples of each term.

8. For a skewed distribution, the most appropriate measure of central tendency is which, the mean, median, or mode? Explain your answer.

9. On a blank sheet of paper, draw the following distribution curves:
   a. Unimodal, symmetric distribution
   b. Positively skewed distribution
   c. Negatively skewed distribution

10. Define and give examples of the following terms:
    a. Positive association
    b. Negative association
    c. Nonlinear association
    d. Dose-response relationship

11. How are a scatter plot and a contingency table helpful in demonstrating an association? Set up a contingency table that would show a hypothetical the association between teenage drinking and automobile crashes.

12. Does a perfect positive correlation coefficient ($r = +1.0$) reflect a stronger or weaker association than a perfect negative correlation ($r = -1.0$)? What do the plus and minus signs mean?

13. Describe a multimodal curve. What is the significance for epidemiology of a multimodal curve? Sketch a multimodal curve.

14. Cases of gastrointestinal illness that occurred during the *Salmonella* Heidelberg epidemic were distributed as a unimodal curve. (Refer back to Figure 2-13.) What is another name for this type of curve? Why is this type of curve important for epidemiology?

15. Confidence interval estimation: Suppose we collect a random sample of 64 blood cholesterol readings from the database of patients at a large health clinic for women. We know that the population standard deviation (σ) is 11.1 mg/dL of blood. The average cholesterol for the sample of women is 206 mg/100 dL of blood. Calculate the 95% confidence interval for μ.

Answer:

$$95\% \text{ CI} = 206 \pm \frac{(1.96)(11.1)}{\sqrt{64}} \quad 95\% \text{ CI}: 203.3 \leftrightarrow 208.7$$

16. According to the National Ambulatory Care Survey, the average annual numbers of visits to physicians for health care among males (ages 15 to 39 years) between 2009 and 2012 were as follows:

    • White, non-Hispanic: 1.64
    • Black, non-Hispanic: 0.89
    • Hispanic: 0.84

    Draw a bar chart using these data. (You can use Excel or another software program.) What can you conclude from the chart? The variable "race" corresponds to what scale of measurement?

Practice Questions for the MCAT® Examination

Epidemiology 101 is a helpful resource for medical school applicants who are preparing for Skill 4: Scientific Inquiry and Reasoning Skills: Data-Based Statistical Reasoning on the MCAT® exam. This chapter contains information for support of Skill 4. The topics included in Skill 4 are shown in italics and reprinted from the website of the American Association of Medical Colleges. (Available at: https://students-residents.aamc.org /applying-medical-school/article/mcat-2015-sirs-skill4/. Accessed September 1, 2016.) The author has created sample questions, which are grouped by topic area. Note that this guide does not cover all of the topics for Skill 4.

• *Using, analyzing, and interpreting data in figures, graphs, and tables*

1. Describe **Figure 2-20**, which presents information on homicide rates. Which of the following statements about the figure is true? (Give the best answer.)
   a. With respect to the total number of homicides, the rates peaked in 2003.
   b. The distribution of rates for the total number of homicides is unimodal.
   c. For age 10–14 years, the distribution for homicides rates is unimodal.
   d. For age 10–14 years, homicides rates have had an increasing trend.

2. Regarding Figure 2-20, the highest homicide rates occurred among:
   a. Males in 1993
   b. Females in 1993
   c. Persons age 15–19 years in 1993
   d. Persons age 20–24 years in 1993

• *Evaluating whether representations make sense for particular scientific observations and data*

3. The Centers for Disease Control and Prevention reported the percentage of children who had abnormal cholesterol levels according to body weight. Among boys, the percentages of abnormal cholesterol levels for normal weight, overweight, and obese persons were approximately 15%, 25% and 45%, respectively. Among girls, the corresponding percentages were approximately 15%, 25%, and 44%, respectively. On the basis of these data, one can conclude the following:
   a. Girls should reduce carbohydrate intake.
   b. Boy should exercise more vigorously than girls.
   c. Gender is not related to abnormal cholesterol.
   d. Both a and b are correct.

4. On the basis of the data in the previous question, how does weight affect abnormal cholesterol levels?
   a. Weight is positively associated with abnormal cholesterol.
   b. Weight is negatively associated with abnormal cholesterol.
   c. Overweight causes abnormal cholesterol levels.
   d. Both a and c are correct.

FIGURE 2-20 Homicide rates among persons age 10–24 years, by sex and age group—United States, 1981–2010.

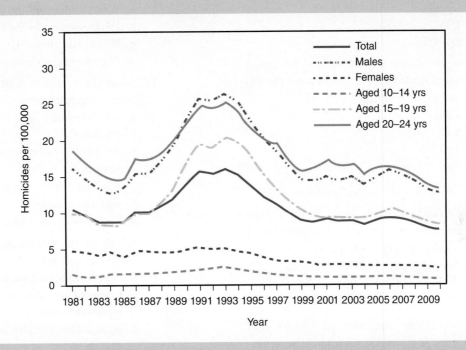

Reprinted from Centers for Disease Control and Prevention. Homicide rates among persons aged 10–24 years—United States, 1981–2010. *MMWR*. 2013;62(27):547.

- *Using measures of central tendency (mean, median, and mode) and measures of dispersion (range, interquartile range, and standard deviation) to describe data*

5. Calculate a mean age of the following sample of ages: {20, 17, 16, 18}
   a. 18.0
   b. 17.7
   c. 16.9
   d. 17.1

6. Calculate the median for the data set: {41, 18, 21, 19, 25, 26, 22, 21}
   a. 19.0
   b. 25.0
   c. 21.0
   d. 21.5

7. Calculate the mode for the data set: {3, 21, 5, 30, 7, 21, 31, 21}
   a. 18
   b. 28
   c. 17
   d. 21

8. What is the range of the data set: {3, 21, 5, 30, 7, 21, 31, 21}
   a. 18
   b. 28
   c. 17
   d. 21

9. The interquartile range of a distribution is defined as:
   a. Q4–Q1
   b. Q2–Q1
   c. Q3–Q1
   d. Q3–Q2

10. Using the deviation score method, calculate a standard deviation of a sample given the following data: $\{n = 36, \sum (X - \overline{X})^2 = 225\}$
    a. 6.25
    b. 6.42
    c. 2.50
    d. 2.54

- *Reasoning about random and systematic error*

11. For a random sample when $\overline{X}$ differs from μ, this difference is most likely a reflection of:
    a. The use of a large sample size (n)
    b. Self-selection by research subjects
    c. Random error that affected the sample
    d. The use of a stratified sample

- *Reasoning about statistical significance and uncertainty (e.g., interpreting statistical significance levels, interpreting a confidence interval)*

12. Calculate the 95% confidence interval for μ given the following information: $\{\overline{X} = 16.3;$ standard error of the mean = 6$\}$
    a. The lower confidence limit is 4.5.
    b. The lower confidence limit is 18.3.
    c. The lower confidence limit is 10.3.
    d. The lower confidence limit is 28.3.

13. We obtain a 95% confidence interval of $\{25.5 \leftrightarrow 30.1\}$. This means that:
    a. It is likely that 95 times out of 100, μ falls within this range.
    b. It is likely that 5 times out of 100, μ falls outside of this range.
    c. It is likely that 100 times out of 100, μ falls within this range.
    d. Both a and b are correct.

14. For a confidence interval (CI), how does changing n affect the length of the interval?
    a. When n increases the CI narrows.
    b. When n increases the CI widens.
    c. When n decreases the CI is less precise.
    d. Both a and c are correct.

15. Select the best statement about a random sample regarding parameter estimation:
    a. All random samples are unbiased estimators.
    b. All random samples are slightly biased estimators.
    c. Random sampling guarantees a representative sample.
    d. Both a and c are correct.

16. Which of the following statements about sample designs is false?
    a. Nonrandom samples are biased.
    b. Convenience samples have unknown representativeness.
    c. Nonrandom samples help in descriptive studies.
    d. None of the statements are false.

- *Using data to explain relationships between variables or make predictions*

17. A medical study reported that the Pearson correlation coefficient (r) between fasting blood sugar level and total cholesterol was 0.70. Assuming that this finding was not due to chance, which of the following statements is most appropriate?
    a. Blood sugar had no relationship with cholesterol.
    b. Blood sugar was inversely related to cholesterol.
    c. Blood sugar had a moderate relationship with cholesterol.
    d. Blood sugar had a one-to-one relationship with cholesterol.

18. Find the value of cell A in the following contingency table (Table 2-10). The number of cases is shown in each cell, with the numbers missing in some cells.
    a. 39
    b. 34
    c. 31
    d. 28

- *Using data to answer research questions and draw conclusions. Identifying conclusions that are supported by research results. Determining the implications of results for real-world situations*

19. Most states, as part of their Graduated Driver Licensing (GDL) program, restrict night driving. Almost one-half of U.S. states with a GDL program impose a night driving restriction that begins at 12:00 AM or later. The Centers for Disease Control and Prevention reported that 57% of fatal crashes among drivers 16 or 17 years of age happened at night before 12:00 AM. A much lower percentage occurred after 12:00 AM. What are the implications of this finding?
    a. Drivers who are 16 or 17 should not be permitted to drive at all.
    b. Drivers who are 16 or 17 should be permitted to drive only during daylight.
    c. Drivers who are 16 or 17 should have driving restrictions earlier at night.
    d. Drivers who are 16 or 17 do not require changes in night driving restrictions.

20. About 35% of adults in poverty status meet federal guidelines for aerobic physical activity. The percentage of adults who meet the guidelines increases with family income level to nearly 70% among people at the highest income levels. Which method is most likely to be effective for encouraging adults in poverty status to participate in aerobic exercise?
    a. In low-income communities, run television ads about the benefits of exercise.
    b. Distribute flyers about the benefits of exercise throughout the community.
    c. Encourage a chain of fitness gyms to open branches in poor communities.
    d. Increase the minimum wage of low-income workers above the poverty level.

TABLE 2-10 Contingency Table

Exposure status	Disease Status		
	Yes	No	Total
Yes	A = ?	B = 6	A + B = ?
No	C = 11	D = 28	C + D = ?
Total	A + C = ?	B + D = ?	A + B + C + D = 76

- *Explaining why income data are usually reported using the median rather than the mean* (from the Psychological, Social, and Biological Foundations of Behavior section)

21. The mean falls to the left of the median in which of the following distributions:
    a. Bimodal distribution
    b. Standard normal distribution
    c. Negatively skewed distribution
    d. Positively skewed distribution

22. A hospital employees' union presented data on doctors' compensation; salary data were compiled on all physicians including medical residents. The distribution of these data were likely to be:
    a. Skewed to the left
    b. Symmetric
    c. Negatively skewed
    d. Positively skewed

The answers to the MCAT practice questions are shown in **Table 2-11**.

TABLE 2-11 Answer Key to MCAT Practice Questions

Question Number	Answer	Question Number	Answer	Question Number	Answer	Question Number	Answer	Question Number	Answer
1	B	6	D	11	C	16	D	21	C
2	A	7	D	12	A	17	C	22	D
3	C	8	B	13	D	18	C		
4	A	9	C	14	D	19	C		
5	B	10	D	15	A	20	D		

REFERENCES

1. Chernick MR, Friis RH. *Introductory Biostatistics for the Health Sciences.* Hoboken, NJ: John Wiley & Sons, Inc.; 2003.

2. Porta M, ed. *A Dictionary of Epidemiology.* 6th ed. New York, NY: Oxford University Press; 2014.

3. Organisation for Economic Cooperation and Development. Glossary of statistical terms. Paris, France: OECD. Available at: https://stats.oecd.org/glossary/detail.asp?ID=2219. Accessed September 3, 2016.

4. Stevens SS. On the theory of scales of measurement. *Science.* 1946;103(2684):677–680.

5. Centers for Disease Control and Prevention. Outbreak of *Salmonella* Heidelberg infections linked to a single poultry producer—13 states, 2012–2013. *MMWR.* 2013;62(27):553–556.

6. Doll R, Peto R. Mortality in relation to smoking: 20 years' observation on male British doctors. *BMJ.* 1976;2(6051):1525–1536.

CHAPTER 3

Epidemiologic Measurements Used to Describe Disease Occurrence

LEARNING OBJECTIVES

By the end of this chapter you will be able to:

- Define three mathematical terms applied to epidemiology and provide examples of each.
- Compare *incidence* and *prevalence* and explain how they are interrelated.
- State one epidemiologic measure of mortality, giving its formula.
- Distinguish between a fertility rate and a birth rate.
- Name the limitations of crude rates and define alternative measures.

CHAPTER OUTLINE

INTRODUCTION

Epidemiologic measurements aid in describing the occurrence of morbidity and mortality in populations. The chapter begins by covering four key mathematical terms that involve the use of fractions and that appear in epidemiologic constructs. You will learn how these terms are applied to fundamental epidemiologic measures of the frequency of diseases in populations and risks associated with exposures to disease agents. This chapter also reveals the different conclusions that can be drawn by examining existing and new cases of disease. Additional topics include basic measures of morbidity and mortality as well as alternative calculations for improving estimates of morbidity and mortality. Finally, you will learn about miscellaneous statistics related to natality and mortality linked to natality. Refer to **Table 3-1** for a list of the major terms and concepts covered in this chapter.

MATHEMATICAL TERMS USED IN EPIDEMIOLOGY

Some important mathematical terms applied to epidemiologic measures are rate, proportion, and percentage; these measures are types of ratios. (Refer to **Figure 3-1**.) The following section defines these terms and gives calculation examples of ratios, proportions, and percentages for mortality from AIDS. The topic of rates will be covered later in the chapter. Data for use in calculating the examples of rates,

TABLE 3-1 List of Important Mathematical and Epidemiologic Terms Used in This Chapter

Mathematical Terms	Epidemiologic Terms: Frequency	Epidemiologic Terms: Risk	Measures Related to Morbidity and Mortality	Measures Related to Natality
Percentage	Count	Attack rate	Case fatality rate	Maternal mortality rate
Proportion	Period prevalence	Incidence rate/ cumulative incidence/ incidence proportion	Crude rate/crude death rate (crude mortality rate)	Infant and perinatal mortality rates/fetal death rate
Rate	Point prevalence	Reference population	Life expectancy	Birth rate
Ratio	Prevalence	Risk factor/population at risk	Specific rate	General fertility rate

proportions, and percentages are given in **Table 3-2**. Following are some data that will be used for the calculations.

Ratio

A **ratio** is defined as "[t]he value obtained by dividing one quantity by another. Rates and proportions (including risk) are ratios…. Ratios are sometimes expressed as percentages."[1] Although a ratio consists of a numerator and a denominator, its most general form does not necessarily have any specified relationship between the numerator and denominator.

A ratio is expressed as follows: ratio = X/Y. Calculation example of a ratio:

Example 1: With respect to AIDS mortality, the sex ratio of deaths (male to female deaths) = X/Y, where: X = 450,451 and Y = 89,895. The sex ratio = 450,451/89,895 = 5 to 1 (approximately).

FIGURE 3-1 Definitions of mathematical terms that are used in epidemiology.

– Ratio (R)	$R = \dfrac{X}{Y}$	X and Y can be any number, including ratios.
– Rate (r)*	$r = \dfrac{X}{\Delta t}$	Type of ratio where the numerator is usually a count, and the denominator is a time elapsed.
– Proportion (p)	$P = \dfrac{A}{A + B}$	Type of ratio where the numerator is part of the denominator.
– Percent (P)	$P = \left(\dfrac{A}{A + B} \right) \times 100$	A proportion is multiplied by 100.

Modified with permission from Aragón T. *Descriptive Epidemiology: Describing Findings and Generating Hypotheses.* Center for Infectious Disease Preparedness, University of California Berkeley School of Public Health. Available at: http://www.iready.org/slides/feb_descriptive.pdf. Accessed August 16, 2016.

TABLE 3-2 Data for Calculations of Rates, Proportions, and Percentages

Cumulative U.S. AIDS mortality, 2002–2006; deaths among adults and adolescents[2]	Males = 450,541 Females = 89,895
Author's hypothetical survey of clinic patients (*n* = 20) regarding intravenous drug use (IDU) in a clinic	Number of IDU users = 19 Number of persons who did not use = 1

Example 2: Referring to the data in Table 3-2, you can observe that the ratio of users of intravenous drugs to nonusers is 19 to 1.

Example 3: In demography, the sex ratio refers to the number of males per 100 females. In the United States, the sex ratio in 2005 was 96.5, meaning that there were more women and girls than men and boys.[3] At the same time, there were considerable variations by state; Alaska and Nevada had the highest sex ratios. In 2010, the U.S. sex ratio increased to 96.7.[4] At birth the sex ratio is approximately 105 males to 100 females. Due to higher mortality among males, the sex ratio deceases with age, a trend shown in **Figure 3-2**. However, from 2000 to 2010, the population of males 60 years and older increased in comparison with the population of females in the same age group. According to the U.S. Census Bureau, this change can be attributed to a narrowing of male-female mortality differences.

Proportion

A **proportion** is a type of ratio in which the numerator is part of the denominator. Proportions may be expressed as percentages.

A proportion is expressed as follows: proportion = A/A + B
Calculation example of a proportion:

Example 1: Proportion of AIDS deaths
Suppose that A = the number of male deaths from AIDS
A = 450,451

FIGURE 3-2 Sex ratio, by age—2000 and 2010.

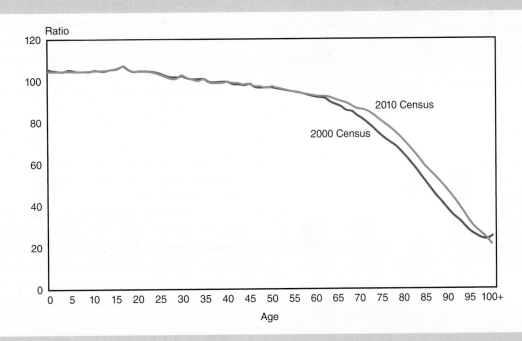

Reprinted from U.S. Census Bureau. Age and Sex Composition: 2010. *2010 Census Briefs.* May 2011:5.

B = the number of female deaths from AIDS

B = 89,895

The proportion of deaths that occurred among males = 450,451/(450,451 + 89,895) = 0.83

Example 2: Proportion of IDU users (data from Table 3-2) Proportion = 19/(19+1) = 0.95

Percentage

A **percentage** is a proportion that has been multiplied by 100. The formula for a percentage is as follows:

percentage = (A/A + B) × 100

Example 1: The percentage of male deaths from AIDS was (0.83 × 100) = 83%.

Example 2: The percentage of IDU users was (0.95 × 100) = 95%.

Example 3: Refer to **Figure 3-3**, which is a graph of the percentage of adults who reported joint pain or stiffness in the United States in 2006. The figure demonstrates that slightly less than one-third of adults had symptoms of joint pain within the preceding 30-day period. The most frequently reported form of pain was knee pain. "During 2006, approximately 30% of adults reported experiencing some type of joint pain during the preceding 30 days. Knee pain was reported by 18% of respondents, followed

by pain in the shoulder (9%), finger (7%), and hip (7%). Joint pain can be caused by osteoarthritis, injury, prolonged abnormal posture, or repetitive motion."[5(p467)]

Let's consider how a proportion (as well as a percentage) can be helpful in describing health conditions. A proportion indicates how important a health outcome is relative to the size of a group. Refer to the following example: suppose there were 10 college dorm residents who had infectious mononucleosis (a virus-caused disease that produces fever, sore throat, and tiredness). How large a problem did these 10 cases represent? To answer this question, one would need to know whether the dormitory housed 20 students or 500 students. If there were only 20 students, then 50% (or 0.50) were ill. Conversely, if there were 500 students in the dormitory, then only 2% (or 0.02) were ill. Clearly, these two scenarios paint a completely different picture of the magnitude of the problem. In this situation, expressing the count as a proportion is indeed helpful. In most situations, it will be informative to have some idea about the size of the denominator. Although the construction of a proportion is straightforward, one of the central concerns of epidemiology is to find and enumerate appropriate denominators to describe and compare groups in a meaningful and useful way.

Rate

Also a type of ratio, a **rate** differs from a proportion because the denominator involves a measure of time. (Refer back to Figure 3-1). The rate measure shown in the figure is the mathematical formula in which elapsed time is denoted in the denominator by the symbol Δt.

Epidemiologic rates are composed of a numerator (the number of events such as health outcomes), a denominator (a population in which the events occur), and a measure of time.[1] This measure of time is the time period during which events in the numerator occur. The denominator consists of the average population in which the events occurred during this same time period.

In epidemiology, rates are used to measure risks associated with exposures and provide information about the speed of development of a disease. Also, rates can be used to make comparisons among populations. More detailed information on rates is provided in the section on crude rates. Medical publications may use the terms ratio, proportion, and rate without strict adherence to the mathematical definitions for these terms. Hence, you must be alert regarding how a measure is defined and calculated.[6]

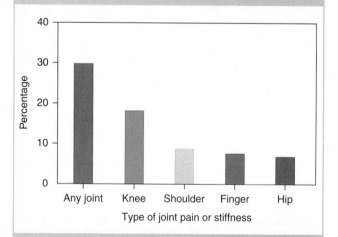

FIGURE 3-3 Percentage of adults reporting joint pain or stiffness, National Health Interview Survey—United States, 2006.

Reprinted from Centers for Disease Control and Prevention. QuickStats: Percentage of adults reporting joint pain or stiffness—National Health Interview Survey, United States, 2006. *MMWR* 2008;57:467.

GENERAL INFORMATION REGARDING EPIDEMIOLOGIC MEASURES

As noted previously, epidemiologic measures represent an application of common mathematical terms such as ratio and proportion to the description of the health of the population. Epidemiologic measures provide the following types of information: (1) the frequency of a disease or condition, (2) associations between exposures and health outcomes, and (3) strength of the relationship between an exposure and a health outcome. **Figure 3-4** gives an overview of the principal epidemiologic measures covered in this chapter; these are count, rate (for example, incidence rate and death rate), risk or odds, and prevalence. Keep in mind that time is a component of rates.

The following considerations are important to the expression of epidemiologic measures:

- Defining the numerator.
  - Case definition (condition)—For epidemiologic measures to be valid, the case of disease or other health phenomenon being studied must be defined carefully and in a manner that can be replicated by others.
  - Frequency—How many cases are there?
  - Severity—Some epidemiologic measures employ morbidity as the numerator and others use mortality.
- Defining the denominator—Does the measure make use of the entire population or a subset of the population? Some measures use the **population at risk**, defined as those members of the population who are capable of developing a disease, for example, people who are not immune to an infectious disease.
- Existing (all cases) versus new cases.

The following sections will define the foregoing terms and concepts.

TYPES OF EPIDEMIOLOGIC MEASURES

A number of quantitative terms, useful in epidemiology, have been developed to characterize the occurrence of disease, morbidity, and mortality in populations. Particularly noteworthy are the terms *incidence* and *prevalence*, which can be stated as frequencies or raw numbers of cases. (These terms are defined later.) In order to make comparisons among populations that differ in size, statisticians divide the number of cases by the population size.

Counts

The simplest and most frequently performed quantitative measure in epidemiology is a count. As the term implies, a **count** refers merely to the number of cases of a disease or other health phenomenon being studied. As shown in **Table 3-3**, an example of a count is the number of cases of infrequently reported notifiable diseases per year.

The previous discussion may leave the reader with the impression that counts, because they are simple measures, are of little value in epidemiology; this is not true, however. In fact, case reports of patients with particularly unusual presentations or combinations of symptoms often spur epidemiologic investigations. In addition, for some diseases even a single case is sufficient to be of public health importance. For example, if a case of smallpox (now eradicated) or Ebola virus disease were reported, the size of the denominator would be irrelevant. That is, in these instances a single case, regardless of the size of the population at risk, would stimulate an investigation.

Measures of Incidence

Measures of incidence are measures of risk of acquiring a disease or measures of the rate at which new cases of disease develop in a population. They may also be used to assess other health outcomes in addition to diseases. The terms covered in this section are incidence, incidence rate, cumulative incidence, incidence density, and attack rate. Incidence measures are central to the study of causal mechanisms with regard to how exposures affect health outcomes. Incidence measures such as cumulative incidence are used to describe the risks associated with certain exposures; they can be used to estimate in a

FIGURE 3-4 Epidemiologic measures—measures of occurrence.

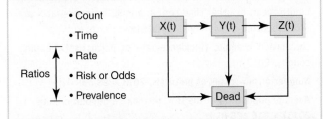

- Count
- Time
- Rate
- Risk or Odds
- Prevalence

Ratios

X(t) → Y(t) → Z(t) → Dead

Reprinted with permission from Aragón T. *Descriptive Epidemiology: Describing Findings and Generating Hypotheses*. Center for Infectious Disease Preparedness, University of California Berkeley School of Public Health. Available at: http://www.idready.org/slides/feb_descriptive.pdf. Accessed August 16, 2016.

TABLE 3-3 Cases of Selected Infrequently Reported Notifiable Diseases (< 1,000 Cases Reported)—United States, 2011–2015

Total Cases Reported by Year					
Disease	2015*	2014	2013	2012	2011
Botulism, foodborne	37	15	4	27	24
Cholera	2	5	14	17	40
Hansen's disease (leprosy)†	89	88	81	82	82
Rabies, human	1	1	2	1	6

†Not reportable in all states.

*Case counts for 2015 are provisional.

Modified data from Centers for Disease Control and Prevention. Notifiable diseases and mortality tables. *MMWR.* 2016;65(24):ND-417.

population "… the probability of someone in that population developing the disease during a specified period, conditional on not dying first from another disease."[7(p23)]

Incidence

The term *incidence* refers to "[t]he number of instances of illness commencing, or of persons falling ill, during a given period in a specified population. More generally, the number of new health-related events in a defined population within a specified period of time."[1] Ways to express incidence include: incidence rate, cumulative incidence, incidence density, and attack rate.

Incidence Rate

The incidence rate is defined as "[t]he RATE at which new events occur in a population."[1] The new events are usually new cases of disease but can be other health outcomes. The incidence rate is a rate because a time period during which the new cases occur is specified and the population at risk is observed. **Figure 3-5** presents the incidence rates for tuberculosis by state in the United States.

The **incidence rate** denotes a rate formed by dividing the number of new cases that occur during a time period by the average number of individuals in the population at risk during the same time period times a multiplier. (Refer to the box, Incidence rate.) The denominator is the average number of persons at risk for the following reason: In most situations, populations are not static because of migration and other

influences on the composition of populations. To overcome this challenge, the population at the midpoint of the year is used as the denominator and is considered to be the average population at risk. The formula for the incidence rate shown in the text box is the formula used commonly in public health.

Incidence rate =

$$\frac{\text{Number of new cases over a time period}}{\text{Average population at risk during the same time period}} \times$$

$$\text{multiplier (e.g., 100,000)}$$

The choice of the multiplier is arbitrary; any convenient multiplier can be chosen.

Population at risk: those members of the population who are capable of developing a disease, e.g., nonimmune persons.

Time period: various time periods can be chosen, e.g., a week, month, year, or other time period; annual incidence rates are often reported in government statistics.

Calculation example (incidence rate of pertussis [whooping cough], 2013):

Number of new cases of pertussis, 2013 = 28,639

Average population of the U.S. (estimated population, July 1, 2013) = 316,128,839

$$\text{Incidence rate} = \left(\frac{28,639}{316,128,839}\right) \times 100,000$$

$$= 9.1 \text{ per } 100,000 \text{ (rounded)}$$

FIGURE 3-5 Rate of tuberculosis cases per 100,000, by state/area—United States, 2013.

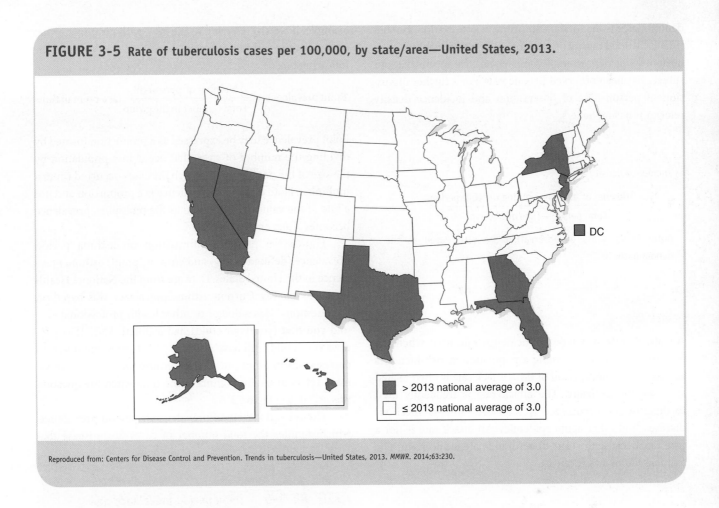

DC

■ > 2013 national average of 3.0

☐ ≤ 2013 national average of 3.0

Reproduced from: Centers for Disease Control and Prevention. Trends in tuberculosis—United States, 2013. *MMWR*. 2014;63:230.

An incidence rate is called **cumulative incidence (incidence proportion)** when *all* individuals in the population are at risk throughout the time period during which they were observed. (Refer to the box, Cumulative incidence.) An example of a population in which all members of the population are at risk is a fixed or closed population (such as the participants in a cohort study) in which no new members are allowed to enter the study after it begins.

Here is a hypothetical calculation example for cumulative incidence: An epidemiologist studies cardiovascular disease among 23,502 male middle-aged alumni of an Ivy League university. Initial medical examinations certify that the alumni have never had a heart attack in the past. During the first year of the research, 111 alums have heart attacks.

$$\text{Cumulative incidence} = \frac{111}{23,502} = .005 \ (0.5\%)$$

In this example the cumulative incidence (incidence proportion) is .005, or 0.5% when expressed as a percentage.

Cumulative incidence (incidence proportion) =

$$\frac{\text{Number of new cases over a time period}}{\text{Total population at risk during the same time period}}$$

Incidence Density

Incidence density is a variation of an incidence rate that is used when the time periods of observation of the members of a population vary from person to person. During a study that takes place over an extended period of time (for example, a cohort study, which is described later in the text), participants may be observed for varying periods of time because some drop out before the study is completed. In order to make use of all participants' data, we calculate incidence density according to the formula shown in the box. The numerator is the number of new cases during the time period and the denominator is the total person-time of observation. Person-time is the total period of time that each individual at risk has been observed. For example, one person-year means that one subject has been observed for one year. For a further discussion of person-time of observation and incidence density, refer to Friis and Sellers.[8]

Incidence density =

$$\frac{\text{Number of new cases during the time period}}{\text{Total person} - \text{Time of observation}}$$

Note: Person-years of observation are often used as the denominator.

Attack Rate

An **attack rate** is a type of incidence rate used when the occurrence of disease among a population at risk increases greatly over a short period of time; attack rate is often related to a specific exposure. The attack rate is frequently used to describe the occurrence of foodborne illness, infectious diseases, and other acute epidemics. An attack rate is not a true rate because the time dimension is often uncertain. The formula for an attack rate is:

Attack rate =

$$\text{Ill} / (\text{Ill} + \text{Well}) \times 100 \text{ during a time period}$$

Calculation example: Fifty-nine people ate roast beef suspected of causing a *Salmonella* outbreak. Thirty-four people fell ill; 25 remained well.

Number ill = 34
Number well = 25
Attack rate = 34/(34 + 25) × 100 = 57.6%

Prevalence

The term **prevalence** (expressed as a proportion) refers to the number of existing cases of a disease or health condition, or deaths in a population at some designated time divided by the number of persons in that population. The two forms of prevalence are point prevalence and period prevalence. **Point** prevalence refers to all cases of a disease, health condition, or deaths that exist at a particular point in time relative to a specific population from which the cases are derived. For

example, if we are referring to illness (morbidity) in a group of people, the formula for point prevalence is shown in the following box.

$$\text{Point prevalence} = \frac{\text{Number of persons ill}}{\text{Total number in the group}} \text{ at a point in time}$$

Point prevalence may be expressed as a proportion formed by dividing the number of cases that occur in a population by the size of the population in which the cases occurred times a multiplier. Note that point prevalence is a proportion and not a rate. If the value of 100 is used as the multiplier, prevalence becomes a percentage.

Figure 3-6 presents information on asthma period prevalence (defined below) and current (point) asthma prevalence in the United States. Data are from the National Health Interview Survey. Current asthma prevalence was based on the questions "Has a doctor or other health professional ever told you that (you/your child) had asthma? AND (Do you/does your child) still have asthma?"[9(p57)] The second question corresponds to point prevalence because the point of assessment refers to having asthma at the time when the question was asked. See Figure 3-6.

The second variety of prevalence is **period prevalence**, which denotes the total number of cases of a disease that

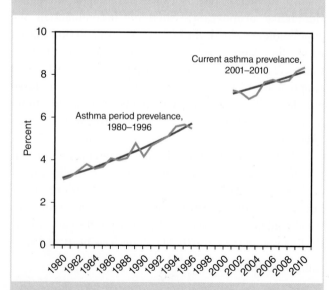

FIGURE 3-6 Asthma period prevalence and current (point) asthma prevalence: United States, 1980–2010.

Adapted from Moorman JE, Akinbami LJ, Bailey CM, et al. National Surveillance of Asthma: United States, 2001–2010. National Center for Health Statistics. *Vital Health Stat.* 2012;3(35)23.

exist during a specified period of time (e.g., a week, month, year, or other interval). An example of period prevalence is asthma period prevalence. The numerator for asthma period prevalence reflects whether a respondent answered affirmatively to the question "[d]uring the past 12 months, did anyone in the family have asthma?"[9(p57)] The time period for this measure is the past year. Figure 3-6 also shows asthma period prevalence.

Lifetime prevalence denotes cases of disease diagnosed at any time during the person's lifetime. Refer to **Figure 3-7** for an illustration of the geographic distribution of lifetime prevalence of asthma in the United States. The data are from the Behavioral Risk Factor Surveillance System. Lifetime asthma prevalence was assessed by asking whether the respondent was ever told by a health professional that they had asthma. The time period was a lifetime.

Prevalence measures are used to describe the scope and distribution of health outcomes in the population. The scope or amount of disease is called the burden of disease in the population. By offering a snapshot of disease occurrence, prevalence data contribute to the accomplishment of two of the primary functions of descriptive epidemiology: to assess variations in the occurrence of disease and to aid in the development of hypotheses that can be followed up by analytic studies.

Populations that differ in size cannot be compared directly by using frequency data, i.e., just the numbers of cases. In order to make such comparisons, prevalence proportions need to be calculated. Then it is possible to compare the proportions of health outcomes among different geographic areas. For example, Figure 3-7 shows how asthma lifetime prevalence (%) varies from state to state.

FIGURE 3-7 Adult self-reported lifetime asthma prevalence.

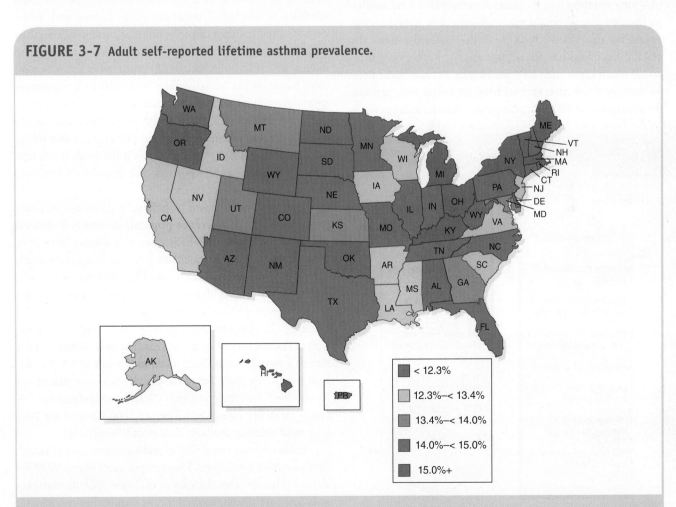

Interrelationships Between Incidence and Prevalence

Incidence and prevalence are interrelated concepts, as demonstrated by **Figure 3-8**. The relationship among incidence, prevalence, and duration of a disease is expressed by the following formula:

$$P \cong ID$$

The prevalence (P) of a disease is proportional to the incidence of the disease times the duration of the disease. Consequently, when the incidence of a disease increases, the prevalence also increases. Other factors that cause the prevalence of a disease to increase are its duration, in-migration of new cases, and development of treatments for the disease, including methods for extending the lives of patients who may not actually be cured. An example of how the duration of a disease affects its prevalence would be two diseases (A—long duration and B—short duration) that have similar incidence rates; we would expect disease A to have a higher prevalence than disease B. In the United States, the incidence of HIV infections has tended to remain constant over time and is much lower than HIV prevalence. Because more people with HIV infection are surviving for longer time periods, the prevalence of HIV is much greater than its incidence.

FIGURE 3-8 Factors influencing observed prevalence.

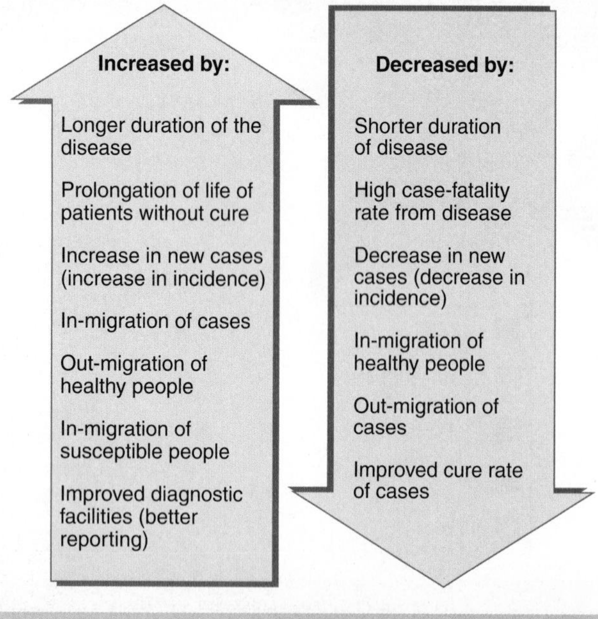

Increased by:

Longer duration of the disease

Prolongation of life of patients without cure

Increase in new cases (increase in incidence)

In-migration of cases

Out-migration of healthy people

In-migration of susceptible people

Improved diagnostic facilities (better reporting)

Decreased by:

Shorter duration of disease

High case-fatality rate from disease

Decrease in new cases (decrease in incidence)

In-migration of healthy people

Out-migration of cases

Improved cure rate of cases

Reprinted with permission from Beaglehole R, Kjellström T. *Basic Epidemiology*. Geneva, Switzerland: World Health Organization; 1993:17.

EPIDEMIOLOGIC MEASURES RELATED TO MORTALITY

Mortality rates (death rates) have trended downward over time in this country. Increasing life expectancy has accompanied this decline in mortality rates. The term **life expectancy** refers to the number of years that a person is expected to live, at any particular year. "Life expectancy at birth represents the average number of years that a group of infants would live if the group was to experience throughout life the age-specific death rates present in the year of birth."[10(p8)] In 2013, life expectancy for the population of the United States was 78.8 years overall, 81.2 years for females, and 76.4 years for males.

Crude Rates/Crude Death Rate

The basic concept of a rate can be broken down into three general categories: crude rates, specific rates, and adjusted rates. A **crude rate** is a type of rate that has not been modified to take into account any of the factors, such as the demographic makeup of the population, that may affect the observed rate. Remember that rates include a time period during which an event occurred. Crude rates are summary rates based on the actual number of events in a population over a given time period. The numerator consists of the frequency of a disease (or other health-related outcome) over a specified period of time, and the denominator is a unit size of population (**Exhibit 3-1**). An example is the crude death rate, which approximates the portion of a population that dies during a time period of interest.[1]

In the formula shown in Exhibit 3-1, the denominator is also termed the **reference population**, which is defined as the population from which cases of a disease have been taken. For example, in calculating the annual **crude death rate** (crude mortality rate) in the United States, one would count all the deaths that occurred in the country during a certain year and assign this value to the numerator. The value for the denominator would be the size of the population of the country during that year. The best estimate of the size of a population is often taken as the size of the population around the midpoint of the year, if such information can be obtained. Referring to Exhibit 3-1, one calculates the U.S. crude mortality rate as 821.5 per 100,000 persons for 2013 (the most recently available data as of this writing).

Rates improve our ability to make comparisons, although they also have limitations. For example, rates of mortality for a specific disease (see the section on cause-specific mortality rates later in this chapter) reduce the standard of comparison to a common denominator, the unit size of population. To illustrate, the U.S. crude death rate for diseases of the heart in 2013 was 193.3 per 100,000. One also might calculate the

EXHIBIT 3-1 Rate Calculation

Rate: A ratio that consists of a numerator and a denominator and in which time forms part of the denominator.

Epidemiologic rates contain the following elements:

- Disease frequency (or frequency of other health outcome)
- Unit size of population
- Time period during which an event occurs

Example (crude death rate, 2013):

Crude death rate =

$$\frac{\text{Number of deaths in a given year}}{\text{Reference population}\left(\text{during midpoint of the year}\right)} \times 100,000$$

(Either rate per 1,000 or 100,000 is used as the multiplier.)

Sample calculation problem (crude death rate in the United States):

Number of deaths in the United States during 2013 = 2,596,993

Population of the United States as of July 1, 2013 = 316,128,839

Crude death rate = (2,596,993/316,128,839) × 100,000 = 821.5 per 100,000

Adapted and reprinted from Friis RH, Sellers TA. *Epidemiology for Public Health Practice*. 5th ed. Burlington, MA: Jones & Bartlett Publishers; 2014:112.

heart disease death rate for geographic subdivisions of the country (also expressed as frequency per 100,000 individuals). These rates then could be compared with one another and with the rate for the United States for judging whether the rates found in each geographic area are higher or lower. For example, the crude death rates in 2013 for diseases of the heart in New York and Texas were 224.1 and 152.0 per 100,000, respectively.[10] On the basis of the crude death rates, it would appear that the death rate was much higher in New York than in Texas or the United States as a whole. This may be a specious conclusion, however, because there may be important differences in population composition (e.g., age differences between populations) that would affect mortality experience. Later in this chapter, the procedure to adjust for age differences or other factors is discussed.

Rates can be expressed in terms of any unit size of population that is convenient (e.g., per 1,000, per 100,000, or per 1,000,000). Many of the rates that are published and routinely used as indicators of public health are expressed according to a particular convention. For example, cancer rates are typically expressed per 100,000 population, and infant mortality is expressed per 1,000 live births. One of the determinants of the size of the denominator is whether the numerator is large enough to permit the rate to be expressed as an integer or an integer plus a trailing decimal (e.g., 4 or 4.2). For example, it would be preferable to describe the occurrence of disease as 4 per 100,000 rather than 0.04 per 1,000, even though both are perfectly correct. Throughout this chapter, the multiplier for a given morbidity or mortality statistic is provided.

Case Fatality Rate

An additional measure covered in this section is the case fatality rate (CFR). The **case fatality rate** refers to the number of deaths due to a disease that occur among people who are afflicted with that disease. The CFR(%), which provides a measure of the lethality of a disease, is defined as the number of deaths due to a specific disease within a specified time period divided by the number of cases of that disease during the same time period multiplied by 100. The formula is expressed as follows:

$$\text{CFR}(\%) = \frac{\text{Number of deaths due to disease "X"}}{\text{Number of cases of disease "X"}} \times 100 \text{ during a time period}$$

The numerator and denominator refer to the same time period. For example, suppose that 45 cases of hantavirus infection occurred in a western U.S. state during a year of interest. Of these cases, 22 were fatal. The CFR would be:

$$\text{CFR}(\%) = \frac{22}{45} \times 100 = 48.9\%$$

An example of an infectious disease that has a high case fatality rate is primary amebic meningoencephalitis, which is extremely rare and nearly always fatal. The causative organism is a type of amoeba (*Naegleria fowleri*) found in bodies of fresh water such as hot springs. This uncommon infection occurs when amoeba-contaminated water enters the nose and the parasites migrate to the brain via the optic nerve.[11]

Proportional Mortality Ratio

The National Vital Statistics Reports (for example, Deaths: Final Data for 2013)[10] provide data on the mortality experience of the United States. From these data, one can compute the crude death rate for the U.S. population as demonstrated previously. In comparison with the crude rate, the proportional mortality ratio (PMR) is used to express the proportion of all deaths that can be attributed to a given cause, for example, diseases of the heart. In 2013, the three leading causes of death were heart disease, cancer, and chronic lower respiratory diseases.

The *proportional mortality ratio PMR(%)* is the number of deaths within a population due to a specific disease or cause divided by the total number of deaths in the population (and multiplied by 100).

Proportional mortality ratio PMR(%) =

$$\frac{\text{Mortality due to a specific cause during a period of time}}{\text{Mortality due to all causes during the same time period}} \times 100$$

Sample calculation: Refer to Table 3-4 for data used in this calculation. In the United States, there were 611,105 deaths due to diseases of the heart in 2013 and 2,596,993 deaths due to all causes in that year. The PMR is (611,105/2,596,993) × 100 = 23.5%.

Table 3-4 presents mortality data for 2013 for the 10 leading causes of death in the United States. In **Figure 3-9** a pie chart illustrates the percentage of total deaths for each of the 10 leading causes of death listed in Table 3-4.

TABLE 3-4 Number and Percentage of Deaths for the 10 Leading Causes of Death in the United States, 2013

Rank	Cause of Death	Number	Percentage of Total Deaths	2013 Crude Death Rate
...	All causes	2,596,993	100.0	821.5
1	Diseases of heart	611,105	23.5	193.3
2	Malignant neoplasms	548,881	22.5	185.0
3	Chronic lower respiratory diseases	149,205	5.7	47.2
4	Accidents (unintentional injuries)	130,557	5.0	41.3
5	Cerebrovascular diseases	128,978	5.0	40.8
6	Alzheimer's disease	84,767	3.3	26.8
7	Diabetes mellitus	75,578	2.9	23.9
8	Influenza and pneumonia	56,979	2.2	18.0
9	Nephritis, nephrotic syndrome, and nephrosis	47,112	1.8	14.9
10	Intentional self-harm (suicide)	41,149	1.6	13.0

Data from Xu JQ, Murphy SL, Kochanek KD, Bastian BA. Deaths: final data for 2013. *National Vital Statistics Reports*. 2016;64(2):5. Hyattsville, MD: National Center for Health Statistics.

FIGURE 3-9 Proportional mortality ratios for 10 major causes of death in the United States, 2013.

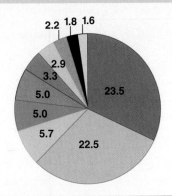

- Diseases of heart
- Malignant neoplasms
- Chronic lower respiratory diseases
- Accidents (unintentional injuries)
- Cerebrovascular diseases
- Alzheimer's disease
- Diabetes mellitus
- Influenza and pneumonia
- Nephritis, nephrotic syndrome, and nephrosis
- International self-harm (suicide)

Data from Xu JQ, Murphy SL, Kochanek KD, Bastian BA. Deaths: Final data for 2013. *National vital statistics reports*; vol 64 no 2. Hyattsville, MD: National Center for Health Statistics. 2016, p. 5.

SPECIFIC RATES

A **specific rate** is a statistic referring to a particular subgroup of the population defined in terms of race, age, or sex. A specific rate also may refer to the entire population but is specific for some single cause of death or illness. The three examples of specific rates discussed in this chapter are cause-specific rates, age-specific rates, and sex-specific rates. You will learn how they can be applied in various situations.

Cause-Specific Rate

The *cause-specific rate* is a measure that refers to mortality (or frequency of a given disease) divided by the population size at the midpoint of a time period times a multiplier. An example of a cause-specific rate is the cause-specific mortality rate, which, as the name implies, is the rate associated with

a specific cause of death. The formula for a cause-specific rate (cause-specific mortality rate) is shown in the text box.

Cause-specific rate (e.g., cause-specific mortality rate) =

$$\frac{\text{Mortality (or frequency of a given disease)}}{\text{Population size at midpoint of time period}} \times 100,000$$

Refer back to Table 3-4 for data used in the following sample calculation of the cause-specific mortality rate for accidents (unintentional injuries) for 2013. In the United States, the number of deaths for accidents (unintentional injuries) was 130,557, whereas the population total on July 1, 2013 was estimated to be 316,128,839. The crude cause-specific mortality rate due to accidents (unintentional injuries) per 100,000 was 130,557/316,128,839 × 100,000 or 41.3 per 100,000.

Age-Specific Rates

An *age-specific rate* refers to the number of cases of disease per age group of the population during a specified time period. Age-specific rates help in making comparisons regarding a cause of morbidity or mortality across age groups. A more precise definition of an age-specific rate is the frequency of a disease (or health condition) in a particular age stratum divided by the total number of persons within that age stratum during a time period. The formula for an age-specific rate is shown in the text box.

AGE-SPECIFIC RATE (R)

Age-specific rate: the number of cases per age group of population (during a specified time period such as a calendar year). The following example pertains to the group age 15 to 24 years, although some other convenient age group could be chosen.

Formula (age-specific death rate [R])

$$R = \frac{\text{Number of deaths among those age 15 to 24 years}}{\text{Number of persons who are age 15 to 24 years}} \times 100,000$$

Sample calculation (deaths from malignant neoplasms): In the United States during 2013, there were 1,496 deaths due to malignant neoplasms among the group age 15 to 24 years, and there were 43,954,402 persons in that age group. The age-specific malignant neoplasm death rate in this age group is 1,496/43,954,402 × 100,000 = 3.4 per 100,000.

FIGURE 3-10 Age-specific hospitalization rates per 10,000 for kidney disease, by age group—National Hospital Discharge Survey, United States, 1980–2005.

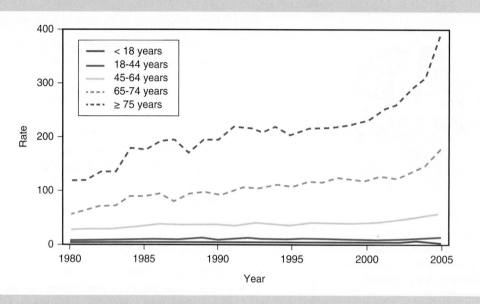

Reprinted from Centers for Disease Control and Prevention. Hospitalization discharge diagnoses for kidney disease—United States, 1980–2005. MMWR. March 2008; 57:311.

Figure 3-10 illustrates data for age-specific rates of hospitalization for kidney disease. For people 45 years of age and older, the age-specific hospitalization rates have shown an increasing trend. The highest rates of hospitalization and the sharpest increase in rates occurred among people age 75 years and older.

Sex-Specific Rates

A sex-specific rate refers to the frequency of a disease in a sex group divided by the total number of persons within that sex group during a time period times a multiplier. The formula for a sex-specific rate is shown in the following text box.

- Estimated number of males in the population as of July 1, 2013: 155,651,602
- Estimated number of females in the population as of July 1, 2013: 160,477,237

The sex-specific crude death rate for males in 2013 per 100,000 was 1,306,034/155,651,602 × 100,000 = 839.1 per 100,000.

The sex-specific crude death rate for females in 2013 per 100,000 was 1,290,959/160,477,237 × 100,000 = 804.4 per 100,000.

Thus, in 2013, the sex-specific crude death rate for males was 839.1 per 100,000 population versus 804.4 per 100,000 population for females.

Sex-specific rate (e.g., sex-specific death rate) =

$$\frac{\text{Number of deaths in a sex group}}{\text{Total number of persons in the sex group}} \times 100,000$$

Sample calculation: In 2013, the following information was recorded about mortality and the population size:

- Number of deaths among males: 1,306,034
- Number of deaths among females: 1,290,959

ADJUSTED RATES

An *adjusted rate* is a rate of morbidity or mortality in a population in which statistical procedures have been applied to permit fair comparisons across populations by removing the effect of differences in the composition of various populations. A factor in rate adjustment is age adjustment. Calculation of age-adjusted rates is a much more involved procedure than that required for crude rates. A weighting process entails the use of detailed information about the age structure of the population for which the rates are being age adjusted. For example, "age-adjusted death rates are constructs that show what the level of mortality would be if no changes occurred in the age composition of the population from year to year."[12(p3)] The direct method of age adjustment involves multiplying the age-specific rates for each subgroup of a population to be standardized by the number in a comparable subgroup of a standard population.

To age adjust the crude mortality rate in the United States, we would use the standard population, which for the United States is the year 2000 population. For example, suppose you wanted to standardize the crude mortality data for the United States for 2003. You would multiply the age-specific death rate for the population under age 1 (700.0 per 100,000) in 2003 by the number in the year 2000 standard population under age 1 (3,794,301). This calculation would need to be repeated for each age stratum. The results for each stratum would then be summed to create a weighted average—the age-adjusted death rate. For additional information regarding the computations involved in age adjustment, refer to *Epidemiology for Public Health Practice*, 5th edition.[8]

According to the National Center for Health Statistics, the age-adjusted death rate in the United States in 2013 was 731.9 deaths per 100,000 U.S. standard population. This figure compares with a crude rate of 821.5 per 100,000 population. In most years since 1980 (with the exception of 1983, 1985, 1988, 1993, 1999, 2005, 2008, and 2013), the age-adjusted death rate in the United States has declined.[10] Refer to **Figure 3-11** for information on trends in age-adjusted and crude mortality rates over time.

Returning to the example in which we compared mortality in New York and Texas, the crude mortality rate for diseases of the heart in 2013 was 224.1 per 100,000 in New York; in Texas, the rate was 152.0 per 100,000. The corresponding age-adjusted rates were 184.8 per 100,000 and 170.7 per 100,000, respectively. The higher crude mortality rate observed in New York in comparison with Texas was due largely to differences in the age structures of the two states. You can see that when the rates were age adjusted, the differences in mortality for diseases of the heart diminished substantially. Consequently, age-adjusted rates permitted a more realistic comparison between the two states than crude rates.

MEASURES OF NATALITY AND MORTALITY LINKED TO NATALITY

Data about natality pertain to birth-related phenomena.[13] Measures of natality include the **crude birth rate** and the fertility rate. Additionally, statisticians compute measures that describe mortality linked to natality. These indices are the maternal mortality rate, fetal mortality rate, and infant mortality rate. This section covers several measures that pertain to the number of births in a population (birth rate) and the fertility of women of childbearing age (fertility rate). Note that by statistical convention, one definition of the childbearing age is 15 to 44 years of age. Related to giving birth is maternal mortality, which occurs during a small number of births in this country. Another fatal outcome is death of the fetus during gestation; such deaths are called fetal mortality. Still another measure tracks death of the newborn during the first year of life. Consult **Table 3-5** for measures presented in this section as well as some of their applications.

Maternal Mortality

Maternal mortality encompasses maternal deaths that result from causes associated with pregnancy. Among the factors related to maternal mortality are race, insufficient healthcare

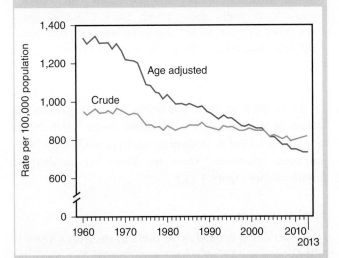

FIGURE 3-11 Crude and age-adjusted death rates: United States, 1960–2013.

Reproduced From: Xu JQ, Murphy SL, Kochanek KD, Bastian BA. Deaths: final data for 2013. *National Vital Statistics Reports.* 2016;64(2):4. Hyattsville, MD: National Center for Health Statistics.

TABLE 3-5 Examples of Measures of Natality and Mortality Linked to Natality

Measure	How Used
Maternal mortality rate	Reflects health disparities such as healthcare access
Infant mortality rate	For international comparisons to identify countries with high rates
Fetal death rate/late fetal death rate	Measures risk of death of the fetus
General fertility rate	Compares populations and subgroups regarding their fertility
Crude birth rate	To project population changes
Perinatal mortality rate	Assesses events that occur during late pregnancy and soon after birth

access, and social disadvantage. The **maternal mortality rate** is the number of maternal deaths ascribed to childbirth divided by the number of live births times 100,000 live births during a year. In 2005, the maternal mortality rate was 15.1 deaths per 100,000 live births (623 total deaths in 2005). The respective maternal mortality rates per 100,000 live births for black and white women were 36.5 and 11.1; the rate for black women was about 3.3 times that for white women.[12]

Maternal mortality rate =

$$\frac{\text{Number of deaths assigned to causes related to childbirth}}{\text{Number of live births}} \times$$

100,000 live births (during a year)

Note: Live births include multiple births.

Infant Mortality Rate

The **infant mortality rate** is defined as the number of infant deaths among infants age 0 to 365 days during a year divided by the number of live births during the same year (expressed as the rate per 1,000 live births). Refer to the text box, Infant mortality rate.

The terms neonatal mortality and postneonatal mortality also are used to describe mortality during the first year of life. The **neonatal mortality rate** is the number of infant deaths under 28 days of age divided by the number of live births during a year. The **postneonatal mortality rate** refers to the number of infant deaths from 28 days to 365 days after birth divided by the number of live births minus neonatal deaths during a year (expressed as rate per 1,000 live births).

Infant mortality (IM) rate =

$$\frac{\text{Number of infant deaths among infants age 0 – 365 days during the year}}{\text{Number of live births during the year}} \times$$

1,000 live births

Sample calculation: In the United States during 2013, there were 23,440 deaths among infants under 1 year of age and 3,932,181 live births. The infant mortality rate was (23,440/3,932,181) × 1,000 = 5.96 per 1,000 live births.

From 2005 to 2013, the infant mortality rate in the United States declined by 13% (6.86 versus 5.96). Infant mortality is related to inadequate health care and poor environmental conditions. There are substantial racial/ethnic variations. (See **Figure 3-12.**)

Fetal Mortality

Fetal mortality is defined as the death of the fetus when it is in the uterus and before it has been delivered. Two measures of fetal mortality are the **fetal death rate** and the **late fetal death rate**. The formulas for these terms are shown in the text box.

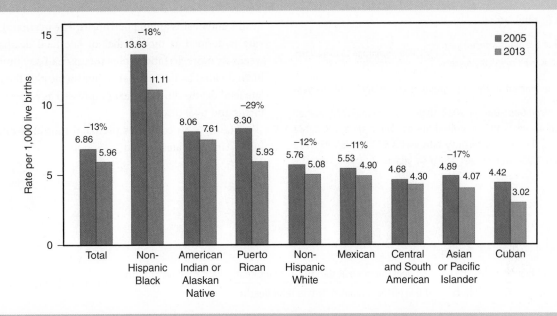

FIGURE 3-12 Infant mortality rates, by race and Hispanic origin of mother—United States, 2005 and 2013.

Reproduced from Mathews TJ, MacDorman MF, Thoma ME. Infant mortality statistics from the 2013 period linked birth/infant death data set. *National Vital Statistics Reports*. 2015;64(9):5. Hyattsville, MD: National Center for Health Statistics.

Fetal Death Rate and Late Fetal Death Rate

Fetal death rate (per 1,000 live births plus fetal deaths) =

$$\frac{\text{Number of fetal deaths after 20 weeks or more gestation}}{\text{Number of live births + number of fetal deaths after 20 weeks or more gestation}} \times 1,000$$

Late fetal death rate (per 1,000 live births plus late fetal deaths) =

$$\frac{\text{Number of fetal deaths after 28 weeks or more gestation}}{\text{Number of live births + number of fetal deaths after 28 weeks or more gestation}} \times 1,000$$

Birth Rates

This section defines the terms *crude birth rate* and *general fertility rate*. The **crude birth rate** refers to the number of live births during a specified period such as a year per the resident population at the midpoint of the year. The birth rate affects the total size of the population.

Crude birth rate =

$$\frac{\text{Number of live births within a given period}}{\text{Population size at the middle of that period}} \times 1,000 \text{ population}$$

Sample calculation: 3,932,181 babies were born in the United States during 2013, when the U.S. population was 316,128,839. The crude birth rate was 3,932,181/316,128,839 = 12.4 per 1,000.

General Fertility Rate (Fertility Rate)

Related to birth rates is the **general fertility rate**, which refers to the number of live births reported in an area during a given time interval divided by the number of women age 15 to 44 years in the area (expressed as rate per 1,000 women age 15 to 44 years). The general fertility rate is referred to more broadly as the fertility rate.

General fertility rate =

$$\frac{\text{Number of live births with in a year}}{\text{Number of women age 15 to 44 years}^*} \times 1{,}000 \text{ women age 15 to 44 years}$$

*Number of women in this age group at the midpoint of the year

Sample calculation: During 2013 there were 62,939,772 women age 15 to 44 years in the United States. There were 3,932,181 live births. The general fertility rate was 3,932,181/62,939,772 = 62.5 per 1,000 women age 15 to 44 years.

Perinatal Mortality

Perinatal mortality (known as definition I from the National Center for Health Statistics) takes into account both late fetal deaths and deaths among newborns. The **perinatal mortality rate** is defined as the number of late fetal deaths (after 28 weeks or more gestation) plus infant deaths within 7 days of birth divided by the number of live births plus the number of late fetal deaths during a year (expressed as rate per 1,000 live births and fetal deaths).

Figure 3-13 compares perinatal mortality rates by race in the United States for 2013.

Perinatal mortality rate =

$$\frac{\text{Number of late fetal deaths (after 28 weeks or more gestation)} + \text{infant deaths within 7 days of birth}}{\text{Number of live births} + \text{number of late fetal deaths}} \times 1{,}000 \text{ live births and fetal deaths}$$

FIGURE 3-13 Perinatal mortality rate, definition I, by race and Hispanic origin of mother—United States, 2013.

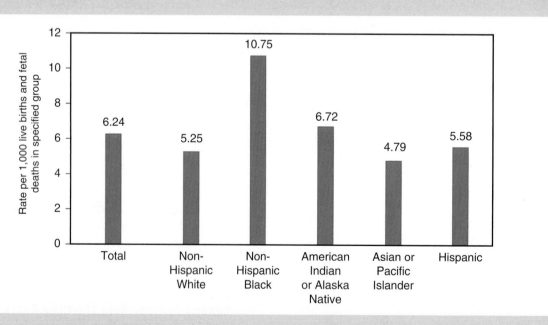

Reproduced from MacDorman MF, Gregory ECW. Fetal and perinatal mortality: United States, 2013. *National Vital Statistics Reports*. 2015;64(8):6. Hyattsville, MD: National Center for Health Statistics.

CONCLUSION

This chapter provided information on measures that are used in epidemiology; these were derived from ratios, such as rates, proportions, and percentages. Types of epidemiologic measures included counts and crude rates as well as case fatality rates, proportional mortality ratios, specific rates, and adjusted rates. These measures are helpful in making descriptive statements about the occurrence of morbidity and mortality and demonstrating risks of adverse health outcomes associated with particular exposures. Two important measures used in epidemiology are prevalence and incidence, which are inter-related terms. Rates are measures that specify a time period during which health events have occurred. A common epidemiologic rate is a crude rate, which allows comparisons of populations that differ in size but not in demographic composition. Specific rates and adjusted rates may be used to overcome some of the problems inherent in crude rates and thus can be used to make comparisons among populations.

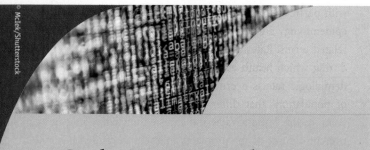

Study Questions and Exercises

1. Define the following terms and give an example of how each one is used in public health:
   a. Maternal mortality rate
   b. Infant mortality
   c. Fetal mortality
   d. Crude birth rate
   e. General fertility rate
   f. Perinatal mortality rate

2. Suppose that an immunization becomes available for an incurable highly fatal disease. A successful immunization campaign has resulted in the immunization of persons who are at risk of the disease. Which of the following measures is likely to be affected? The case-fatality rate, the mortality rate, or, no change in either would occur.

3. Describe what is meant by the term *ratio*. Compare and contrast rates, proportions, and percentages. Give an example of each one.

4. An epidemiologist presented information regarding the annual prevalence (number of cases per 1,000) of adolescent pregnancy to a local health planning board. The epidemiologist compared data for the local county with data for the United States as a whole. One of the members of the planning board objected that this comparison was not valid because the county is much smaller than the entire country. Do you agree with the objection?

5. How does a prevalence proportion (expressed as number of cases per unit size of population) differ from an incidence rate?

6. Distinguish between period prevalence and incidence. What is the definition of lifetime prevalence? Explain the meaning of the formula, $P \cong ID$.

7. Define the term *crude rate*, giving an example. What are the advantages of using crude rates instead of frequency data such as counts?

8. Define the term *adjusted rate*. What is one of the main purposes of adjusted rates? Compare the advantages and disadvantages of crude and adjusted rates. What is meant by age adjustment? Describe the applications of age-adjusted rates.

9. What types of information are found by using specific rates, such as cause-specific, age-specific, and sex-specific rates, instead of crude rates?

10. Many communities and jurisdictions throughout the United States have legalized recreational use of marijuana. Suppose you are asked to conduct a questionnaire study of the prevalence of marijuana use in a community where use of marijuana is legal. Propose interview questions to assess the following measures of prevalence: point prevalence, period prevalence (one-year time period), and lifetime prevalence.

11. Explain the following measures of incidence and compare their applications: incidence rate, cumulative incidence rate, incidence density, and attack rate.

12. In 2010, the sex ratio among the age group 70-79 years was 81.0. The sex ratio among the age group 100 years and older was 20.7. How might one account for this decline in the sex ratio?

13. Refer back to Table 3-3. What quantitative measure is shown in the table? Describe the annual trends in the cases of infrequently reported notifiable diseases.

14. Calculate the incidence rate (per 100,000 population) of primary and secondary syphilis (combined) in 2013 from the following data:

Number of reported cases in 2013: 17,357

Estimated population of the United States as of July 1, 2013: 316,128,839

15. **Table 3-6** provides hypothetical data regarding the prevalence of diabetes in two counties in the United States.

    Based on 2020 prevalence (percentage), which of the two counties had a higher burden of disease from diabetes?

16. Refer to Exhibit 3-1. Calculate the crude death rate (per 100,000) from the following data:

    Number of deaths in the United States during 1990 = 2,148,463

    Population of the United States as of July 1, 1990 = 248,709,873

    How did the crude death rate in 2013 compare with the crude death rate in 1990?

17. Calculate the infant mortality rate (per 1,000 live births) from the following data:

    Number of infant deaths under 1 year in the United States during 1991 = 36,766

    Number of live births during 1991 = 4,111,000

    How did the infant mortality rate in 2013 compare with the infant mortality rate in 1991? (Note: refer to the text for 2013 data.)

18. Calculate the crude birth rate (per 1,000 population) from the following data:

    Number of live births during 1991 = 4,111,000

    Population of the United States as of July 1, 1991 = 252,688,000

    How did the crude birth rate in 2013 compare with the crude birth rate in 1991? (Note: refer to text for 2013 data.)

19. Calculate the general fertility rate (per 1,000 women aged 15-44) from the following data:

    Number of live births during 1991 = 4,111,000

    Number of women (15 to 44 years of age) in the United States as of July 1, 1991 = 59,139,000

    How did the general fertility rate in 2013 compare with the general fertility rate in 1991? (Note: refer to text for 2013 data.)

    Questions 20 through 22 refer to **Table 3-7**.

20. What is the sex ratio for total injuries?

21. What is the crude mortality rate per 100,000 population?

22. What is (a) the cause-specific mortality rate for injuries, and (b) the case fatality rate (%) for injuries?

TABLE 3-6 Hypothetical Data for Diabetes

	Estimated Total Population on July 1, 2020	Total Number of Cases of Diabetes in 2020
County A	11,020,000	356,289
County B	3,900,000	253,612

TABLE 3-7 Hypothetical Data for Unintentional Injuries

	Total Injuries	Fatal Injuries	Nonfatal Injuries	Number in Population	Total Deaths from All Causes
Men	73	3	70	2,856	9
Women	41	2	39	2,981	8

Answers to calculation problems

14. 5.5 per 100,000
15. County B (6.5% versus 3.2%)
16. The crude death rate declined from 863.8 per 100,000 to 821.5 per 100,000.
17. The infant mortality rate decreased from 8.95 to 5.86.
18. The crude birth rate declined from 16.3 per 1,000 to 12.4 per 1,000.
19. The general fertility rate declined from 69.5 per 1,000 to 62.5 per 1,000.
20. 1.78 to 1, male to female
21. 291.2 per 100,000
22. (a) 85.7 per 100,000; (b) 4.4%

Young Epidemiology Scholars (YES) Exercises

The Young Epidemiology Scholars: Competitions website provides links to teaching units and exercises that support instruction in epidemiology. The YES program, discontinued in 2011, was administered by the College Board and supported by the Robert Wood Johnson Foundation. The exercises continue to be available at the following website: http://yes-competition.org/yes /teaching-units/title.html. The following exercises relate to topics discussed in this chapter and can be found on the YES competitions website.

1. Bayona M, Olsen C. Measures in Epidemiology
2. Huang FI, Baumgarten M. Adolescent Suicide: The Role of Epidemiology in Public Health
3. McCrary F, St. George DMM. Mortality and the Trans-Atlantic Slave Trade

REFERENCES

1. Porta M, ed. *A Dictionary of Epidemiology*. 6th ed. New York, NY: Oxford University Press; 2014.
2. Centers for Disease Control and Prevention. HIV/AIDS surveillance report, 2006. Vol. 18. Atlanta, GA: U.S. Department of Health and Human Services, Centers for Disease Control and Prevention; 2008:1–55.
3. U.S. Census Bureau. Age and sex distribution in 2005. Population profile of the United States: dynamic version. Available at: http://www.census.gov/population/pop-profile/dynamic/AgeSex.pdf. Accessed September 30, 2016.
4. U.S. Census Bureau. Age and sex composition: 2010. *2010 Census Briefs*; May 2011.
5. Centers for Disease Control and Prevention. QuickStats: Percentage of adults reporting joint pain or stiffness—National Health Interview Survey, United States, 2006. *MMWR*. 2008;57:467.
6. Hennekens CH, Buring JE. *Epidemiology in Medicine*. Boston, MA: Little, Brown; 1987.
7. Morgenstern H, Thomas D. Principles of study design in environmental epidemiology. *Environ Health Perspect*. 1993;101(Suppl 4):23–38.
8. Friis RH, Sellers TA. *Epidemiology for Public Health Practice*. 5th ed. Burlington, MA: Jones & Bartlett Learning; 2014.
9. Moorman JE, Akinbami LJ, Bailey CM, et al. National Surveillance of Asthma: United States, 2001–2010. *National Center for Health Statistics*. Vital Health Stat 3(35).
10. Xu JQ, Murphy SL, Kochanek KD, Bastian BA. Deaths: final data for 2013. *National Vital Statistics Reports*. 2016;64(2). Hyattsville, MD: National Center for Health Statistics.
11. Centers for Disease Control and Prevention. Primary amebic meningoencephalitis—Arizona, Florida, and Texas, 2007. *MMWR*. 2008;57:573–577.
12. Kung HC, Hoyert DL, Xu JQ, Murphy SL. Deaths: final data for 2005. *National Vital Statistics Reports*. 2008;56(10). Hyattsville, MD: National Center for Health Statistics.
13. Schneider D, Lilienfeld DE. *Lillienfeld's Foundations of Epidemiology*. 4th ed. New York, NY: Oxford University Press; 2015.

© Oleg Baliuk/Shutterstock

CHAPTER **4**

Data and Disease Occurrence

LEARNING OBJECTIVES

By the end of this chapter you will be able to:

- Define the term *big data* and give one example of its epidemiologic applications.
- State three factors that affect the quality of epidemiologic data.
- Differentiate between vital statistics data and reportable disease statistics.
- List four data sources that are used in epidemiologic research.
- Describe the role of international organizations in disseminating epidemiologic data.

CHAPTER OUTLINE

INTRODUCTION

You probably have not given much thought to epidemiologic data. However, this is a cutting-edge topic that has extreme importance for our country and modern society. In the present chapter you will learn how high-quality data are linked to the accomplishment of important functions such as performance of essential public health services, especially program and policy evaluation. A mastery of data-related skills can help you bring needed assets to public health and commercial venues.

This chapter extends the coverage of quantitative measures by providing information about sources of data that are used for epidemiologic research. Previously, you learned about epidemiologic measures derived from ratios, rates, proportions, and percentages. The epidemiologic measures that were described included counts and crude rates as well as case fatality rates, proportional mortality ratios, specific rates, and adjusted rates. All of these measures are used to describe morbidity and mortality in populations. In addition, the terms *incidence* and *prevalence* were defined. The present chapter will link these concepts with data sources.

Two vital concerns of epidemiology are, first, the quality of data available for describing the health of populations and, second, whether these data are being applied in an appropriate manner. Specifically, you will learn appropriate and inappropriate uses for particular types of data. For example, it is not feasible to calculate some epidemiologic measures without a qualified data source. This chapter will come in handy when you are seeking data for computing basic indices of morbidity and mortality. The information presented will also aid you in evaluating associations between exposures and health outcomes derived from epidemiologic research. Refer to **Table 4-1** for a list of important terms used in this chapter.

EPIDEMIOLOGY IN THE ERA OF BIG DATA

Increasingly, you have heard about big data. What exactly is meant by "**big data**?" This somewhat ambiguous term refers to vast electronic storehouses of information that include Internet search transactions, social media activities, data from health insurance programs, and electronic medical records from receipt of healthcare services. These data are relevant to epidemiology because they may cover entire populations or, at least, very large numbers of people. In addition, number crunchers can analyze big data to discover patterns of variables (distributions and determinants) associated with diseases. By combining big data, epidemiologists have new insights into the determinants of morbidity and mortality. However, the uses of big data have weaknesses as well as strengths.

Three qualities, known as the **three Vs**, characterize big data: volume, variety, and velocity.[1] **Figure 4-1** illustrates these terms, which are defined in **Table 4-2**. The vast troves of accumulated data include people's social media accounts, online activities, and purchases in stores. It is technically possible to combine this information with health data, visits to doctors, hospital stays, and health insurance programs. The procedure known as **data linkage** is used to join data elements contained in databases by tying them together with a common identifier. Refer to **Figure 4-2** for an illustration of this process. Other data with potential for linkage include real-time transmissions from cellular telephones and the output from fitness tracking devices.

Some firms (often called data brokers) specialize in big data analytics and data mining. The process of **data mining** involves gathering and exploring large troves of data in order to discern heretofore unrecognized patterns and associations in the data. For example, a political organization asked a Silicon Valley firm to identify voters who favored tighter immigration controls. The ironic answer turned out to be "Chevy truck drivers who like Starbucks."[2]

Google and Facebook track the activity of Internet users, as do online retailers. An illustration of applying the methodology of big data to health research is Google's introduction of Google Flu Trends (GFT) in the fall of 2008. The objective of GFT was to provide an early warning for influenza in advance of surveillance information from the Centers for Disease Control and Prevention (CDC).[3] Subsequently, GFT was found to substantially overestimate the prevalence of influenza,[4] thereby highlighting one of the limitations of using big data to predict disease

TABLE 4-1 List of Important Terms Used in This Chapter

Data Acquisition	Criteria for Data Quality	Data Sources
Big data	Appropriate uses of data	American Community Survey
Data linkage	Availability of data	Morbidity surveys of the population
Data mining	Completeness of population coverage	Public health surveillance
MEDLINE	External validity	Registry data
Online retrieval	Nature of the data	Reportable disease statistics
Three Vs of big data	Personally identifiable information	U.S. Census Bureau
WHOSIS	Representativeness of data	Vital events

FIGURE 4-1 The three defining features of big data.

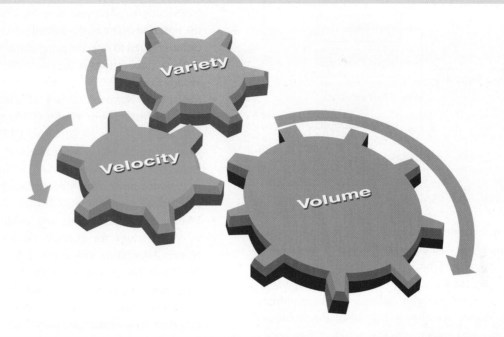

Data from Roski J, Bo-Linn GW, Andrews TA. Creating value in health care through big data: opportunities and policy implications. *Health Affairs*. 2014;33(7):1115-1122.

occurrence. Other data analytic firms have used transit data to visualize travel patterns in order to pinpoint delays and congestion in public transit systems.[5] This is a daunting task because public transit systems often are vast (especially in large cities) and generate huge quantities of data. These examples are only a few illustrations of how big data are being used by technology companies (think Apple and Uber) as well as other commercial and nonprofit organizations.

TABLE 4-2 The Three Vs of Big Data

The Three Vs	Definition
Volume	"Massive amounts of data strain the capacity and capability of traditional data storage, management, and retrieval systems such as data warehouses. Big data requires flexible and easily expandable data storage and management solutions."
Variety	"Health care data today come in many formats, such as the structured and free-text data captured by EHRs, diagnostic images, and data streaming from social media and mobile applications."
Velocity	"Most traditional health IT infrastructures are not able to process and analyze massive amounts of constantly refreshed, differently formatted data in real time. Big-data infrastructure makes it possible to manage data more flexibly and quickly than has been the case,…"

Data from Roski J, Bo-Linn GW, Andrews TA. Creating value in health care through big data: opportunities and policy implications. *Health Affairs*. 2014;33(7):1116.

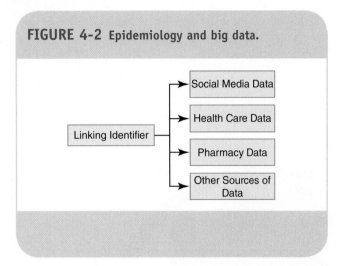

FIGURE 4-2 Epidemiology and big data.

However, in addition to their promise of breakthroughs, the applications of big data are accompanied by caveats for epidemiologic research. One is the concern for personal privacy when the data are accessed in ways not originally intended by the individual who makes a purchase online or goes to the doctor. Another is that all of the rigorous criteria of science and epidemiologic research design need to be upheld. These include considerations regarding the reliability and validity of data, correct use of study designs, and recognition of the criteria of causal inference. Also, errors such as misidentification of cases can occur when records are combined through record linkage. In addition, patterns of data points that have been linked by data mining may represent only relationships and not necessarily causal associations.

ONLINE SOURCES FOR RETRIEVAL OF EPIDEMIOLOGIC INFORMATION

The process of **online retrieval** involves the acquisition of information from websites that are available to the public as well as from proprietary sites. Extensive resources are available for online retrieval of epidemiologic information, and the number of websites seems to be growing exponentially. Among the numerous websites that may be researched for data and other pertinent epidemiologic information are the following:

- Google (www.google.com. Accessed June 30, 2016): The Google site facilitates rapid access to epidemiologic documents and links. You can use Google most effectively when you create appropriate search terms. One may search for reports in written text

format as well as for images and access to other materials.
- Centers for Disease Control and Prevention (CDC) (www.cdc.gov/. Accessed June 30, 2016): This site is the portal to many of the federal government's publications related to infectious and chronic diseases. One of these publications is the *Morbidity and Mortality Weekly Report.*
- MEDLINE, National Library of Medicine (NLM), National Institutes of Health (NIH) (www.nlm.nih. gov/. Accessed June 30, 2016): **MEDLINE** is a site for performing bibliographic searches of health-related literature. You can search for citations to health-related literature on PubMed (www.ncbi.nlm.nih.gov/ pubmed/. Accessed June 30, 2016).
- Websites of organizations and publications related to epidemiology, for example, the American Public Health Association (www.apha.org/. Accessed June 30, 2016): The American Public Health Association publishes the *American Journal of Public Health.* A second example is the Society for Epidemiologic Research (www.epiresearch.org/. Accessed June 30, 2016), which sponsors the *American Journal of Epidemiology.* Professional organizations such as these sponsor health-related conferences, which provide learning opportunities about epidemiology.
- World Health Organization Statistical Information System (**WHOSIS**) (www.who.int/whosis/en/. Accessed June 30, 2016): The World Health Organization website provides data on the occurrence of morbidity and mortality from a worldwide perspective.

Navigate through the web and access these sites. Not only are they interesting in themselves, but also they will link you to many other related websites.

FACTORS THAT AFFECT THE QUALITY OF EPIDEMIOLOGIC DATA

The quality of epidemiologic data is a function of the sources from which they were derived as well as how completely the data cover their reference populations. Data quality affects the permissible applications of the data and the types of statistical analyses that may be performed. Four questions that should be raised with respect to the quality of epidemiologic data are the following:

- What is the **nature of the data**, including sources and content? Examples of data that this chapter will cover are vital statistics (data from recording births and deaths), surveillance data, reportable disease statistics, and data from case registries. Other data that are important for epidemiologic research are the results of specialized surveys, records from healthcare and insurance programs, and information from international organizations.

- How available are the data? The term **availability of the data** refers to the investigator's access to data (e.g., patient records and databases in which personally identifying information has been removed). Release of personally identifiable information is prohibited in the United States and many other developed countries. In the United States, epidemiologic data that might identify a specific person may not be released without the person's consent. The Health Insurance Portability and Accountability Act of 1996 (HIPAA) protects personal information contained in health records. Thus, individual medical records that disclose a patient's identity, reveal his or her diagnoses and treatments, or list the source of payment for medical care are confidential. On the other hand, data banks that collect information from surveys may release epidemiologic data as long as individuals cannot be identified.

- How complete is the population coverage? **Completeness of population coverage** refers to the degree to which the data reflect a population of interest to a researcher. The completeness of the population coverage affects the representativeness of the data. The term **representativeness** (also known as external validity) refers to the generalizability of the findings to the population from which the data have been taken. Some data sources (for example, mortality statistics) cover the population extensively. Other data sources, such as those from health clinics, medical centers, health maintenance organizations (HMOs), and insurance plans, may exclude major subsets of the nonserved or noncovered population.

- What are the **appropriate uses of the data**? In some instances the data may be used only for cross-sectional analyses. In others, the data may be used primarily for case-control studies. And in still others, the data may provide information about the incidence of disease and may be used to assess risk status. These issues will be revisited in the chapter on epidemiologic study designs.

U.S. CENSUS BUREAU

Measures of morbidity and mortality require accurate information about the size and characteristics of the population. The U.S. Census Bureau offers a plethora of data regarding the characteristics of our country. **Figure 4-3** portrays the bureau's logo with the date of Census 2020. One of the applications of census data is the clarification of denominators used in epidemiologic measures, such as rates and proportions. Also, descriptive and other epidemiologic studies classify health outcomes according to sociodemographic variables; consequently, accurate information about these characteristics is needed.

You can obtain data and related products from the U.S. Census Bureau by accessing the Census website (www.census.gov) and the American FactFinder (http://factfinder.census.gov/faces/nav/jsf/pages/using_factfinder.xhtml. Accessed June 30, 2016.). The census provides a wealth of data that can be used to define the denominator in epidemiologic measures. These data include official estimates of the total population size and subdivisions of the population by geographic area. The **U.S. Census Bureau** conducts a census of the population every 10 years (the decennial census—e.g., 1980, 1990, 2000, 2010, 2020, and beyond) and calculates estimates of the population size during the nondecennial years.

In order to keep U.S. population estimates current with changes due to births, deaths, and migration, the Census Bureau provides annual estimates. The bureau creates annual estimates by starting with the population base, for example, the population size on April 1, 2010, and adds the number

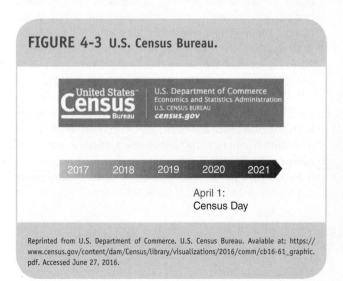

FIGURE 4-3 U.S. Census Bureau.

Reprinted from U.S. Department of Commerce. U.S. Census Bureau. Avaiable at: https://www.census.gov/content/dam/Census/library/visualizations/2016/comm/cb16-61_graphic.pdf. Accessed June 27, 2016.

of births and the net number of migrants and then subtracts the number of deaths. This same procedure is followed over successive years and produces estimates with a high degree of accuracy.[6] Census 2010 employed a short form only; detailed information collected previously by the long questionnaire is now part of the Census Bureau's American Community Survey.[7] (Refer to **Exhibit 4-1** for additional information about the 2010 Census.)

THE VITAL REGISTRATION SYSTEM AND VITAL EVENTS

Vital events are deaths, births, marriages, divorces, and fetal deaths. The vital registration system in the United States collects information routinely on these events. The legal authority for the registration of vital events within the United States is held by individual states, five U.S. territories (e.g., Puerto Rico), the Commonwealth of the Northern Mariana Islands, New York City, and Washington, D.C. These jurisdictions are charged with keeping records of vital events and providing certificates of marriage and divorce as well as birth and death certificates. In many instances, certificates that document vital events are also available from local health departments in the United States.

Deaths

Data are collected routinely on all deaths that occur in the United States. Mortality data have the advantage of being almost totally complete because deaths are unlikely to go unrecorded in the United States. In many instances, the funeral director completes the death certificate. Then the attending physician completes the section on date and cause of death. If the death occurred as the result of unintentional injury, suicide, or homicide, or if the attending physician is unavailable, then the medical examiner or coroner completes and signs the death certificate. Finally, the local registrar checks the certificate for completeness and accuracy and sends a copy to the state registrar. The state registrar also checks for completeness and accuracy and sends a copy to the National Center for Health Statistics (NCHS), which compiles and publishes national mortality rates (e.g., in National Vital Statistics Reports).

Death certificate data in the United States include information about the decedent shown in **Table 4-3**. An example of a death certificate and additional information regarding the kinds of data collected are shown in **Figure 4-4**.

Mortality data are one of the most commonly used indices in public health. Although available and fairly complete,

---

EXHIBIT 4-1   About the 2010 Census

The 2010 Census represented the most massive participation movement ever witnessed in our country. Approximately 74% of the households returned their census forms by mail; census workers, walking neighborhoods throughout the United States, counted the remaining households. National and state population totals from the 2010 Census were released on December 21, 2010. Redistricting data, which include additional state, county, and local counts, were released starting in February 2011.

For the 2000 Census, additional questions were asked of a sample of persons and housing units (generally one in six households) on topics such as income, education, place of birth, and more. Information on those topics is now available as part of the **American Community Survey.**

For the 2010 Census, 10 questions were asked of every person and housing unit in the United States. Information is available on:

- Age
- Hispanic or Latino origin
- Household relationship
- Race
- Sex
- Tenure (whether the home is owned or rented)
- Vacancy characteristics

Since 1975, the Census Bureau has had the responsibility to produce small-area population data needed to redraw state legislative and congressional districts. Other important uses of Census data include the distribution of funds for government programs, such as Medicaid; planning the right locations for schools, roads, and other public facilities; helping real estate agents and potential residents learn about neighborhoods; and identifying trends over time that can help predict future needs. Most census data are available for many levels of geography, including states, counties, cities and towns, ZIP Code Tabulation Areas, census tracts, blocks, and more.

Adapted and reprinted from United States Census Bureau. Available at: http://factfinder.census.gov/faces/nav/jsf/pages/programs.xhtml?program=dec. Accessed June 28, 2016.

TABLE 4-3 Typical Data Recorded in Death Certificates

Demographic characteristics	Date and place of death— hospital or elsewhere
• Age	• Cause of death
• Sex	• Immediate cause
• Race	• Contributing factors

the certificate may list the cause of death as heart failure or pneumonia, each of which could be a complication of diabetes. Another factor that detracts from the accuracy of death certificates is lack of standardization of diagnostic criteria employed by various physicians in different hospitals and settings. Yet another problem is the stigma associated with certain diseases. For example, if the decedent died as a result of HIV infection or alcoholism and was a long-time friend of the attending physician, the physician may be reluctant to specify this information on a document that is available to the general public.

Birth Statistics

Birth statistics include live births and fetal deaths. Presumably, birth and fetal death statistics are nearly complete in their coverage of the general population. (Refer to **Table 4-4** for a list of information collected by certificates of live birth and reports of fetal death.) One of the uses of birth

death certificates may not be entirely accurate regarding the assigned cause of death. When an older person with a chronic illness dies, the primary cause of death may be unclear. Death certificates list multiple causes of mortality as well as the underlying cause. However, assignment of the cause of death sometimes may be arbitrary. In illustration, diabetes may not be given as the immediate cause of death; rather,

FIGURE 4-4 U.S. Standard Certificate of Death*

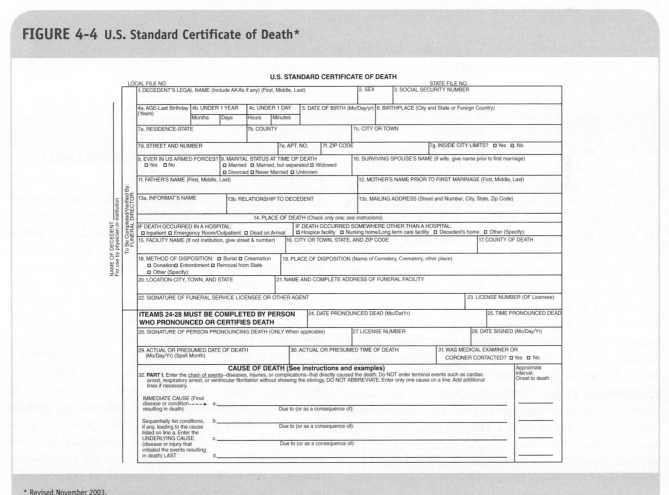

* Revised November 2003.

Reprinted from Centers for Disease Control and Prevention. Available at: http://www.cdc.gov/nchs/data/dvs/DEATH11-03final-acc.pdf. Accessed August 11, 2016.

TABLE 4-4 Examples of Information Collected by Birth and Fetal Death Certificates

Variable	U.S. Certificate of Live Birth	U.S. Report of Fetal Death
Name	Child's name	Name of fetus (optional)
Disposition (e.g., burial)	Not applicable	Disposition of fetus
Location	Facility name	Where delivered
Mother identifying information	Name, age, and place of residence	Name, age, and place of residence
Mother	Height, weight, number of previous live births	Height, weight, number of previous live births
Conditions contributing to fetal death	Not applicable	Initiating cause and other causes (e.g., pregnancy complications, fetal anomalies)
Risk factors in pregnancy	Diabetes, hypertension, infections	Diabetes, hypertension, infections
Congenital anomalies	Anencephaly, cleft palate, Down syndrome	Anencephaly, cleft palate, Down syndrome
Father	Name and age	Name and age

certificate data is for calculation of birth rates; information also is collected about a range of conditions that may affect the neonate, including conditions present during pregnancy, congenital malformations, obstetric procedures, birth weight, length of gestation, and demographic background of the mother. Some of the data may be unreliable, reflecting possible inconsistencies and gaps in the mother's recall of events during pregnancy. Still another concern is that some malformations and illnesses may not be detected at the time of birth (for example, because the newborn appears to be normal). Many of the foregoing deficiencies of birth certificates also apply to the data contained in certificates of fetal death. In addition, state to state variations in requirements for fetal death certificates further reduce their utility for epidemiologic studies. Nevertheless, birth and fetal death certificate data have been used in many types of epidemiologic research. One of these is research topics concerning environmental influences on congenital malformations. For example, these data have been used to search for clusters of birth defects in geographic areas where mothers may have been exposed to possible teratogens (agents that cause fetal malformation), such as pesticides or toxic pollutants.

DATA FROM PUBLIC HEALTH SURVEILLANCE PROGRAMS: THREE EXAMPLES

Three examples of public health surveillance programs are those for communicable and infectious diseases, noninfectious diseases, and risk factors for chronic disease. **Public health surveillance** refers to the systematic and continuous gathering of information about the occurrence of diseases and other health phenomena. As part of the surveillance process, personnel analyze and interpret the data they have collected and distribute the data and associated findings to planners, health workers, and members of the public health community.

The public health community has been concerned with the possibility of using surveillance systems for detecting diseases associated with bioterrorism as well as early detection of disease outbreaks in general. **Figure 4-5** shows a worker protected against biological disease agents. The term *syndromic surveillance* describes a procedure "… to identify illness clusters early, before diagnoses are confirmed and reported to public health agencies, and to mobilize a rapid response, thereby reducing morbidity and mortality."[8] Epidemiologists think of

FIGURE 4-5 A CDC laboratorian at work in a maximum containment, or "hot lab."

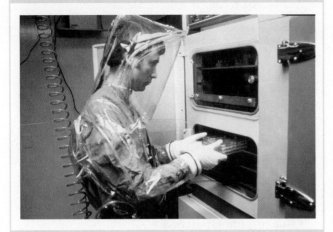

Reprinted from Centers for Disease Control and Prevention. Public Health Image Library, ID# 5538. Available at: http://phil.cdc.gov/phil/home.asp. Accessed March 8, 2016.

syndromic surveillance as an early warning system for disease outbreaks.

Surveillance programs operate at the local, national, and international level. Here are some examples of surveillance systems:

- Communicable and infectious diseases. In the United States, healthcare providers and related workers send reports of diseases (known as notifiable and reportable diseases) to local health departments, which in turn forward them to state health departments and then to the CDC. The CDC reports the occurrence of internationally quarantinable diseases (e.g., plague, cholera, and yellow fever) to the World Health Organization.
- Noninfectious diseases. Surveillance programs often focus on the collection of information related to chronic diseases, such as asthma.
- Risk factors for chronic diseases. The Behavioral Risk Factor Surveillance System (BRFSS) was established by the Centers for Disease Control and Prevention to collect information on behavior-related risk factors for chronic disease. One of the tasks of the BRFSS is the monitoring of health-related quality of life in the United States.

Figure 4-6 gives an overview of a simplified surveillance system, which shows how reports of cases of disease (e.g., infectious diseases) move up the hierarchy. Potential reporting sources are physicians and other healthcare providers as well as workers in clinical laboratories and other health-related facilities. Data recipients include county health departments at the primary level, state health departments at the secondary level, and federal agencies at the tertiary level. Data recipients at all of these levels are involved in feedback and dissemination of information required for appropriate public health action. **Exhibit 4-2** and the section on reportable disease statistics describe these activities in more detail.

Reportable and Notifiable Disease Statistics

By legal statute, physicians and other healthcare providers must report cases of certain diseases, known as reportable and notifiable diseases, to health authorities. **Reportable disease statistics** are statistics derived from diseases that physicians and other healthcare providers must report to government agencies according to legal statute. Such diseases are called reportable (notifiable) diseases. They are usually infectious and communicable diseases that might endanger a population; examples are sexually transmitted diseases, rubella, tetanus, measles, plague, and foodborne disease. In addition, individual states may elect to maintain reports of communicable and noncommunicable diseases of local concern. To supplement the notifiable disease surveillance system, the CDC operates a surveillance system for several noteworthy diseases such as salmonellosis, shigellosis, and influenza. For example, reports of influenza are tracked from October through May.

Examples of nationally notifiable infectious diseases are shown in **Table 4-5**. Some of the diseases and conditions are reportable in some states only; others are reportable in all states. The list changes every so often. For more information regarding United States and state requirements, refer to "Mandatory Reporting of Infectious Diseases by Clinicians, and Mandatory Reporting of Occupational Diseases by Clinicians," a publication of the Centers for Disease Control and Prevention.[9]

The major deficiency of reportable and notifiable data for epidemiologic research purposes is the possible incompleteness of population coverage. First, not every person who develops a disease that is on this list of notifiable conditions may seek medical attention; in particular, persons who are afflicted with asymptomatic and subclinical illnesses are unlikely to visit a physician. For example, an active case of typhoid fever will go unreported if the affected individual is unaware that he or she has the disease. Typhoid Mary (whose case will be discussed in the chapter on infectious diseases) illustrated this phenomenon. Another factor associated with lack of complete population coverage is the occasional

FIGURE 4-6 Simplified flow chart for a generic surveillance system.

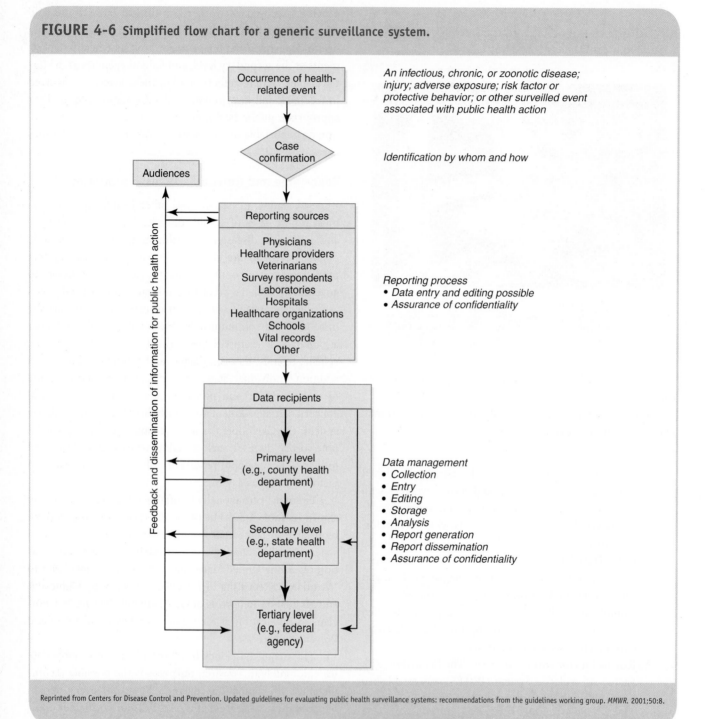

failure of overwhelmed healthcare providers to fill out the required reporting forms. This shortcoming can occur if responsible individuals do not keep current with respect to the frequently changing requirements for disease reporting in a local area. Also, as discussed earlier, a physician may be unwilling to risk compromising the confidentiality of the physician–patient relationship, especially as a result of concern and controversy about reporting cases of diseases that carry social stigma. For example, incompleteness of HIV reporting may stem from the potential sensitivity of the diagnosis. The author, who previously was associated with a local health department, observed that widespread and less

EXHIBIT 4-2 National Notifiable Diseases Surveillance System History

In 1878, Congress authorized the U.S. Marine Hospital Service (i.e., the forerunner of the Public Health Service [PHS]) to collect morbidity reports regarding cholera, smallpox, plague, and yellow fever from U.S. consuls overseas; this information was to be used for instituting quarantine measures to prevent the introduction and spread of these diseases into the United States. In 1879, a specific congressional appropriation was made for the collection and publication of reports of these notifiable diseases. The authority for weekly reporting and publication of these reports was expanded by Congress in 1893 to include data from states and municipal authorities. To increase the uniformity of the data, Congress enacted a law in 1902 directing the Surgeon General to provide forms for the collection and compilation of data and for the publication of reports at the national level. In 1912, state and territorial health authorities—in conjunction with PHS—recommended immediate telegraphic reporting of five infectious diseases and the monthly reporting, by letter, of 10 additional diseases. The first annual summary of The Notifiable Diseases in 1912 included reports of 10 diseases from 19 states, the District of Columbia, and Hawaii. By 1928, all states, the District of Columbia, Hawaii, and Puerto Rico were participating in national

reporting of 29 specified diseases. At their annual meeting in 1950, the State and Territorial Health Officers authorized a conference of state and territorial epidemiologists whose purpose was to determine which diseases should be reported to PHS. In 1961, CDC assumed responsibility for the collection and publication of data concerning nationally notifiable diseases.

The list of nationally notifiable infectious diseases and conditions is revised periodically. An infectious disease or condition might be added to the list as a new pathogen emerges, or a disease or condition might be removed as its incidence declines. Public health officials at state and territorial health departments collaborate with CDC staff in determining which infectious diseases and conditions should be considered nationally notifiable. The Council of State and Territorial Epidemiologists (CSTE), with input from CDC, makes recommendations annually for additions and deletions to the list. The list of infectious diseases and conditions considered reportable in each jurisdiction varies over time and across jurisdictions.

Data on selected notifiable infectious diseases are published weekly in the *Morbidity and Mortality Weekly Report* (*MMWR*) and at year-end in the annual *Summary of Notifiable Diseases, United States*.

Adapted and reprinted from Centers for Disease Control and Prevention. National Notifiable Diseases Surveillance System. History and background. Available at: https://www.cdc.gov/nndss/history.html. Accessed June 28, 2016; Centers for Disease Control and Prevention. Summary of notifiable infectious diseases and conditions—United States, 2013. *MMWR*. October 23, 2015;62(53):1–119.

dramatic conditions such as streptococcal pharyngitis (sore throat) sometimes are unreported. More severe and unusual diseases, such as diphtheria, are almost always reported. Referring to Table 4-5, you will see that anthrax is an example of a nationally notifiable disease. **Figure 4-7** provides an illustration of a person who has contracted anthrax.

Chronic Disease Surveillance: The Example of Asthma

Asthma, a highly prevalent disease that incurs substantial medical and economic costs, is associated with inflammatory lung and airway conditions that can result in breathing difficulty, coughing, chest tightness, and other pulmonary symptoms. Severe asthma symptoms can be life threatening. Asthma surveillance programs provide data necessary for the development and evaluation of healthcare services for afflicted persons. The California Department of Health Services has established an asthma surveillance system that "uses data from a wide variety of sources to describe the burden of asthma in the state. Surveillance data include, but are not limited to: the number

of people with asthma, frequency of symptoms, use of routine health care, visits to the emergency department and hospital, costs of healthcare utilization, and deaths due to asthma."[10(p3)]

The Asthma Surveillance Pyramid (refer to **Figure 4-8**) describes the range of asthma outcomes. "The bottom of the pyramid represents asthma prevalence, or all people with asthma. This is the largest group in the pyramid and refers to the lowest level of asthma severity. Each successively higher level in the pyramid represents an increased level of asthma severity and a smaller proportion of people affected. Outside the pyramid are quality of life, cost, pharmacy, and triggers; these are four factors that impact all of the other outcomes of the pyramid."[10(p10)]

Behavioral Risk Factor Surveillance System

The Behavioral Risk Factor Surveillance System (BRFSS) is a noteworthy program used by the United States to monitor at the state level behavioral risk factors that are associated with chronic diseases. (See **Figure 4-9** for the logo of the BRFSS and **Exhibit 4-3** for a description of the program.) Public health experts regard the BRFSS as one of America's leading

TABLE 4-5 Examples of Nationally Notifiable Conditions—United States, 2016

- Anthrax
- Botulism
- Gonorrhea
- Hepatitis A, hepatitis B, hepatitis C
- Human immunodeficiency virus (HIV) infection (acquired immune deficiency syndrome (AIDS) has been reclassified as HIV Stage III) (AIDS/HIV)
- Meningococcal disease
- Mumps
- Syphilis
- Tuberculosis
- Viral hemorrhagic fever (includes Ebola virus)
- Zika virus disease

Data from Centers for Disease Control and Prevention. National Notifiable Diseases Surveillance System (NNDSS). 2016 Nationally Notifiable Conditions. Available at: https://www.cdc.gov/nndss/conditions/notifiable/2016/. Accessed June 28, 2016.

FIGURE 4-7 Patient with anthrax, one of the nationally notifiable diseases.

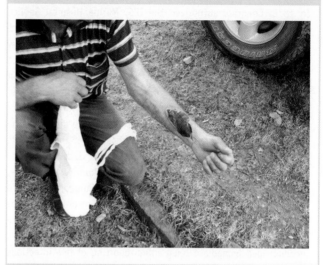

Reprinted from Centers for Disease Control and Prevention. Public Health Image Library #19826. Accessed June 27, 2016.

FIGURE 4-8 The Asthma Surveillance Pyramid: a description of California's asthma data.

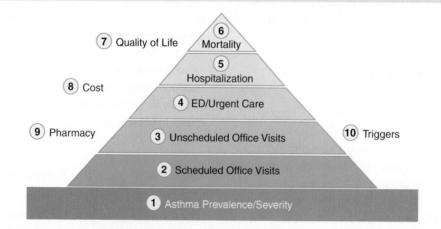

Reproduced from Centers for Disease Control and Prevention. "A Public Health Reponse to Asthma," PHTN Satellite Broadcast, Course Materials 2001.

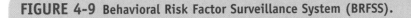

FIGURE 4-9 Behavioral Risk Factor Surveillance System (BRFSS).

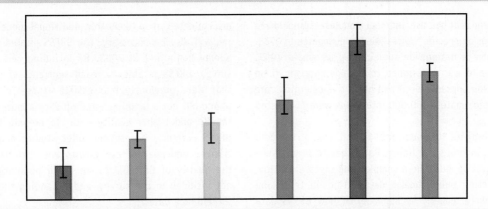

Reprinted from Centers for Disease Control and Prevention. BRFSS prevalence & trends data. Available at: http://www.cdc.gov/brfss/brfssprevalence/. Accessed June 27, 2016.

EXHIBIT 4-3 Behavioral Risk Factor Surveillance System

The Behavioral Risk Factor Surveillance System (BRFSS) is the nation's premier system of health-related telephone surveys that collect state data about U.S. residents regarding their health-related risk behaviors, chronic health conditions, and use of preventive services. Established in 1984 with 15 states, BRFSS now collects data in all 50 states as well as the District of Columbia and three U.S. territories. BRFSS completes more than 400,000 adult interviews each year, making it the largest continuously conducted health survey system in the world. By collecting behavioral health risk data at the state and local level, BRFSS has become a powerful tool for targeting and building health promotion activities.

A Brief History

By the early 1980s, scientific research clearly showed that personal health behaviors played a major role in premature morbidity and mortality. Although national estimates of health risk behaviors among U.S. adult populations had been periodically obtained through surveys conducted by the National Center for Health Statistics (NCHS), these data were not available on a state-specific basis. This deficiency was viewed as a critical obstacle to state health agencies trying to target resources to reduce behavioral risks and their consequent illnesses. National data may not be applicable to the conditions found in any given state; however, achieving national health goals required state and local agency participation.

About the same time that personal health behaviors received wider recognition in relation to chronic disease morbidity and mortality, telephone surveys emerged as an acceptable method for determining the prevalence of many health risk behaviors among populations. In addition to their cost advantages, telephone surveys were especially desirable at the state and local level, where the necessary expertise and resources for conducting area probability sampling for in-person household interviews were not likely to be available.

As a result, surveys were developed and conducted to monitor state-level prevalence of the major behavioral risks among adults associated with premature morbidity and mortality. The basic philosophy was to collect data on actual behaviors, rather than on attitudes or knowledge, that would be especially useful for planning, initiating, supporting, and evaluating health promotion and disease prevention programs.

To determine feasibility of behavioral surveillance, initial point-in-time state surveys were conducted in 29 states from 1981–1983. In 1984, the CDC established the BRFSS, and 15 states participated in monthly data collection. Although the BRFSS was designed to collect state-level data, a number of states from the outset stratified their samples to allow them to estimate prevalence for regions within their respective states. CDC developed a standard core questionnaire for states to use to provide data that could be compared across states. Initial topics included smoking, alcohol use, physical inactivity, diet,

(Continues)

EXHIBIT 4-3 Behavioral Risk Factor Surveillance System (Continued)

hypertension, and seat belt use. Optional modules—standardized sets of questions on specific topics—were implemented in 1988.

BRFSS became a nationwide surveillance system in 1993. The questionnaire was redesigned to include rotating fixed core and rotating core questions and up to five emerging core questions. Approximately 100,000 interviews were completed in 1993.

BRFSS mark[ed] its 30th year in 2013 and remains the gold standard of behavioral surveillance. Public health surveillance in the future will be much more complex and involve multiple ways of collecting public health data. Although telephone surveys will likely remain the mainstay of how BRFSS data

are collected, it is likely that additional modes of interviewing will also be necessary. The BRFSS piloted the Cell Phone Survey beginning in 2008. By including cell phones in the survey, BRFSS is able to reach segments of the population that were previously inaccessible—those who have a cell phone but not a landline—and produce a more representative sample and higher quality data. To prepare for the future, BRFSS currently has several pilot studies and research initiatives underway. These efforts are critical for improving the quality of BRFSS data, reaching populations previously not included in the survey, and expanding the utility of the surveillance data.

Adapted and reprinted from Centers for Disease Control and Prevention, Behavioral Risk Factor Surveillance System. About BRFSS. Available at: http://www.cdc.gov/brfss/about/and http://www.cdc.gov/brfss/about/about_brfss.htm. Accessed June 28, 2016.

sources of behavioral risk factors, for example, smoking and lifestyle. It is also the world's largest ongoing health survey.

However, because the BRFSS is operated at the state level, the data may not be adequate for analyses at finer levels of aggregation such as counties. Moreover, sufficient information may not be available regarding health topics not specifically addressed by the BRFSS. As a result, some states operate local versions of the BRFSS. An example is the California Health Interview Survey (CHIS), which provides information on the health and demographic characteristics of California residents who reside in geographic subdivisions of the state. From time to time, CHIS adds special topics that are of interest to Californians. CHIS is housed at the UCLA Center for Health Policy Research at the University of California, Los Angeles. Data from the BRFSS and CHIS may be downloaded from their respective websites.

CASE REGISTRIES

A **registry** is a centralized database for collection of information about a disease. Registries, maintained for many types of conditions, including cancer, are used to track patients and to select cases for case-control studies. The term register refers to the document that is used to collect the information.[11]

An example of a cancer registry is the National Program of Cancer Registries (NPCR), which is administered by CDC. This program "… collects data on the occurrence of cancer; the type, extent, and location of the cancer; and the type of initial treatment."[12] The NPCR covers 96% of the U.S. population through its support of cancer registries in

45 states, the District of Columbia, and U.S. territories and jurisdictions.

A second example of a registry is the Surveillance, Epidemiology, and End Results (SEER) Program. The National Cancer Institute (NCI) operates the SEER program, which comprises an integrated system of registries in strategic locations across the United States. At present, SEER covers about 28% of the U.S. population. Examples of information collected include demographic characteristics of cancer patients, their primary tumor site, cancer markers (for example, estrogen receptors), cancer staging, treatments, and survival.[13] **Figure 4-10** shows the location of SEER program cancer registries. **Figure 4-11** illustrates the sequence of surveillance of data flow in the SEER program.

Together, the National Program of Cancer Registries and SEER cover the complete U.S. population. Researchers, public health officials, and policy makers regard the data collected by these registries as essential to their work. Another registry is the California Cancer Registry operated by the State of California. (Refer to the case study for a description of how this registry is using real-time electronic submission of cancer data.) **Table 4-6** gives an overview of some of the possible uses of data from a cancer registry.

DATA FROM THE NATIONAL CENTER FOR HEALTH STATISTICS

The scope of information available from the National Center for Health Statistics (NCHS) is extensive. Examples of data available from the NCHS through its population surveys are

FIGURE 4-10 SEER program registries.

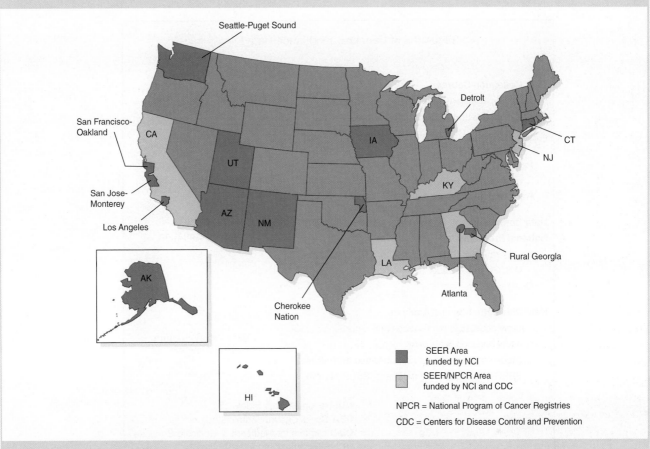

Reprinted from National Cancer Institute. Data flow in NCI's SEER registries September 2011. Available at: http://seer.cancer.gov/about/factsheets/SEER_Data_Flow_.pdf. Accessed August 11, 2016.

CASE STUDY: INNOVATIONS AT THE CALIFORNIA CANCER REGISTRY

The State of California funds the California Cancer Registry, which has been in operation since 1988 and has compiled data on about 4.5 million people with cancer. However, the existing reporting mechanism necessitates that information may be up to 2 years old. For this reason, the registry has implemented a new real-time data collection system for gathering information about cancer. The new system will improve the timeliness and accuracy of reporting through the use of standardized electronic forms. Real-time data could help doctors identify those treatments that are the most effective so that their cancer patients could be directed to these therapies. Cancer patients would also be better informed about optimal care for their conditions. Timely information might also be helpful in alerting patients to ongoing clinical trials for cancer treatments. In the past, the registry has played a crucial role in identifying cancer clusters and projecting survival rates for the various forms of cancer. It has also helped to identify health disparities such as differences in screening and outcomes among sociodemographic groups. Implementation of the real-time system is consistent with the many changes that technology has brought about in health care.

Data from Gorman A. Logging cancer data from the get-go. *The Orange County Register*. August 7, 2016.

FIGURE 4-11 The temporal sequence of cancer surveillance data flow.

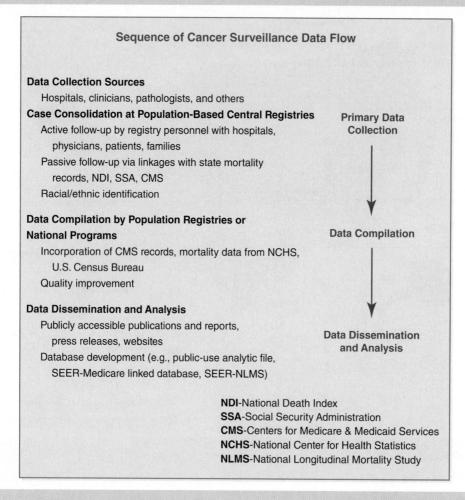

Sequence of Cancer Surveillance Data Flow

Data Collection Sources
    Hospitals, clinicians, pathologists, and others
Case Consolidation at Population-Based Central Registries
    Active follow-up by registry personnel with hospitals,
        physicians, patients, families
    Passive follow-up via linkages with state mortality
        records, NDI, SSA, CMS
    Racial/ethnic identification

Data Compilation by Population Registries or
National Programs
    Incorporation of CMS records, mortality data from NCHS,
        U.S. Census Bureau
    Quality improvement

Data Dissemination and Analysis
    Publicly accessible publications and reports,
        press releases, websites
    Database development (e.g., public-use analytic file,
        SEER-Medicare linked database, SEER-NLMS)

Primary Data Collection

Data Compilation

Data Dissemination and Analysis

NDI-National Death Index
SSA-Social Security Administration
CMS-Centers for Medicare & Medicaid Services
NCHS-National Center for Health Statistics
NLMS-National Longitudinal Mortality Study

Reprinted from National Cancer Institute. Data flow in NCI's SEER registries; September 2011. Available at: http://seer.cancer.gov/about/factsheets/SEER_Data_Flow_.pdf. Accessed August 11, 2016.

TABLE 4-6 Uses of Data from Cancer Registries

- Monitor cancer trends over time.
- Show cancer patterns in various populations and identify high-risk groups.
- Guide planning and evaluation of cancer control programs.
- Help set priorities for allocating health resources.
- Advance clinical, epidemiologic, and health services research.

Adapted and reprinted from Centers for Disease Control and Prevention. National program of cancer registries (NPCR). Available at: http://www.cdc.gov/cancer/npcr/about.htm. Accessed July 22, 2016.

given in **Table 4-7**. Note that both the National Health Interview Survey (NHIS) and the National Health and Nutrition Examination Survey (NHANES) are examples of **morbidity surveys of the population**. The surveys can be designed to elicit information about issues that may not be picked up by other routinely available sources, for example, reportable disease statistics. The NHANES collects information from physical examinations. Such data may disclose undiagnosed conditions not counted by other data collection methods.

National Health Interview Survey

The NCHS conducts the NHIS, which has been in operation since 1957.[14] **Figure 4-12** shows the logo of the NHIS. Data from the NHIS are used for monitoring how well the nation is progressing toward specific health objectives as well as

TABLE 4-7 National Center for Health Statistics Surveys

	National Health Interview Survey (NHIS)	National Health and Nutrition Examination Survey (NHANES)	National Survey of Family Growth
Data source and methods	Personal interviews	Personal interviews, physical examinations, laboratory tests, nutritional assessment, DNA repository	Personal interviews, men and women 15–44 years of age
Selected data items	• Health status and limitations • Utilization of health care • Health insurance • Access to care • Selected health conditions • Poisonings and injuries • Health behaviors • Functioning/disability • Immunizations	• Selected diseases and conditions including those undiagnosed or undetected • Nutrition monitoring • Environmental exposures monitoring • Children's growth and development • Infectious disease monitoring • Overweight and diabetes • Hypertension and cholesterol	• Contraception and sterilization • Teenage sexual activity and pregnancy • Infertility, adoption, and breastfeeding • Marriage, divorce, and cohabitation • Fatherhood involvement

Data from Centers for Disease Control and Prevention. National Center for Health Statistics. Population surveys. Available at: http://www.cdc.gov/nchs/surveys.htm. Accessed June 28, 2016.

FIGURE 4-12 The National Health Interview Survey.

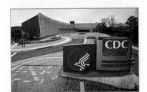

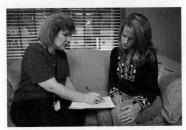

Photos courtesy of CDC/ James Gathany

for tracking people's health status and access to health care. The goal of the survey is to collect data from a representative sample of the U.S. population. During each survey wave, interviewers contact up to 40,000 households and obtain data on as many as 100,000 respondents. The interview consists of a set of unvarying core items plus additional questions that change from year to year. Refer again to Table 4-7 for information regarding topics covered by the NHIS. The NCHS releases datasets that contain results from the NHIS and also publishes related documents.

National Health and Nutrition Examination Survey

NHANES is also under the administrative purview of the NCHS, which is housed within the Centers for Disease Control and Prevention.[15] The National Health Survey Act of 1956 provided for the creation of studies to characterize illness and disability in the United States. NHANES evolved from this act. The special feature of NHANES is the collection of information from physical examinations coupled with interviews. A mobile examination center is used for performing physical examinations, laboratory tests, and interviews. The latter may also be conducted in the respondent's home. As of 1999, NHANES has operated as a continuous survey with data released in 2-year cycles. The interviews and examinations performed during the 2-year cycle of 2009–2010 each involved slightly more than 10,000 individuals. Table 4-7 gives additional information regarding NHANES.

National Vital Statistics System (NVSS)

As noted previously, vital events include births, deaths, marriages, divorces, and fetal deaths. The NVSS is employed by the NCHS to collect and distribute information about vital events in the United States.[16] The NCHS contracts with jurisdictions that are responsible for registering vital events and has promoted the development of standardized forms such as death certificates used for reporting vital events. The NCHS relies on information from the NVSS to publish *Vital Statistics of the United States* and *National Vital Statistics Reports* (NVSR). An example of an NVSR publication is *Births: Preliminary Data for 2014.*[17] **Figure 4-13** reports data on cesarean deliveries in the United States—information

obtained from the NVSS and printed in *Births: Preliminary Data for 2014.* NVSS-related programs include the Linked Birth and Infant Death Data Set, the National Survey of Family Growth, and the National Death Index.

DATA FROM INTERNATIONAL ORGANIZATIONS

Two examples of organizations that provide international and foreign data regarding diseases and health are the World Health Organization (WHO; www.who.int), mentioned earlier, and the European Union.

Figure 4-14 illustrates the WHO headquarters. Programs and information collection supported by WHO include:

- Global infectious disease surveillance. WHO has created a "network of networks" that link existing surveillance systems, such as those operated at the local and national levels in WHO member states. In addition, International Health Regulations, published

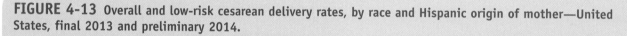

FIGURE 4-13 Overall and low-risk cesarean delivery rates, by race and Hispanic origin of mother—United States, final 2013 and preliminary 2014.

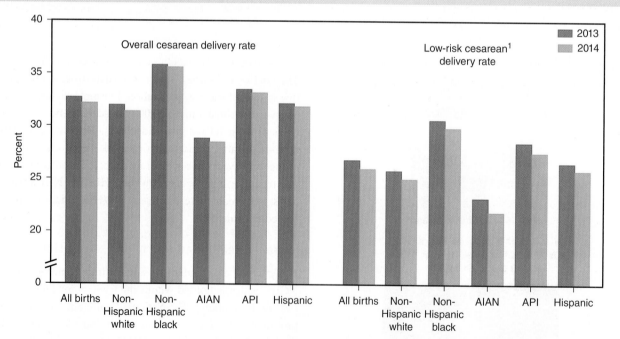

[1]Defined as singleton, term (37 or more weeks of completed gestation based on obsteric estimate), vertex (not breech) cesarean deliveries to women having a first birth.
NOTE: AIAN is American Indian or Alaska Native; API is Asian Pacific Islander.
SOURCE: CDC/NCHS, National Vital Statistics System.

Reprinted from Hamilton BE, Martin JA, Osterman MJK, Curtin SC. Births: preliminary data for 2014. *National Vital Statistics Reports.* 2015;64(6):1. Hyattsville, MD: National Center for Health Statistics.

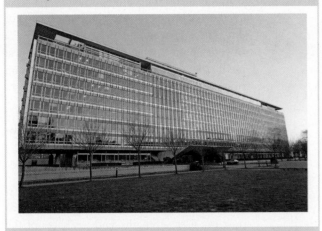

FIGURE 4-14 World Health Organization Headquarters, Geneva, Switzerland.

© Martin Good/Shutterstock

by WHO, legally mandate the reporting by WHO member states of three diseases of international importance—plague, cholera, and yellow fever.[18]

- WHOSIS. This interactive database yields data on 70 health indicators for 193 WHO member states.[19]
- Mortality data. Who collects data on levels and causes of mortality for children and adults.

The European Union provides statistics that cover a range of topics including public health. Access the website called "Eurostat: your key to European statistics" by using the following link: http://ec.europa.eu/eurostat. (Accessed June 30, 2016.) Some of the public health data available from this site and applicable to the member states of the European Union are related to social and health inequalities (e.g., death rates and suicide rates) and determinants of health (e.g., salmonellosis and smoking). This interactive website permits the user to develop customized tables, graphs, and maps.

MISCELLANEOUS DATA SOURCES

Several additional examples of data sources are provided here in order to flesh out the richness of potential information for epidemiologic research. While many of these sources have contributed valuable information, they also may have limitations with respect to completeness of population coverage due to their highly selective nature, methodological limitations, and availability to researchers. These sources of data include the following:

- Patient databases from provider groups, health insurance plans, and other insurers
- Clinical data (e.g., from clinical laboratories, physicians' records, hospitals, and special clinics)
- School health records
- Information from absenteeism reports
- Armed forces records

CONCLUSION

Epidemiology is a quantitative discipline that requires data for descriptive and analytic studies. Epidemiologists have increased their awareness of the potential of big data for illuminating morbidity and mortality in the population. Extensive data resources are available for retrieval online. Many health-related organizations operate websites that can be accessed by data professionals, students, and the public. A central concern of epidemiology is data quality, which can be assessed by applying several criteria discussed in this chapter. Epidemiologists use data from a variety of sources including the vital registration system of the United States, public health surveillance systems, case registries, the NCHS, and international data sources. The goal of this chapter has been to share information about the value of data sources for public health and epidemiology. Hopefully, this chapter has encouraged you to contemplate how mastery of data-retrieval skills could enhance your career in public health.

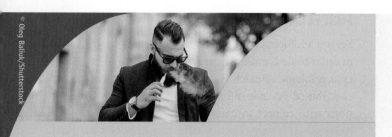

Study Questions and Exercises

1. Define the following terms and give an example of each one:

   a. Vital events
   b. Public health surveillance
   c. Syndromic surveillance
   d. Reportable and notifiable diseases
   e. Registry

2. This chapter provides examples of websites where you might obtain epidemiologic data. Identify a health topic that may interest you and conduct a search of the Internet in order to find some new examples of websites that might be relevant to your interest.

3. Describe the types of information that can be obtained from the vital registration system of the United States.

4. What is the purpose of surveillance systems? Describe the components of a surveillance system. Discuss the limitations of data collected from surveillance systems.

5. Describe the Behavioral Risk Factor Surveillance System. How does it differ from a surveillance system for infectious diseases?

6. What is one of the major types of case registries? Describe uses of data from the SEER program.

7. Describe data collection programs operated by the NCHS. What are some of the major differences between NHIS and the NHANES. In your opinion, what do you think is the best method to obtain health-related information from study participants?

8. Refer to Table 4-5 (notifiable diseases). Select three diseases that interest you. Access the Pub-Med website (www.ncbi.nlm.nih.gov/pubmed/) and develop of bibliography of five epidemiologic references on each disease.

9. Create a table in which you compare and contrast the uses, strengths, and weakness of the following types of data: mortality data, birth statistics, surveillance data, and morbidity survey of the population, for example NHIS.

10. Define the term *big data*. Using you own ideas, state what data sources might be included in big data. What do you believe are some of the advantages and disadvantages of using big data for epidemiologic research?

Young Epidemiology Scholars (YES) Exercises

The Young Epidemiology Scholars: Competitions website provides links to teaching units and exercises that support instruction in epidemiology. The YES program, discontinued in 2011, was administered by the College Board and supported by the Robert Wood Johnson Foundation. The exercises continue to be available at the following website: http://yes-competition.org/yes/teaching-units/title.html. The following exercises relate to topics discussed in this chapter and can be found on the YES competitions website.

1. Kaelin MA, St. George DMM. Descriptive Epidemiology of Births to Teenage Mothers.

REFERENCES

1. Roski J, Bo-Linn GW, Andrews TA. Creating value in health care through big data: opportunities and policy implications. *Health Affairs*. 2014;33(7):1115–1122.

2. Halper E. Privacy at risk in hunt for data on voters. *Los Angeles Times*. January 28, 2016.

3. Lohr S. Google flu trends: the limits of big data. *The New York Times*. Available at: http://bits.blogs.nytimes.com/2014/03/28/google-flu-trends-the-limits-of-big-data/?_r=0. Accessed June 29, 2016.

4. Lazer D, Kennedy R, King G, Vespignani A. The parable of Google flu: traps in big data analysis. *Science*. 2014;343:1203–1205.

5. Lien T. Start-up makes sense of transit data. *Los Angeles Times*. February 28, 2016.

6. U.S. Census Bureau. Methodology for the United States population estimates: vintage 2014. Available at: https://www.census.gov/popest/methodology/2014-natstcopr-meth.pdf. Accessed July 23, 2016.

7. U.S. Census Bureau. American Community Survey. Available at: https://www.census.gov/history/www/programs/demographic/american_community_survey.html. Accessed June 30, 2016.

8. Henning KJ. Overview of syndromic surveillance: what is syndromic surveillance? *MMWR*. 2004;53(Suppl):5–11.

9. Chorba TL, Berkelman RL, Safford SK, et al. Mandatory reporting of infectious diseases by clinicians, and mandatory reporting of occupational diseases by clinicians. *MMWR Recomm Rep*. 1990;39(RR-9):1–17.

10. Milet M, Lutzker L, Flattery J. *Asthma in California: a surveillance report*. Richmond, CA: California Department of Public Health, Environmental Health Investigations Branch; May 2013.

11. Terracini B, Zanetti R. A short history of pathology registries, with emphasis on cancer registries. *Soz Praventivmed*. 2003;48(1):3–10.

12. Centers for Disease Control and Prevention. National program of cancer registries (NPCR). Available at: http://www.cdc.gov/cancer/npcr/about.htm. Accessed July 22, 2016.

13. National Institutes of Health, National Cancer Institute. SEER Surveillance, Epidemiology, and End Results Program. NIH Publication No. 12-4722. March 2012.

14. Centers for Disease Control and Prevention. National Center for Health Statistics. *National Health Interview Survey*. Hyattsville, MD: National Center for Health Statistics.

15. Zipf G, Chiappa M, Porter KS, et al. National Health and Nutrition Examination Survey: plan and operations, 1999–2010. National Center for Health Statistics. *Vital Health Stat*. 2013;1(56).

16. Centers for Disease Control and Prevention. National Center for Health Statistics. About the National Vital Statistics System. Available at: http://www.cdc.gov/nchs/nvss/about_nvss.htm. Accessed June 29, 2016.

17. Hamilton BE, Martin JA, Osterman MJK, Curtin SC. Births: preliminary data for 2014. *National Vital Statistics Reports*. 2015;64(6):1. Hyattsville, MD: National Center for Health Statistics.

18. World Health Organization. Global infectious disease surveillance. Fact Sheet No 200. Available at: http://www.who.int/mediacentre/factsheets/fs200/en/. Accessed June 29, 2016.

19. World Health Organization. WHO Statistical Information System (WHOSIS). Available at: http://www.who.int/whosis/en. Accessed July 22, 2016.

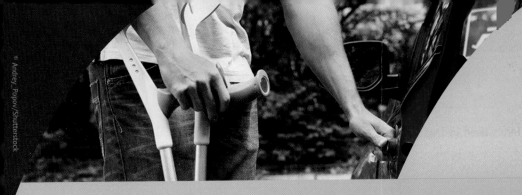

CHAPTER **5**

Descriptive Epidemiology: Patterns of Disease— Person, Place, Time

LEARNING OBJECTIVES

By the end of this chapter you will be able to:

- Define the term *descriptive epidemiology*.
- Name two examples of uses of descriptive epidemiology.
- Compare three types of descriptive epidemiologic studies.
- Describe the process of epidemiologic inference in the context of descriptive epidemiology.
- Give two examples each of person, place, and time variables and describe how they relate to the distribution of health outcomes.

CHAPTER OUTLINE

INTRODUCTION

Human health and disease are unequally distributed throughout populations. This generalization applies to differences among population groups subdivided according to age and other demographic characteristics, among different countries, within a single country, and over time. For example, income inequality is reflected in differences in life expectancy between the wealthiest Americans (longer lives) and those at the bottom of the economic ladder (shorter lives). Among racial and ethnic groups, black men who are living in poverty have lower life expectancies in comparison with members of the same racial group who exceed the poverty level.

When specific diseases, adverse health outcomes, or other health characteristics are more prevalent among one group than among another, or more prevalent in one country than in another, the logical question that follows is "Why?" To answer the question "Why," one must consider "three Ws"—Who was affected? Where did the event occur? When did the event occur?

In Chapter 4 you will learn about person, place, and time, which are the three major epidemiologic descriptive variables. Then you will explore how they are used in descriptive epidemiologic studies in order to address the three Ws. The types of descriptive epidemiologic research including cross-sectional studies will be covered. An important takeaway from Chapter 4 will be strengths and weakness of descriptive epidemiology. Table 5-1 lists the terms related to descriptive epidemiology and subcategories of variables that make up person, place, and time.

TABLE 5-1 List of Important Terms Used in This Chapter

Descriptive Epidemiology	Major Descriptive Epidemiologic Variables		
Study Design Terms	Person	Place	Time
Case reports	Age	International	Clustering
Case series	Health disparities	Localized patterns	Cyclic trends
Cross-sectional study	Race	Spatial clustering	Point epidemic
Descriptive epidemiology	Sex	Urban-rural	Secular trends
Descriptive epidemiologic study	Socioeconomic status	Within country	Temporal clustering

WHAT IS DESCRIPTIVE EPIDEMIOLOGY?

The field of **descriptive epidemiology** classifies the occurrence of disease according to the variables of person (who is affected), place (where the condition occurs), and time (when and over what time period the condition has occurred). A **descriptive epidemiologic study** is one that is "… concerned with characterizing the amount and distribution of health and disease within a population."[1(p741)] Descriptive epidemiology provides valuable information for the prevention of disease, design of interventions, and conduct of additional research. Descriptive epidemiologic studies set the stage for more focused investigations into questions raised. Such investigations include evaluating observed trends, planning for needed services, and launching more complex research.

Consider the example of a descriptive epidemiologic study of children who were exclusively breastfed. The practice of breastfeeding has been recommended for reinforcing the health of babies and mothers and promoting mother–child bonding. **Table 5-2** provides the characteristics (a descriptive epidemiologic statement) of babies who were breastfed. Data were collected by the National Immunization Survey.[2] The survey defined exclusive breastfeeding "… as *only* breast milk—*no* solids, no water, and no other

liquids." Note that the table shows person variables: sex and race/ethnicity (of child) and the mother's age, education, marital status, and socioeconomic status (as measured by income-to-poverty ratio). A place variable (location of residence of mother) is shown also. According to the survey, the income-to-poverty ratio was the "[r]atio of self-reported family income to the federal poverty threshold value depending on the number of people in the household." The category unmarried included "… never married, widowed, separated, [and] divorced." The variable metropolitan area was defined according to definitions used by the U.S. Census Bureau.

What can you infer from this example? The table indicates that approximately 43% of infants in the United States are breastfed exclusively through 3 months of age and that the percentage drops to about 22% through the age of 6 months. Other observations include the following: non-Hispanic black mothers tend to engage in breastfeeding less often than other racial/ethnic groups and lower frequencies of breastfeeding occur among women (in comparison with the rest of the study population) who are younger, have lower levels of education and income, and are unmarried. The reader may want to speculate about the reasons for the results that are displayed and develop hypotheses for interventions to increase breastfeeding.

TABLE 5-2 Rates of Exclusive Breastfeeding by Sociodemographic Characteristics, among Children Born in 2012

	Sample Size	Exclusive Breastfeeding through 3 Months	Exclusive Breastfeeding through 6 Months
Characteristic	n	% ± half 95% CI[a]	% ± half 95% CI
U.S. national overall percentage	14,768	43.3 ± 1.6	21.9 ± 1.4
Sex			
Male	7,554	41.5 ± 2.1	20.6 ± 1.8
Female	7,214	45.2 ± 2.3	23.3 ± 2.0
Race/ethnicity			
Hispanic	2,749	40.3 ± 3.8	20.8 ± 3.3
Non-Hispanic white	8,546	48.0 ± 1.9	24.4 ± 1.7
Non-Hispanic black	1,460	33.4 ± 4.1	13.9 ± 2.9
Non-Hispanic Asian	662	46.5 ± 7.5	26.9 ± 7.1
Education			
Less than high school	1,559	32.8 ± 4.5	16.1 ± 3.9
High school graduate	2,696	33.5 ± 3.1	16.3 ± 2.5
Some college or technical school	3,814	41.2 ± 3.2	19.5 ± 2.7
College graduate	6,699	57.2 ± 2.2	30.6 ± 2.2
Age of mother			
Under 20	103	28.3 ± 13.1	8.0 ± 7.7
20–29	5,315	37.8 ± 2.4	18.8 ± 2.1
30 or older	9,350	47.8 ± 2.1	24.5 ± 1.8
Income-to-poverty ratio			
Less than 100	3,768	31.7 ± 2.9	15.6 ± 2.3

(continues)

TABLE 5-2 Rates of Exclusive Breastfeeding by Sociodemographic Characteristics, among Children Born in 2012 (*continued*)

	Sample Size	Exclusive Breastfeeding through 3 Months	Exclusive Breastfeeding through 6 Months
100–199	2,880	40.5 ± 3.3	19.9 ± 2.8
200–399	3,920	54.5 ± 3.0	27.1 ± 3.0
400–599	2,317	53.7 ± 3.8	30.2 ± 3.9
600 or greater	1,883	54.4 ± 4.3	27.9 ± 4.1
Marital status			
Married	10,534	51.5 ± 1.9	27.2 ± 1.7
Unmarried	4,234	29.7 ± 2.6	13.2 ± 2.1
Residence			
Metropolitan	4,679	44.5 ± 2.5	21.4 ± 2.1
Nonmetropolitan	1,540	37.1 ± 4.4	19.3 ± 4.2

[a]Breastfeeding rates presented in this table are based on dual-frame (landline and cellular telephone) samples from 2013 and 2014 National Immunization Surveys. Reproduced from: Centers for Disease Control and Prevention. Breastfeeding among U.S. children born 2002–2012, CDC National Immunization Surveys. Available at: http://www.cdc.gov/breastfeeding/data/nis_data/rates-any-exclusive-bf-socio-dem-2012.htm. Accessed August 8, 2016.

USES OF DESCRIPTIVE EPIDEMIOLOGIC STUDIES

As you may have inferred from the foregoing example, descriptive epidemiologic studies aid in the realization of general aims, which are shown in the following text box.

Aims of descriptive epidemiology

1. Permit evaluation of trends in health and disease.
2. Provide a basis for planning, provision, and evaluation of health services.
3. Identify problems to be studied by analytic methods, and suggest areas that may be fruitful for investigation.

Adapted from Friis RH, Sellers TA. *Epidemiology for Public Health Practice.* 5th ed. Burlington, MA: Jones & Bartlett Learning; 2014:159.

Permit Evaluation of Trends in Health and Disease

This objective includes monitoring of known diseases as well as the identification of emerging problems. Comparisons are made among population groups, geographical areas, and time periods. In the breastfeeding example, investigators reported that infants who resided in metropolitan areas were breastfed more frequently than infants who resided outside of metropolitan areas; in addition, infants from families with lower income levels (less than 100% of the income-to-poverty ratio) were breastfed less frequently than infants from families with higher income levels. These findings highlighted the relationships between the frequency of breastfeeding and both residential locations and income levels as potential emerging problems.

Provide a Basis for Planning, Provision, and Evaluation of Health Services

Data needed for efficient allocation of resources often come from descriptive epidemiologic studies. The breastfeeding example demonstrated that race (non-Hispanic blacks), age of mother (mothers who were younger than 20 years of age), and marital status (unmarried) were associated with lower frequency of breastfeeding. An implication of this descriptive study is that an intervention program to increase the frequency of breastfeeding might target pregnant, unmarried, younger black women.

Identify Problems to Be Studied by Analytic Methods and Suggest Areas that May Be Fruitful for Investigation

Among the phenomena identified by the breastfeeding study was a reduction in breastfeeding after infants reached 3 months of age. This observation raises the question: "What caused the drop-off in breastfeeding?" You might hypothesize that when mothers return to work or other activities, breastfeeding becomes inconvenient. You might be able to think of many other hypotheses as well. The next step would be to design a more complex study—an analytic study to explore the hypotheses that have been raised. Examples of these types of studies are case-control, cohort, and experimental designs. (See Chapter 7.)

TYPES OF DESCRIPTIVE EPIDEMIOLOGIC STUDIES

Three types of descriptive epidemiologic studies are individual case reports, case series, and cross-sectional studies (e.g., a survey of a population). Case reports and case series are among the most basic types of descriptive studies.

Case Reports

Case reports are accounts of a single occurrence of a noteworthy health-related incident or small collection of such events. (Refer to the text box: Injuries Associated with Bison Encounters.) The following section provides examples of case reports.

Injuries Associated with Bison Encounters—Yellowstone National Park, 2015

American bison *(Bison bison)* are the largest terrestrial mammals in the Western Hemisphere. Yellowstone is home to the largest U.S. bison population on public land, with an estimated 4,900 bison in July 2015. Mating season occurs from July to September, coinciding with Yellowstone's peak tourism season. Mature bull aggressiveness increases during mating

season. Yellowstone promulgates regulations that prohibit visitors from "… willfully approaching, remaining, viewing, or engaging in any activity within 300 ft (91 m) of bears or wolves, or within 75 ft (23 m) of any other wildlife, including nesting birds, or within any distance that disturbs, displaces, or otherwise interferes with the free unimpeded movement of wildlife, or creates or contributes to a potentially hazardous condition or situation."

During May through July 2015, five injuries associated with bison encounters occurred. Case reports were reviewed to evaluate circumstances surrounding these injuries to inform prevention. The five people injured during 2015 (four Yellowstone visitors and one employee) ranged in age from 16 to 68 years (median = 43 years); four were female. Every incident occurred in developed areas, such as hiking trails or geyser basins. Two people were gored, and three were tossed into the air. Four people required hospitalization, three of whom were transported by helicopter ambulance. There were no deaths.

All encounters resulted from failure to maintain the required distance of 75 ft (23 m) from bison. Four injuries occurred when three or more people approached the bison. Two people were injured while walking on hiking trails. Three people sustained injuries while taking photographs at a distance of approximately 3 to 6 ft (1–2 m) from bison, including two who turned their back on the bison to take the photograph; one person reported taking a cell phone self-portrait (selfie), which necessitated getting close to the animal.

Adapted and reprinted from Centers for Disease Control and Prevention. *MMWR*. 2016;65(11):293.

Case reports, such as the one that described bison encounters, can highlight the need for investigations by public health authorities, enforcement of public health laws and practices, and in-depth epidemiologic research. Case reports are abundant in the medical literature, for example, *Morbidity and Morbidity Weekly Report (MMWR)*. Some examples are the following.

Adverse Reactions to Cosmetic Surgery

Cosmetic surgery and related procedures are typically (but not invariably) performed on healthy individuals. The use of cosmetic procedures to enhance beauty is becoming increasingly popular in many parts of the United States among all classes of people, no longer just affluent VIPs. Sometimes these procedures, which are often invasive, incur the risk of serious complications or even death.

The Centers for Disease Control and Prevention (CDC) published three case reports of women who developed adverse reactions (acute kidney failure) to injections of cosmetic soft-tissue fillers, which are substances used to improve the appearance of bodily areas such as lips and buttocks. The injections were administered by an unlicensed and unsupervised practitioner at the same clinic (known as facility A) in North Carolina.[3] These adverse reactions necessitated extended hospitalizations and hemodialysis. Follow-up interviews, investigations, and inspections of facility A were conducted. Subsequently, the Guilford County (North Carolina) Health Director mandated that facility A cease administration of all injections and initiated legal action against the unlicensed practitioner.

Rabid Dog Imported from Egypt

An animal rescue organization imported a large group of dogs and cats from Egypt to the United States for distribution and adoption nationally. In June 2015, one of the dogs placed in a foster home in Virginia developed symptoms of rabies, which was confirmed by laboratory testing. Investigations determined that the animal's vaccination certificate had been falsified. This incident suggests that imported domestic animals may carry the risk of not having adequate vaccination against rabies.[4]

Case Series

In comparison with a case report, a **case series** is a larger collection of cases of disease, often grouped consecutively and listing common features such as the characteristics of affected patients. A sample case series was developed for primary amebic meningoencephalitis (PAM), a highly fatal disease associated with infection by *Naegleria fowleri*. The *Naegleria* workgroup (formed by the CDC and the Council of State and Territorial Epidemiologists) reviewed all cases of PAM that were reported in the United States between 1937 and 2007. Preliminary findings were that a total of 121 cases occurred during the approximately 70-year time period. The largest number of cases reported in any 1 year (2007) was six. About 93% of the people afflicted were male (median age = 12 years). The primary exposure source was described as freshwater (untreated and warm) in lakes and rivers.[5] **Figure 5-1** demonstrates the number of PAM cases distributed according to the year in which they were reported.

Cross-Sectional Studies

More complex than case reports and case series are **cross-sectional studies**. This type of investigation is defined as one "… that examines the relationship between diseases (or

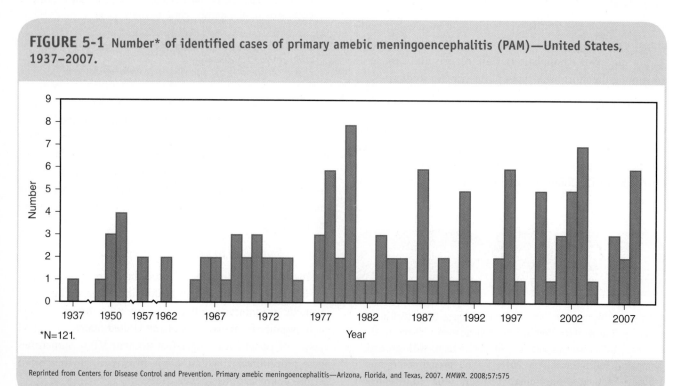

FIGURE 5-1 Number* of identified cases of primary amebic meningoencephalitis (PAM)—United States, 1937–2007.

*N=121.

Year

other health outcomes) and other variables of interest as they exist in a defined population at one particular time. The presence or absence of disease and the presence or absence of the other variables… are determined in each member of the study population or in a representative sample at one particular time."[6]

Thus, a cross-sectional study is a type of prevalence study in which exposures and distributions of disease are determined at the same time, although it is not imperative for the study to include both exposure and disease. A cross-sectional study may focus only on the latter.[1] Cross-sectional designs make a one-time assessment (similar to a snapshot) of the prevalence of disease in a study group that in most situations has been sampled randomly from the parent population of interest. As is true of descriptive studies in general, cross-sectional studies may be used to formulate hypotheses that can be followed up in analytic studies.

Here is an example of a cross-sectional study: The Behavioral Risk Factor Surveillance System (BRFSS) conducts an ongoing survey (using random digit dialing techniques) of civilian, noninstitutionalized U.S. residents age 18 years and older. This section presents sleep data gathered by BRFSS during 2014.

An interesting public health question is whether Americans are getting enough sleep. As the pace of our lives quickens, legitimate concerns have been raised about the quality of our sleep patterns. **Figure 5-2** shows a sleepy commuter. Insufficient sleep has been linked to risk of chronic diseases (for example, obesity and cardiovascular disease). Fatigued individuals are at greater risk of injuries when performing demanding tasks, such as driving.

Data from the 2014 survey examined the prevalence of adults who had healthy sleep patterns.[7] Healthy sleep duration was defined as having 7 hours or more of sleep each night. The survey question was: "On average, how many hours of sleep do you get in a 24-hour period?" **Table 5-3** presents the results for respondents who had an average of 7 or more hours of sleep at night; the findings are distributed according to the variables of age group, race/ethnicity, sex, employment status, and education level.

Regarding sleeping for at least 7 hours each night (the recommended amount of sleep), Table 5-3 shows that approximately 65% of the total sample reported meeting this criterion. Conversely, about one-third of the sample did not have adequate sleep levels. Among all age groups in the survey, people age 65 years and older had the highest prevalence of recommended sleep levels. A lower

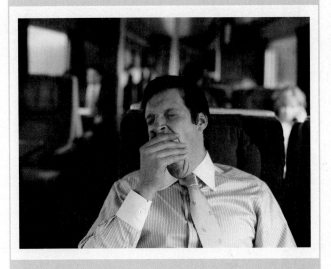

FIGURE 5-2 Sleep deprivation.

© Digital Vision/Getty

prevalence of recommended sleep levels was reported for non-Hispanic blacks as well as American Indians/Alaska Natives and Native Hawaiian/Pacific Islanders. (The latter two groups are not shown in the table.)

Refer to **Figure 5-3** for information regarding national variations in the achieving of recommended levels of sleep. States with lower levels of recommended sleep duration tended to be clustered in the southeastern United States and along the Appalachians; these same geographical regions also have high levels of chronic health issues such as obesity. Other states that fell below recommended levels were located in the upper Midwest, for example, Michigan.

Epidemiologic Inferences from Descriptive Data

Descriptive epidemiology and descriptive studies provide a basis for generating hypotheses; thus studies of this type connect intimately with the process of epidemiologic inference. The process of inference in descriptive epidemiology refers to drawing conclusions about the nature of exposures and health outcomes and formulating hypotheses to be tested in analytic research. **Figure 5-4** illustrates the process of epidemiologic inference.

Refer to the center panel of the figure, which suggests that epidemiologic inference is initiated with observations.

TABLE 5-3 Adults* Who Reported 7 or More Hours of Sleep per 24-Hour Period, by Selected Characteristics—Behavioral Risk Factor Surveillance System, United States, 2014

Characteristic	Number (unweighted)	Percentage**†	(95% CI)†
Age group (yrs)			
18–24	23,234	67.8	(66.8–68.7)
25–34	42,084	62.1	(61.3–62.9)
35–44	52,385	61.7	(60.9–62.5)
45–64	173,357	62.7	(62.2–63.1)
≥ 65	153,246	73.7	(73.2–74.2)
Race/ethnicity			
White, non-Hispanic	348,988	66.8	(66.4–67.1)
Black, non-Hispanic	33,535	54.2	(53.3–55.2)
Hispanic	29,044	65.5	(64.5–66.4)
Sex			
Men	185,796	64.6	(64.2–65.0)
Women	258,510	65.2	(64.8–65.7)
Employment status			
Employed	220,751	64.9	(64.4–65.3)
Unemployed	19,300	60.2	(58.8–61.6)
Retired	130,478	60.9	(54.4–67.1)
Unable to work	31,953	51.0	(49.4–52.5)
Homemaker/student	37,393	69.5	(68.5–70.5)
Education level			
High school diploma	125,462	62.4	(61.8–63.0)
Some college	120,814	62.4	(61.8–62.9)
College graduate or higher	161,088	71.5	(71.0–71.9)
Total	**NA**	**64.9**	**(64.6–65.2)**

*n = 444,306

**Age-adjusted

†Weighted

Adapted and reprinted from Centers for Disease Control and Prevention. Prevalence of healthy sleep duration among adults—United States, 2014. *MMWR*. 2016;65(6):139.

FIGURE 5-3 Age-adjusted percentage of adults who reported 7 or more hours of sleep per 24-hour period, by state—Behavioral Risk Factor Surveillance System, United States, 2014.

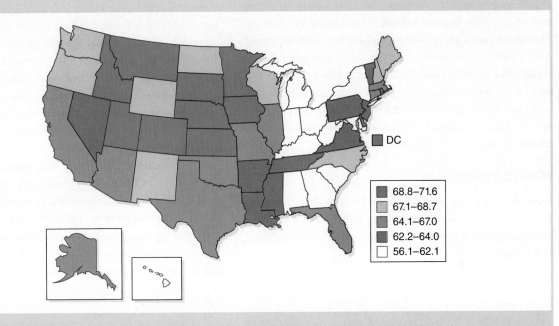

■	68.8–71.6
■	67.1–68.7
■	64.1–67.0
■	62.2–64.0
□	56.1–62.1

Reprinted from Centers for Disease Control and Prevention. Prevalence of healthy sleep duration among adults–United States, 2014. *MMWR.* 2016;65(6):140.

FIGURE 5-4 Process of epidemiologic inference (how epidemiologists think about data).

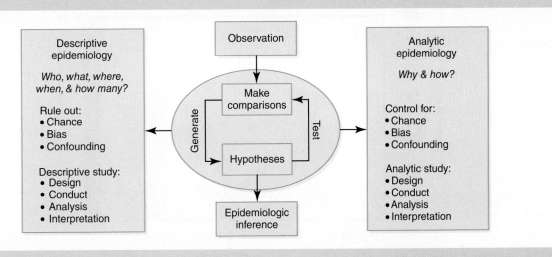

Reprinted with permission from Aragón T. *Descriptive epidemiology: describing findings and generating hypotheses.* Center for Infectious Disease Preparedness, University of California Berkeley School of Public Health. Available at: http://www.idready.org/slides/feb_descriptive.pdf. Accessed August 16, 2008.

The observation(s) made in descriptive epidemiology (left-hand panel) culminate in hypotheses. As discussed previously, descriptive epidemiology aims to characterize health phenomena according to person, place, and time (who, where, and when). This process involves quantifying the findings (how many cases) and providing insights into what happened. After conducting a descriptive study, the epidemiologist must evaluate the findings carefully in order to rule out chance factors, biases, and confounding. (These terms are defined later in the text.) The right-hand panel is titled "analytic epidemiology," which is concerned with testing hypotheses in order to answer the questions "why?" and "how?"

PERSON VARIABLES

Examples of person variables covered in this chapter are age, sex, race, and socioeconomic status. Other person variables include marital status, nativity (place of origin), migration, and religion.

Age

Age is perhaps the most important factor to consider when one is describing the occurrence of virtually any disease or illness because age-specific disease rates usually show greater variation than rates defined by almost any other personal attribute. (For this reason, public health professionals often use age-specific rates when comparing the disease burden among populations.) As age increases, overall mortality increases, as do the incidence of and mortality from many chronic diseases. For example, in the United States in 2013, age-specific death rates for malignant neoplasms (cancers) demonstrated substantial age-related increases, from 2.2 per 100,000 population at ages 5 to 14 years to 1,635.4 cases per 100,000 at age 85 years and older.[8] Similarly, age-adjusted incidence rates for invasive cancers show steep increases with age.[9] Invasive cancers are cancers that have spread and are not localized to a single site. The increasing trend for invasive cancers is shown in **Figure 5-5**.

The causes of morbidity and mortality differ according to stage of life. During childhood, among unvaccinated people, infectious diseases such as mumps and chickenpox occur most commonly. Teenagers are affected by unintentional injuries, violence, and substance abuse. Among younger adults, unintentional injury is the leading cause of death. And finally, among older adults, morbidity and mortality from chronic diseases such as diabetes, heart disease, and cancer take hold.

Another example of an age association is the relationship between age of mother and rates of diabetes, which increase the risk of complications of pregnancy. Mothers who give birth when they are older have higher rates of diabetes than

FIGURE 5-5 Age-adjusted incidence rates of invasive cancers by age group, 2012.

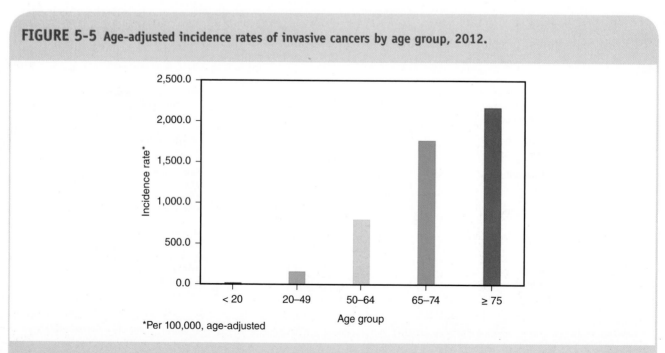

*Per 100,000, age-adjusted

Data from Centers for Disease Control and Prevention. Invasive cancer incidence and survival—United States, 2012. *MMWR.* 64(49);2014:1355.

mothers who give birth at younger ages. In 1990, the rate of diabetes among mothers younger than age 20 was less than 10 per 1,000 births. In comparison, the rate was more than six times higher among mothers who were age 40 years and older. By 2004, the corresponding rates had increased to about 10 per 1,000 and 80 per 1,000, respectively.[10] In 2014, those respective rates were approximately 22 and 138.[11]

A final illustration concerns age differences in birth rates for teenage mothers. In 2004, the overall teenage birth rate was 41.1 per 1,000 females age 15 to 19 years. At that time, the birth rate (22.1 per 1,000) was lower for teenagers age 15 to 17 years than the rate (70.0 per 1,000 females) for older teenagers age 18 to 19 years.[10] In 2014, the birth rate for teenagers age 15 to 19 years was 24.2 per 1,000 females age 10 to 19 years.[11] **Figure 5-6** shows the declining trend in teenage birth rates by age group from 1990 to 2014.

Sex

Numerous epidemiologic studies have shown **sex** differences in a wide array of health phenomena, including mortality and morbidity. Regarding sex differences in mortality (with some exceptions), the population age-adjusted death rate has declined in the United States since 1980.[12] Males generally have higher all-cause age-specific mortality rates than females from birth to age 85 and older; the ratio of male to female age-adjusted death rates in 2005 was 1.4 to 1.

Sex differences occur in mortality from chronic diseases such as cancer. **Figure 5-7** displays leading sites of cancer incidence and mortality estimated for 2016. The cancer diagnoses with the highest incidence are prostate cancer for males (21% of all new cases) and breast cancer for females (29% of all new cases).[13] For both males and females, cancer of the lung and bronchus are the leading cause of cancer mortality.

Race/Ethnicity

The United States is becoming increasingly racially and ethnically diverse. Scientists have proposed that **race** is a social and cultural construct, rather than a biological construct.[14] Race and ethnicity are, to some extent, ambiguous characteristics that tend to overlap with nativity and religion. Nativity refers to the place of origin of the individual or his or her relatives. A common subdivision used in epidemiology is

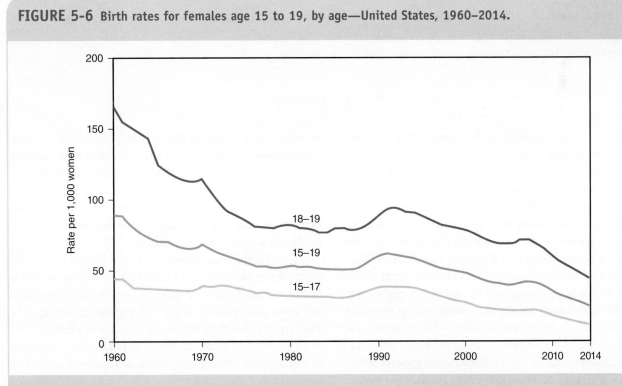

FIGURE 5-6 Birth rates for females age 15 to 19, by age—United States, 1960–2014.

Reprinted from Hamilton BE, Martin JA, Osterman MJK, et al. Births: final data for 2014. *National Vital Statistics Reports.* 2015;64(12):5. Hyattsville, MD: National Center for Health Statistics.

FIGURE 5-7 Leading sites of new cancer cases and deaths—2016 estimates.

Estimated new cases		Estimated deaths	
Male	**Female**	**Male**	**Female**
Prostate 180,890 (21%)	Breast 246,660 (29%)	Lung & bronchus 85,920 (27%)	Lung & bronchus 72,160 (26%)
Lung & bronchus 117,920 (14%)	Lung & bronchus 106,470 (13%)	Prostate 26,120 (8%)	Breast 40,450 (14%)
Colon & rectum 70,820 (8%)	Colon & rectum 63,670 (8%)	Colon & rectum 26,020 (8%)	Colon & rectum 23,170 (8(%)
Urinary blader 58,950 (7%)	Uterine corpus 60,050 (7%)	Pancreas 21,450 (7%)	Pancreas 20,330 (7%)
Melanoma of the skin 46,870 (6%)	Thyroid 49,350 (6%)	Liver & intrahepatic bile duct 18,280 (6%)	Ovary 14,240 (5%)
Non-hodgkin lymphoma 40,170 (5%)	Non-hodgkin lymphoma 32,410 (4%)	Leukemia 14,130 (4%)	Uterine corpus 10,470 (4%)
Kidney & ranal pelvis 39,650 (5%)	Melanoma of the skin 29,510 (3%)	Esophagus 12,720 (4%)	Leukemia 10,270 (4%)
Oral cavity & pharynx 34,780 (4%)	Leukemia 26,050 (3%)	Urinary blader 11,820 (4%)	Liver & intrahepatic bile duct 8,890 (3%)
Leukemia 34,090 (4%)	Pancreas 25,400 (3%)	Non-hodgkin lymphoma 11,520 (4%)	Non-hodgkin lymphoma 8,330 (3%)
Liver & intrahepatic bile duct 28,410 (3%)	Kidney & renal pelvis 23,050 (3%)	Brain & other nervous system 9,440 (3%)	Brain & other nervous system 6,610 (2%)
All sites 841,390 (100%)	All sites 843,820 (100%)	All sites 314,290 (100%)	All sites 281,400 (100%)

Reproduced from American Cancer Society. *Cancer facts and figures 2016*. Atlanta, GA: American Cancer Society; 2016, 20.

foreign-born versus native-born. In Census 2000 and continuing with Census 2010, the U.S. Census Bureau classified race into five major categories: white; black or African American; American Indian and Alaska Native; Asian; and Native Hawaiian and other Pacific Islander.

To a degree, race tends to be synonymous with ethnicity because people who come from a particular racial stock also may have a common ethnic and cultural identification. Also, assignment of some individuals to a particular racial classification on the basis of observed characteristics may be difficult. Often, one must ask the respondent to elect the racial group with which he or she identifies. The responses one elicits from such a question may not be consistent: Individuals may change ethnic or racial self-identity or respond differently on different occasions, depending on their perception of the intent of the race question. Classification of persons of mixed racial parentage also may be problematic.[15] Census 2000 allowed respondents to check a multiracial category, which was used for the first time. Changes in the definitions of racial categories affect the denominators (i.e., the numbers in a particular racial subgroup) of rates used to track various health outcomes and the consequent assessments of unmet needs and social inequalities in health.[16]

In 2016, the total population of the United States—the third most populous country on the globe—was estimated to be 324 million. Figure 5-8 demonstrates the estimated racial and ethnic composition of the U.S. population during 2014. The largest percentage of the population was white (73.8%). Blacks made up 12.6% of the U.S. population. According to the Census Bureau, Hispanics and Latinos can be of any race; as a result, they are not shown in the figure as a separate group.

FIGURE 5-8 Racial/ethnic distribution of the population—United States, 2014 estimates.*

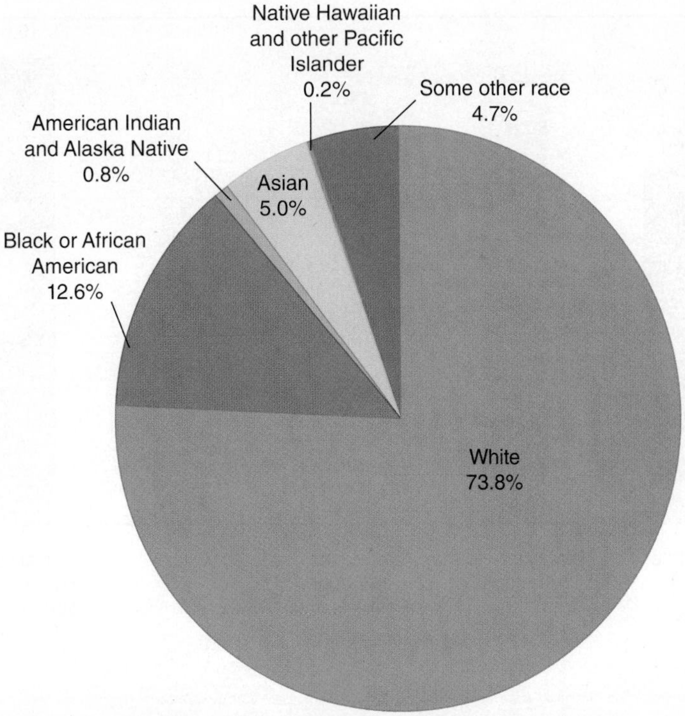

Native Hawaiian
and other Pacific
Islander
0.2%

Some other race
4.7%

American Indian
and Alaska Native
0.8%

Asian
5.0%

Black or African
American
12.6%

White
73.8%

* Data is for individuals who declare only one race.

Data from U.S. Census Bureau. American FactFinder. Available at: http://factfinder.census.gov/faces/nav/jsf/pages/index.xhtml. Accessed April 20, 2016.

America's diversity yields many examples of racial and ethnic differences in health characteristics. The following section lists three conditions that show such variations.

- Asthma: Individuals who classified themselves as Asian or as Hispanic/Latino had a lower percentage of self-reported asthma (ever had asthma) than either non-Hispanic whites or non-Hispanic blacks. Refer to **Figure 5-9** for information on other racial/ethnic groups.
- No usual source of medical care: For people diagnosed with diabetes, serious heart conditions, and hypertension, non-Hispanic whites and non-Hispanic blacks reported less frequently than Hispanics that they had no usual source of care (**Figure 5-10**).
- Difficulties in physical functioning: Native Hawaiians and Pacific Islanders had the largest percentages of adults (age 18 years and older) who had such difficulties (**Figure 5-11**).

- Gonorrhea incidence: During 2010 through 2014, non-Hispanic blacks had the highest incidence of gonorrhea. However, the incidence of gonorrhea among blacks declined during this period, although in 2014 it remained above the incidence for other racial and ethnic groups. In 2014, non-Hispanic blacks had a gonorrhea incidence that was about eleven times greater than that reported for non-Hispanic whites (**Figure 5-12**).

Socioeconomic Status

Socioeconomic status (SES) is defined as a "[d]escriptive term for a person's position in society,..."[6] SES is often formulated as a composite measure of three interrelated dimensions: a person's income level, education level, and type of occupation. In some instances, income level alone is used as an indicator of SES; in other cases, two or more of the foregoing dimensions are combined into composite

FIGURE 5-9 Age-adjusted percentage of adults age 18 years and older with asthma, by race/ethnicity.

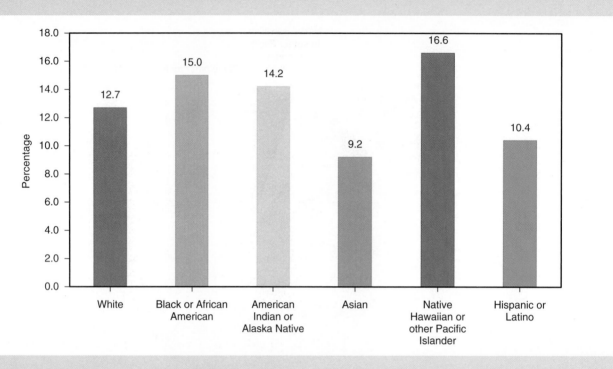

Data from Centers for Disease Control and Prevention. National Center for Health Statistics. *Summary Health Statistics: National Health Interview Survey, 2014*. Table A-2a, 1.

FIGURE 5-10 No usual source of care among adults 45 to 64 years of age, by selected diagnosed chronic conditions and race and Hispanic origin—United States, 2004–2005.

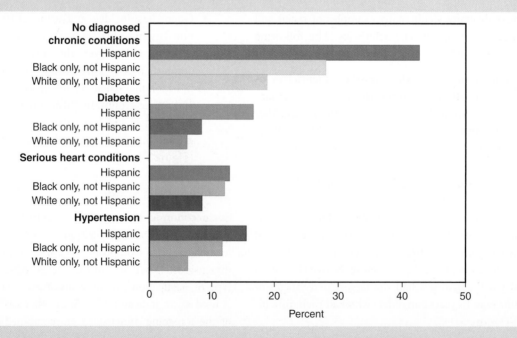

Reprinted from National Center for Health Statistics. *Health, United States, 2007. With chartbook on trends in the health of Americans*. Hyattsville, MD: National Center for Health Statistics; 2007:69.

FIGURE 5-11 Age-adjusted percentages of difficulties in physical functioning among adults age 18 or over, by race—United States, 2014.

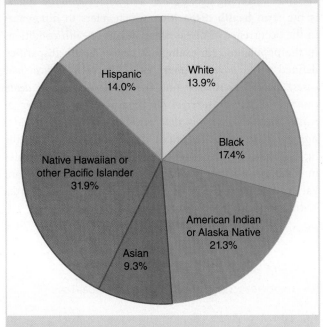

Data from Centers for Disease Control and Prevention. National Center for Health Statistics. *Summary Health Statistics: National Health Interview Survey, 2014*, Table A-10a, 1.

variables. A three-factor measure would classify persons with high SES as those at the upper levels of income, education, and employment status (e.g., the "learned professions"). The social class gradient (variability in SES from high to low and vice versa) is strongly and inversely associated with levels of morbidity and mortality. Those who occupy the lowest SES positions are confronted with excesses of morbidity and mortality from numerous causes (from mental disorders, to chronic and infectious diseases, to the consequences of adverse lifestyles).

One of the dimensions of SES—income—may be expressed in several ways in order to assess its impact on health outcomes. For example, poverty is a measure based on before-tax income from sources such as earnings, unemployment compensation, interest, and Social Security. Poverty exists when a single person or family has an income that is below a threshold set by the U.S. Census Bureau. For a single person younger than age 65 years, the poverty level in 2015 was annual income below the threshold of $12,331. Poverty status also can be computed for families; the poverty level is a function of the total income of a family in relationship to the poverty threshold. The threshold for poverty in a family is determined by summing the poverty thresholds provided by the U.S. Census Bureau for each adult and child living in a family. In 2015,

FIGURE 5-12 Rates of reported cases of gonorrhea, by race/ethnicity—United States, 2010–2014.

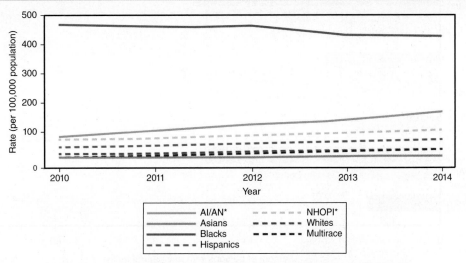

*AI/AN = American Indians/Alaska Natves; NHOPI = Native Hawaiians/other Pacific islanders.
NOTE: Includes 43 states reporting race/ethnicity data in office of Management and Budget compliant formats during 2010-2014.

Reprinted from Centers for Disease Control and Prevention. *Sexually Transmitted Disease Surveillance 2014*. Atlanta, GA: U.S. Department of Health and Human Services; 2015. 23.

the poverty threshold for a five-person family that comprises two adults and three children was $28,286. The ratio of income to poverty is the ratio of an individual's or family's income to their poverty threshold. If the five-person family had an annual income of $29,000 in 2015, their income-to-poverty ratio was $29,000/$28,286 or 1.02; this ratio can also be expressed as 102% of poverty. Similarly, all poverty ratios can also be expressed as percentages; to illustrate, 200% of poverty refers to an income that is twice the poverty threshold.[17]

An example of the association between poverty and health outcomes is provided by access to dental care. Refer to **Figure 5-13**, which presents U.S. data for 2005 for persons who made no dental visits during the past year. The respondents were classified according to four poverty levels. At all age levels, as the percentage of poverty level increased, there was a stepwise decrease in the number of persons who made no dental visits. Among all age groups shown, the largest percentage of persons who made no dental visits was for those below 100% of the poverty level.

Related to the topic of race (as well as other demographic variables including age, gender, and socioeconomic status) is the term **health disparities**, which refers to differences in the occurrence of diseases and adverse health conditions in the population. An example is cancer health disparities, defined as "… *adverse differences in cancer incidence (new cases), cancer prevalence (all existing cases), cancer death (mortality), cancer survivorship, and burden of cancer or related health conditions that exist among specific population groups in the United States.*"[18] Currently, blacks have the highest age-adjusted overall cancer incidence and death rates in comparison with four other racial/ethnic groups (Asian/Pacific Islander, Hispanic/Latino, American Indian/Alaska Native, and white).

FIGURE 5-13 No dental visit in the past year among persons with natural teeth, by age and percentage of poverty level—United States, 2005.

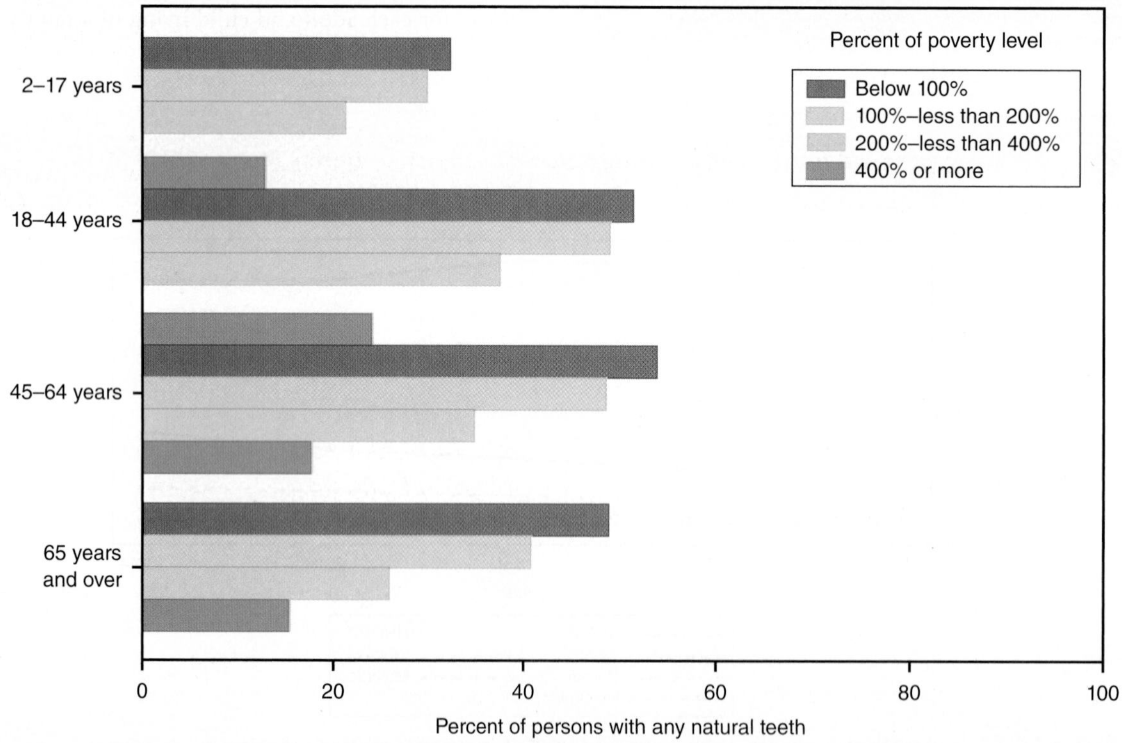

Reprinted from National Center for Health Statistics. *Health, United States, 2007. With chartbook on trends in the health of Americans.* Hyattsville, MD: National Center for Health Statistics; 2007:85.

PLACE VARIABLES

Morbidity and mortality vary greatly with respect to place (geographic regions that are being compared). Some possible comparisons according to place are international, national (within-country variations such as regional and urban-rural comparisons), and localized occurrences of disease.

International

The World Health Organization (WHO), which sponsors and conducts ongoing surveillance research, is the premier source of information about international variations in rates of disease. WHO statistical studies portray international variations in infectious and communicable diseases, malnutrition, infant mortality, suicide, and other conditions. As might be expected, both infectious and chronic diseases show great variation from one country to another. Some of these differences may be attributed to climate, cultural factors, national dietary habits, and access to health care.

Such variations are reflected in great international differences in life expectancy. The U.S. Central Intelligence Agency reported the ranked life expectancy at birth in 2014 for 224 countries.[19] The three countries with the highest life expectancy were Monaco (89.6 years), Macau (technically not a country; 84.5 years), and Japan (84.5 years); the United States ranked 42 (79.6 years). The countries ranked as having the three lowest life expectancies were Guinea-Bissau (49.9 years), South Africa (49.6 years), and Swaziland (49.4 years, the lowest). Life expectancy in many European countries, including Italy, France, and Germany, exceeded that of the United States. The United States' neighboring country, Canada, ranked fourteenth in life expectancy worldwide (81.7 years).

An example of an infectious disease that shows international variations and decreasing incidence is polio, which at one time occurred worldwide. Polio is a viral infection that either is asymptomatic or produces a nonspecific fever in the majority of cases; about 1% of cases produce a type of paralysis known as flaccid paralysis. Immunization programs have helped to eradicate indigenous wild polio cases in the Western Hemisphere, Europe, and many other parts of the world. In 2002, polio was endemic in parts of Africa, Afghanistan, Pakistan, and on the Indian subcontinent. From these endemic areas, polio spread to several African and Middle Eastern countries where the wild polio virus was reestablished. As a result of polio eradication programs, transmission of polio continued only in Afghanistan, Pakistan, India, and Nigeria by 2006. From then until 2011, outbreaks recurred in 39 formerly polio-free countries. Despite these setbacks, since

2011 progress has been made toward eradication of polio. In 2014, polio was eliminated from India. The only remaining countries with endemic polio are Afghanistan, Nigeria, and Pakistan. In 2013, only 407 polio cases were reported worldwide. **Figure 5-14** compares the countries with polio between 1988 and 2014. You can see how the number of countries with endemic polio was reduced dramatically.

National (Within Country)

Many countries, especially large ones, demonstrate within-country variations in disease frequency. Regional differences in factors such as climate, latitude, and environmental pollution affect the prevalence and incidence of diseases. In the United States, comparisons of disease occurrence are made by geographic region (north, east, south, and west), state, or county. An example of state-level variation is the percentage of adults who self-reported a history of stroke. In 2010, the states with the highest percentages included those in the southern United States (e.g., Louisiana and Alabama) and Nevada.[20] The age-adjusted prevalence of stroke in the country was 2.6%. (Refer to **Figure 5-15**.)

Urban-Rural Differences

Urban and rural sections of the United States show variations in morbidity and mortality related to environmental and lifestyle issues. Urban diseases and causes of mortality are more likely to be those spread by person-to-person contact, crowding, and inner-city poverty or associated with urban pollution. Children's lead poisoning is an example of a health issue that occurs among urban residents who may be exposed to lead-based paint from decaying older buildings.

Agriculture is a major category of employment for the residents of rural areas. Farm workers often are exposed to hazards such as toxic pesticides and unintentional injuries caused by farm equipment. **Figure 5-16** shows the distribution of nonfatal occupational farming injuries by state during 1993–1995 (the most recent data available). The highest rate of injuries occurred in Mississippi (14.5 per 100 full-time workers).

One group of employees who are at risk of health hazards associated with farming is migrant workers. Often they reside in crowded, substandard housing that exposes them to infectious agents found in unsanitary milieus. Many of these workers labor under extremely arduous conditions and lack adequate rest breaks, drinking water, and toilet facilities.

Localized Patterns of Disease

Localized patterns of disease are those associated with specific environmental conditions that may exist in a particular geographic area. Illustrations include lung cancer associated

FIGURE 5-14 Countries that never eliminated polio, 1988 versus 2014.

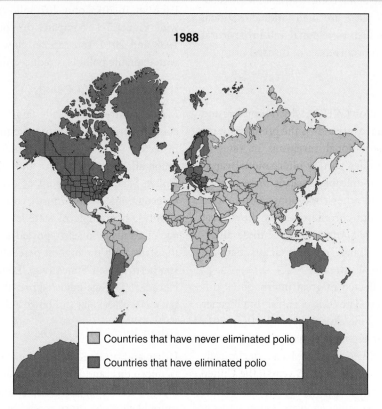

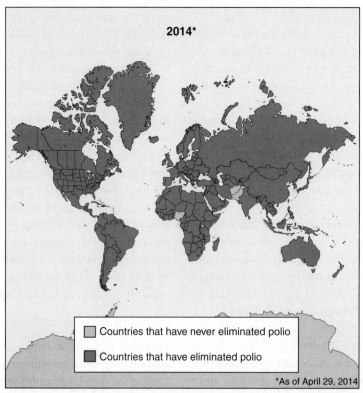

FIGURE 5-15 Age-adjusted prevalence of stroke among noninstitutionalized adults age 18 years or greater, by state—Behavioral Risk Factor Surveillance System, United States, 2010.

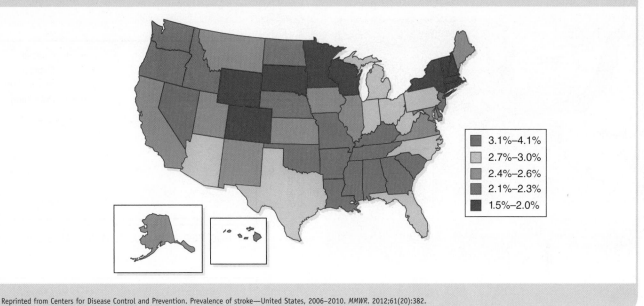

3.1%–4.1%
2.7%–3.0%
2.4%–2.6%
2.1%–2.3%
1.5%–2.0%

Reprinted from Centers for Disease Control and Prevention. Prevalence of stroke—United States, 2006–2010. *MMWR*. 2012;61(20):382.

FIGURE 5-16 Rates of nonfatal occupational farming injuries by state, 1993–1995.

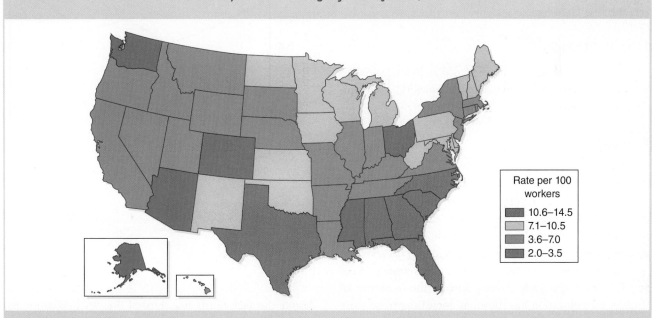

Rate per 100 workers

10.6–14.5
7.1–10.5
3.6–7.0
2.0–3.5

Reprinted from Centers for Disease Control and Prevention, National Institute for Occupational Safety and Health. *Worker Health Chartbook, 2004*. DHHS (NIOSH) Publication No. 2004-146. Cincinnati, OH: National Institute for Occupational Safety and Health; 2004:203.

with radon gas found in some geographic areas and arsenic poisoning linked to high levels of naturally occurring arsenic in the water. Local environmental conditions also may support disease vectors that may not survive in other areas.

(Vectors are intermediaries—insects or animals—involved in the transmission of disease agents.)

An example of a localized pattern of disease is provided by dengue fever, a viral disease transmitted by a species of

FIGURE 5-17 Jurisdictions affected by dengue fever outbreak—Texas-Mexico border, 2005.

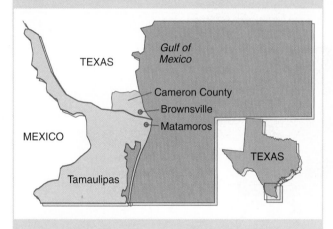

Reprinted from Centers for Disease Control and Prevention. Dengue hemorrhagic fever—U.S.-Mexico border, 2005. *MMWR.* 2007;56:785.

FIGURE 5-18 Age-adjusted suicide rates among people age 10 to 24 years, by sex and mechanism—United States, 1994–2012.

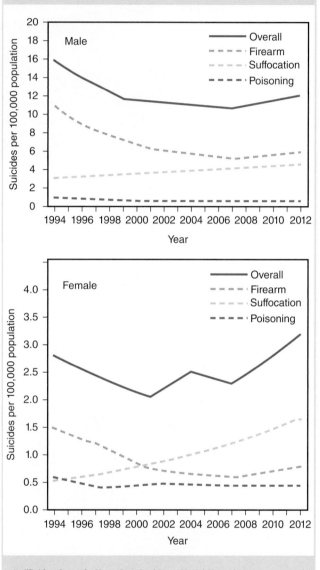

Modified from Centers for Disease Control and Prevention. Suicide trends among persons aged 10–24 years—United States, 1994–2012. *MMWR.* 2016;64(8):203.

mosquito (a vector) that is present along the border that separates Texas from Mexico near the Gulf of Mexico. Localized populations of the mosquitoes are thought to have contributed to an outbreak of dengue fever in 2005. The affected areas are shown in **Figure 5-17**.

TIME VARIABLES

Some types of disease occurrence according to time variables are secular trends, cyclic fluctuation (seasonality), point epidemics, and clustering.

Secular Trends

Secular trends refer to gradual changes in the frequency of diseases or other health-related conditions over long time periods. **Figure 5-18** reports trends in annual suicide rates between 1994 and 2012 among males and females age 10 to 24 years. Over that time period suicide rates were higher among males than among females.[21] Suicides by firearms and by suffocation were the leading mechanisms among males and females, respectively. Among females the frequency of suicides by suffocation has shown an increasing trend since about 1994.

Here is an example of the absence of a secular trend. Hypertension (high blood pressure) is a risk factor for stroke, cardiovascular disease, kidney disease, and other adverse health outcomes. Effective regimens and medications are available for the treatment and control of the condition;

despite this fact, nearly one-third of the U.S. population has hypertension.[22] Among all adults, this level did not change very much (only slight variations in age-adjusted prevalence) between 1999–2000 and 2013–2014 as shown in **Figure 5-19**, which tracks the age-adjusted prevalence of hypertension. On a more optimistic note, more people are bringing their high blood pressure under control.

FIGURE 5-19 Age-adjusted trends in hypertension and controlled hypertension among adults age 18 years and over—United States, 1999–2014.

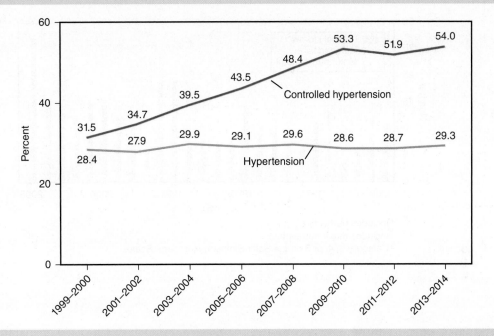

Reprinted from Yoon SS, Fryar CD, Carroll MD. Hypertension prevalence and control among adults: United States, 2011–2014. NCHS Data Brief. 2015; (220):5. Hyattsville, MD: National Center for Health Statistics.

Cyclic (Seasonal) Trends

Many phenomena (e.g., weather and health related) show cyclic trends. What is meant by a cyclic trend? **Cyclic trends** are increases and decreases in the frequency of a disease or other phenomenon over a period of several years or within a year.

Severe weather events in the Atlantic basin of the United States show cyclic trends, demonstrating a high level of seasonal activity since 1995. (Refer to **Figure 5-20**.) The 2005 season when Hurricane Katrina struck was the most active hurricane season on record.

With respect to health-related events, many infectious diseases (for example, pneumonia and influenza) and chronic diseases (for example, coronary heart disease) manifest cyclical patterns of occurrence, with increases and decreases during the year. Mortality from pneumonia and influenza peaks during February, decreases during March and April, and reaches its lowest level during the early summer. Enteroviruses are common viruses that affect human beings globally and are linked to a spectrum of illnesses that range from minor to severe; detections of enterovirus infections have increased in frequency during the summer months within

the past two decades. (See **Figure 5-21**.) Deaths from unintentional injuries (for example, drownings) have seasonal patterns, as do fatal coronary events.

Point Epidemics

A **point epidemic** may indicate the response of a group of people circumscribed in place to a common source of infection, contamination, or other etiologic factor to which they were exposed almost simultaneously.[23] An example was demonstrated by an outbreak of *Vibrio* infections that followed Hurricane Katrina in 2005.

Vibrio is a genus of bacteria that can affect the intestines (producing enteric diseases) and can cause wound infections. One of the illnesses caused by *Vibrio* is cholera (agent: toxigenic *Vibrio cholerae*). Cases of illnesses from toxigenic *V. cholerae* were not identified in the Katrina outbreak. In addition to *V. cholerae*, some other types of *Vibrio* are nontoxigenic *V. cholerae*, *V. parahaemolyticus* (can cause intestinal disorders), and *V. vulnificus* (can cause wound infections). These bacteria can be transmitted through contaminated food and water and by many other mechanisms. During floods, public health

FIGURE 5-20 Number of tropical storms, hurricanes, and major hurricanes, by year—Atlantic Basin, 1980–2005.

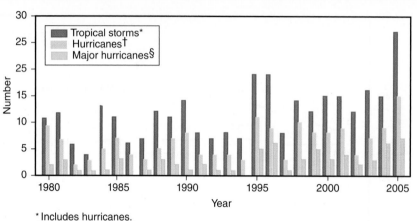

* Includes hurricanes.
† Includes major hurricanes.
§ Category 3, 4, or 5 on the Saffir-Simpson Hurricane Scale.

Reprinted from Centers for Disease Control and Prevention. Public health response to Hurricanes Katrina and Rita—United States, 2005. *MMWR.* 2006;55:231.

FIGURE 5-21 Percentage of enterovirus reports, by month of specimen collection—United States, 1983–2005.

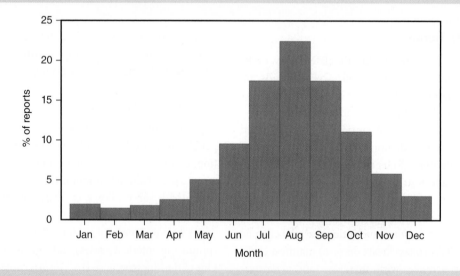

Reprinted from Khetsuriani N, LaMonte-Fowlkes A, Oberste MS, Pallansch MA. Centers for Disease Control and Prevention. Enterovirus surveillance—United States, 1970–2005. In: Surveillance Summaries, September 15, 2006. *MMWR.* 2006;55 (No. SS-8):17.

officials need to monitor the presence of infectious disease agents such as *Vibrio* in the drinking-water supply.

Figure 5-22 shows the distribution of cases of *Vibrio*-associated illnesses after Hurricane Katrina in 2005. The figure demonstrates that 5 people died and 22 people were hospitalized for *Vibrio* illness; these cases occurred among residents of Louisiana and Mississippi. The first hospital admission occurred on August 29 and the last on September 5.

FIGURE 5-22 Cases of post-Hurricane Katrina *Vibrio* illness among residents of Louisiana and Mississippi,* by date of hospital admission—United States, August 29–September 11, 2005.

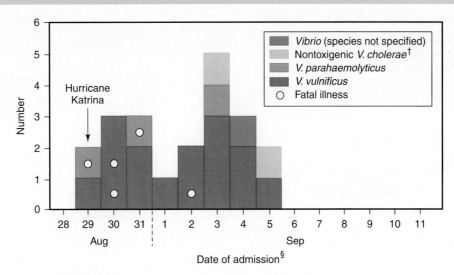

* N = 22; Alabama, a third state under surveillance, reported no cases.
† Nontoxigenic *V. cholerae* illnesses represent infections entirely distinct from the disease cholera, which is caused by toxigenic *V. cholerae* serogroup O1 or O139.
§ Date of admission was not available for one Louisiana resident. In cases that did not require hospitalization, the date represents the first contact with a healthcare provider for the illness.

Reprinted from Centers for Disease Control and Prevention. *Vibrio* illnesses after Hurricane Katrina—multiple states, August–September 2005. *MMWR.* 2005;54:928.

The frequency of cases peaked on September 3. Most of these cases were wound associated and are believed to have been the result of an infection acquired by contact with floodwaters.

Clustering

An example of a pattern derived from descriptive studies is disease **clustering**, which refers to "[a] closely grouped series of events or cases of a disease or other health-related phenomena with well-defined distribution patterns in relation to time or place or both. The term is normally used to describe aggregation of relatively uncommon events or diseases (e.g., leukemia, multiple sclerosis)."[6] Clustering may suggest common exposure of the population to an environmental hazard; it also may be purely spurious—due to the operation of chance. One cause of spurious clustering is called the Texas sharpshooter effect (see box).

Clustering can refer to spatial clustering and temporal clustering. **Spatial clustering** indicates cases of disease (often uncommon diseases) that occur in a specific geographic region, a common example being a cancer cluster. **Temporal** **clustering** denotes health events that are related in time, such as the development of maternal postpartum depression a few days after a mother gives birth. Another example of temporal clustering is postvaccination reactions such as syncope (fainting); the number of such reactions increased among females age 11 to 18 years during 2007. (Refer to **Figure 5-23**.)

Texas sharpshooter effect

A traveler passing through a small town in Texas noted a remarkable display of sharpshooting. On almost every barn he passed there was a target with a single bullet hole that uncannily passed through the center of the bull's-eye. He was so intrigued by this that he stopped at a nearby gas station to ask about the sharpshooter. With a chuckle, the attendant told him that the shooting was the work of Old Joe. Old Joe would first shoot at the side of a barn and then paint targets centered over his bullet holes so that each shot appeared to

FIGURE 5-23 Number of postvaccination syncope* episodes reported to the Vaccine Adverse Event Reporting System, by month and year of report—United States, January 1, 2004–July 31, 2007.

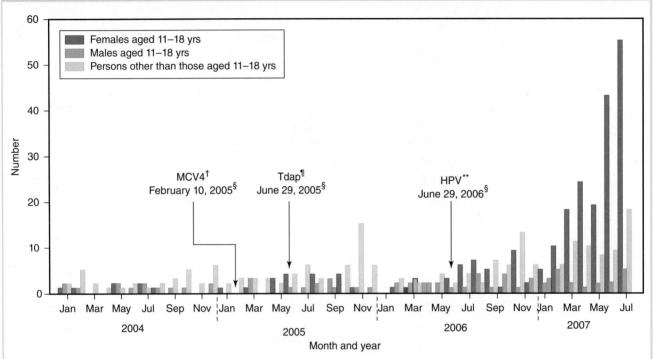

* Includes persons aged ≥ 5 years who had syncope onset after vaccination on the same date.
† Meningococcal conjugate vaccine.
§ Date on which the Advisory Committee on Immunization Practices decided to add this newly licensed adolescent vaccine to the Vaccines for Children Program.
¶ Tetanus toxoid, reduced diphtheria toxoid, and acellular pertussis vaccine.
** Quadrivalent human papillomavirus recombinant vaccine. HPV vaccine is licensed only for females.

Reprinted from Centers for Disease Control and Prevention. Syncope after vaccination—United States, January 2005–July 2007. *MMWR.* 2008;57:458.

pass through the center of the target.... In a random distribution of cases of cancer over a geographic area, some cases will appear to occur very close together just on the basis of random variation. The occurrence of a group of cases of a disease close together in time and place at the time of their diagnosis is called a cluster.

Reprinted from Grufferman S. Methodologic approaches to studying environmental factors in childhood cancer. *Environ Health Perspect.* 1998;106(Suppl. 3):882.

CONCLUSION

Descriptive epidemiology classifies the occurrence of disease according to the variables of person, place, and time. Descriptive epidemiologic studies aid in generating

hypotheses that can be explored by analytic epidemiologic studies. Another use of descriptive epidemiology is to prioritize adverse health outcomes for interventions. This chapter presented information on several types of descriptive studies including case reports, case series, and cross-sectional studies. The Behavioral Risk Factor Surveillance System (BRFSS) is an example of an ongoing cross-sectional study of health characteristics of the population of the United States. Person variables discussed in the chapter were age, sex, race/ethnicity, and socioeconomic status. Place variables included the following types of comparisons: international, national (within country), urban-rural, and localized patterns. Time variables encompassed secular time trends, cyclic trends, point epidemics, and clustering. Descriptive epidemiology is an important component of the process of epidemiologic inference.

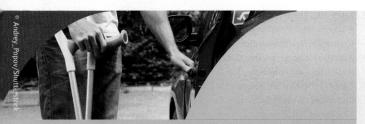

Study Questions and Exercises

1. Refer back to Table 5-2, which presents characteristics of infants who were exclusively breastfed. Describe the results shown in the table. Suppose you wanted to conduct a survey of breastfeeding in your own community:
   a. How would you choose the participants?
   b. What questionnaire items would you include in the survey?
   c. What type of study design is a survey?

2. State three uses for descriptive epidemiologic studies. How could descriptive epidemiologic studies examine the following health issues?
   a. The obesity epidemic in the United States
   b. Increases in the prevalence of type 2 diabetes among adolescents
   c. Abuse of prescription narcotic drugs

3. Define the terms *case reports* and *case series*. Indicate how they are similar and how they differ. Search the Internet for examples of case reports and case series of disease.

4. Refer back to Table 5-3, which gives the percentage of adults who reported insufficient sleep. Provide a detailed account of the findings presented in the table. What additional information would you like to have in order to determine the reasons why people have insufficient sleep?

5. Refer back to the section on sex differences. How did the top five types of invasive cancer differ in incidence between males and females? Can you hypothesize reasons for these differences?

6. What are some examples of racial/ethnic classifications used to describe health characteristics? Name two conditions that vary according to race/ethnicity.

7. What is meant by the term *health disparities*? What do you think could be done about them from the societal and public health points of view?

8. How does life expectancy at birth in the United States compare with that in other countries? Do you have any suggestions for improving life expectancy in the United States? What could be done to raise the life expectancies of residents in the countries that have the three lowest levels?

9. Name three characteristics of time that are used in descriptive epidemiologic studies and give an example of each one.

10. The prevalence of hypertension has remained essentially unchanged for nearly a decade. Propose a descriptive epidemiologic study to explore the reasons for this phenomenon.

Young Epidemiology Scholars (YES) Exercises

The Young Epidemiology Scholars: Competitions website provides links to teaching units and exercises that support instruction in epidemiology. The YES program, discontinued in 2011, was administered by the College Board and supported by the Robert Wood Johnson Foundation. The exercises continue to be available at the following website: http://yes-competition.org/yes/teaching-units/title.html. The following exercises relate to topics discussed in this chapter and can be found on the YES competitions website.

1. Kaelin MA, St. George DMM. Descriptive Epidemiology of Births to Teenage Mothers.
2. Olsen C, St. George DMM. Cross-Sectional Study Design and Data Analysis.

REFERENCES

1. Friis RH, Sellers TA. *Epidemiology for Public Health Practice*. 5th ed. Burlington, MA: Jones & Bartlett Learning; 2014.

2. Centers for Disease Control and Prevention. Breastfeeding among U.S. children born 2002–2012, CDC National Immunization Surveys. Available at: http://www.cdc.gov/breastfeeding/data/nis_data/rates-any -exclusive-bf-socio-dem-2012.htm. Accessed August 8, 2016.

3. Centers for Disease Control and Prevention. Acute renal failure associated with cosmetic soft-tissue filler injections—North Carolina, 2007. *MMWR*. 2008;57:453–456.

4. Sinclair JR, Wallace RM, Gruszynski K, et al. Rabies in a dog imported from Egypt with a falsified rabies vaccination certificate—Virginia, 2015. *MMWR*. 2015;64(49):1359–1362.

5. Centers for Disease Control and Prevention. Primary amebic meningoencephalitis—Arizona, Florida, and Texas, 2007. *MMWR*. 2008;57:573–577.

6. Porta M, ed. *A Dictionary of Epidemiology*. 6th ed. New York, NY: Oxford University Press; 2014.

7. Centers for Disease Control and Prevention. Prevalence of healthy sleep duration among adults—United States, 2014. *MMWR*. 2016;65(6):137–141.

8. Xu JQ, Murphy SL, Kochanek KD, Bastian BA. Deaths: final data for 2013. *National Vital Statistics Reports*. 2016;64(2). Hyattsville, MD: National Center for Health Statistics.

9. Centers for Disease Control and Prevention. Invasive cancer incidence and survival—United States, 2012. *MMWR*. 2015;64(49):1353–1358.

10. Martin JA, Hamilton BE, Sutton PD, et al. Births: final data for 2004. *National Vital Statistics Reports*. 2006;55(1). Hyattsville, MD: National Center for Health Statistics.

11. Hamilton BE, Martin JA, Osterman MJK, et al. Births: final data for 2014. *National Vital Statistics Reports*. 2015;64(12). Hyattsville, MD: National Center for Health Statistics. Supplemental tables. Available at: http://www.cdc.gov/nchs/data/nvsr/64/nvsr64_12tables.pdf. Accessed July 25, 2016.

12. Kung HC, Hoyert DL, Xu JQ, Murphy SL. Deaths: final data for 2005. *National Vital Statistics Reports*. 2008;56(10). Hyattsville, MD: National Center for Health Statistics.

13. American Cancer Society. *Cancer Facts and Figures 2016*. Atlanta, GA: American Cancer Society; 2016.

14. Fine MJ, Ibrahim SA, Thomas SB. The role of race and genetics in health disparities research (editorial). *Am J Public Health*. 2005;95:2125–2128.

15. McKenney NR, Bennett CE. Issues regarding data on race and ethnicity: the Census Bureau experience. *Pub Health Rep*. 1994;109:16–25.

16. Krieger N. Counting accountably: implications of the new approaches to classifying race/ethnicity in the 2000 census (editorial). *Am J Public Health*. 2000;90:1687–1689.

17. U.S. Census Bureau. Poverty: How the Census Bureau measures poverty. Available at: https://www.census.gov/topicsincome-poverty/poverty /guidance/poverty-measures.html. Accessed July 25, 2016.

18. National Cancer Institute. Factsheet: Cancer health disparities: questions and answers. Available at: http://www.cancer.gov/about-nci /organization/crchd/cancer-health-disparities-fact-sheet. Accessed July 25, 2016.

19. Central Intelligence Agency. Rank order—country comparison: life expectancy at birth. *The World Factbook*; 2016. Available at: https://www. cia.gov/library/publications/the-world-factbook/rankorder/2102rank. html. Accessed July 30, 2016.

20. Centers for Disease Control and Prevention. Prevalence of stroke—United States, 2006–2010. *MMWR*. 2012;61(20):379–382.

21. Centers for Disease Control and Prevention. Suicide trends among persons aged 10–24 years—United States, 1994–2012. *MMWR*. 2016;64(8):201–205.

22. Yoon SS, Fryar CD, Carroll MD. Hypertension prevalence and control among adults: United States, 2011–2014. *NCHS Data Brief*. 2015; (220). Hyattsville, MD: National Center for Health Statistics.

23. MacMahon B, Pugh TF. *Epidemiology Principles and Methods*. Boston, MA: Little, Brown; 1970.

CHAPTER **6**

Association and Causality

LEARNING OBJECTIVES

By the end of this chapter you will be able to:

- Describe the history of changing concepts of disease causality.
- Compare and contrast noncausal and causal associations.
- Distinguish between deterministic and stochastic models of causality.
- Name at least three of the criteria of causality, giving examples of each one.
- State one example of how chance affects associations among variables.

CHAPTER OUTLINE

INTRODUCTION

One often encounters articles in the popular media about the latest findings of epidemiologic research. Many of these engaging stories pertain to dietary issues. An example is the role of chemicals in food (particularly "nonorganic" foods) in causing cancer. Another popular topic is how taking nutritional supplements can improve your health—keep your eyesight keen, prevent heart attacks, help your joints to move more smoothly, etc. Or, a pronouncement declares that drinking coffee is bad for your health, while it is permissible (and even desirable) to consume alcohol in moderation. These statements are often taken from the findings of epidemiologic studies.

This chapter will launch an in-depth discussion of analytic epidemiology by presenting concepts related to association and causality. You should keep in mind that one of the goals of analytic epidemiology (using epidemiology to study the etiology of diseases) is to determine potential causal associations between exposures and health outcomes. As part of studying about the etiology of diseases, epidemiologists infer causal associations regarding exposure factors and diseases. Remember that the author distinguished between analytic epidemiology and descriptive epidemiology (using epidemiologic methods to describe the occurrence of diseases in the population). You will learn the background information needed to assert that associations between exposures and disease found in research are causal, for example, the assertion that smoking causes lung cancer. This information includes applying the criteria for assessing causality and taking into account factors that can affect the validity of observed associations. This chapter will enable you to take a critical look at research and evaluate findings that become translated into media articles. Refer to **Table 6-1** for an overview of terms covered in this chapter.

TABLE 6-1 List of Important Terms Used in This Chapter

History of Disease Causation	Associations among Variables	Causality	Assessing the Operation of Chance
Contagion	Association	Criteria of causality	Clinically significant
Environmental influences	Causal association	Deterministic model	Confidence interval estimate
Germ theory	Direct association	Multivariate	Inference
Miasma	Exposure	(multifactorial, multiple)	p-value
Spontaneous generation	Hypothesis	causality	Parameter
Witchcraft	Indirect association	Exposure	Point estimate
Wrath of the gods	Method of difference	Necessary cause	Power
	Method of concomitant variation	Operationalization	Sample
	Noncausal association	Stochastic process	Statistic
	Null hypothesis	Sufficient cause	Statistical significance
	Operationalization	Sufficient component	parameter
	Statistically independent	cause model	Statistic
	Statistically independent		
	Theories		

DISEASE CAUSALITY IN HISTORY

In classical times, people were mystified about the causes of disease. Can you imagine how frightening it was to live in a time when epidemics periodically swept over cities leaving a high body count in their paths? The earliest accounts of epidemics attributed them to magical explanations. Eventually, environmental factors became more widely recognized as possible causes for disease outbreaks. Later, miasma theories gained acceptance and held sway for several centuries. Finally, the germ theory of disease took hold and became the predecessor of contemporary theories of disease transmission. **Table 6-2** gives an overview of the history of disease causality.

Witchcraft, Demons, and Gods

In early history, supernatural or magical explanations such as **witchcraft** were used to account for transmission of infectious diseases.[1] For example, the ancients attributed devastating epidemics to the **wrath of the gods**; some believed that disease outbreaks were a punishment by the gods for people's sins. Others attributed diseases to demons and evil spirits, which could be removed by exorcism. Still others thought that comets and earthquakes caused epidemics.

Environmental Influences

Among a group of classical philosophers, the focus shifted from the supernatural to the influence of environmental factors, and environmental factors gained transcendence in theories of the causes of disease. In his influential writings, the Greek philosopher Hippocrates argued that **environmental influences** such as climate, geographic location, and water quality were associated with diseases. For example, during certain times of the year, one might contract malaria from contact with low-lying marshy areas—a thesis that was linked to the environment and not supernatural forces.

TABLE 6-2 Causes of Disease from a Historical Perspective

Supernatural Explanations (Examples)		Early Scientific Explanations		Germ Theory of Disease
Witchcraft	Comets	The environment	Spontaneous generation	Louis Pasteur's discoveries
Wrath of the gods	Earthquakes	Miasmas	Contagion	Robert Koch's postulates

Theory of Contagion

The 16th-century poet, physician, and mathematician Girolamo Fracastoro (1478–1553) expounded the theory of contagion for the spread of infections. The theory of **contagion** proposed "… that infections are caused by transferable seed-like beings, seminaria or germs, which could cause infection."[1(p59)] The modes for transmitting disease could include direct contact, indirect contact, and airborne transmission; these modes are aligned remarkably with modern knowledge.

Miasmas

During the Middle Ages, the miasma theory of disease came into fashion and persisted for centuries into the 1800s.[2] According to this theory, a **miasma** was an airborne toxic vapor composed of malodorous particles from decomposing fetid materials. **Figure 6-1** communicates the notion of a miasma that contaminated soldiers on the battlefield and caused them to become ill with cholera.

This theory of miasmas was consistent with the view of 18th century social reformers who observed that epidemics often were concentrated in the unhygienic and economically depressed neighborhoods in England. Often these densely packed urban areas had poorly ventilated homes, were filthy, and were sullied by pools of sewage, rotting carcasses of animals, and mounds of decaying garbage. "Early Victorian Britain, as every good schoolchild knows, was filthy, or parts of it were. While the hearth and home of the middle classes, that great site of 'bourgeois domesticity' were kept scrupulously clean, the urban industrial slums of the working classses overflowed with filth, especially human excrement."[3] The famous English social reformer and sanitarian Edwin Chadwick (1800–1890) advocated for improving environmental health by increasing drainage to eliminate stagnant pools and increasing ventilation in homes.

The miasma theory of disease also held sway in accounting for cholera epidemics in London during the mid-1800s.[4] However, John Snow (the "father of epidemiology") departed from the orthodoxy of his time by alleging that cholera was a waterborne disease. Snow investigated a deadly cholera outbreak that occurred London in 1849. In line with Snow's view was the illustration in **Figure 6-2**, which highlights the frightening organisms that might be

FIGURE 6-1 Cholera tramples the victors and the vanquished both.

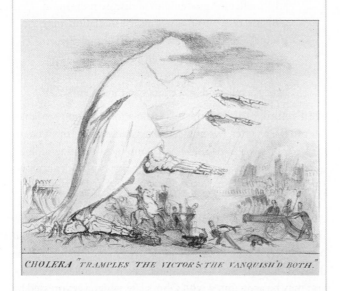

FIGURE 6-2 A microscopic view of a drop of water from the Thames River (London, England).

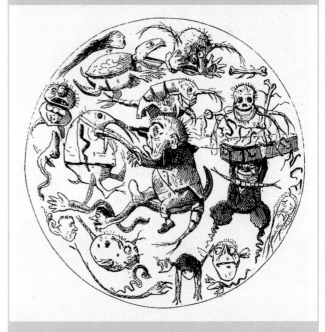

found in a microscopic view of a drop of Thames water. *Punch* magazine published this illustration in 1850.

Spontaneous Generation

The theory of **spontaneous generation** postulated that simple life forms such as microorganisms, insects, and small animals could arise spontaneously from nonliving materials. For example, it had been observed that maggots seem to be produced by decaying meat and mice arose from grain. The creation of both maggots and mice was attributed to spontaneous generation of life forms.

Germ Theory of Disease

Louis Pasteur and Robert Koch are examples of scientists who advanced the **germ theory of disease**, which linked microorganisms to the causation of disease. With the germ theory of disease, the French chemist Louis Pasteur (1822–1895) was able to debunk the theory of spontaneous generation. In his laboratory, shown in **Figure 6-3**, he was able to demonstrate that microbes could grow in a flask that contained nutrients.

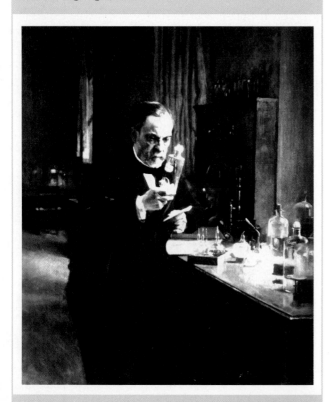

FIGURE 6-3 Pasteur, standing in his laboratory examining a glass bottle, 1885.

Reproduced from U.S. National Library of Medicine. NLM Image ID: B020592 Available at: http://resource.nlm.nih.gov/101425977. Accessed August 13, 2016.

Pasteur observed that microorganisms present in the air would grow when they came into contact with the culture medium but would not grow when they were prevented from reaching the nutrients in the flask. Another scientist who fostered the germ theory was the German scientist Robert Koch (1843–1910), who developed four postulates (Koch's postulates) for the transmission of bacterial diseases such as tuberculosis.

DETERMINISTIC AND PROBABILISTIC CAUSALITY IN EPIDEMIOLOGY

One of the ongoing concerns of epidemiology is to be able to assert that a causal association exists between an exposure factor and a disease (or other adverse health outcome) in the host. The word **association** refers to a linkage between or among variables. The term **exposure** denotes contact with factors that usually may be linked to adverse outcomes such as specific forms of morbidity and mortality. The issue of causality in epidemiologic studies is complex. The term *cause* has been defined a number of different ways in epidemiology. Causal inference in epidemiology has underpinnings in the history of philosophy. In their classic epidemiology textbook, MacMahon and Pugh stated:

> [T]he word *cause* is an abstract noun and, like *beauty*, will have different meanings in different contexts. No definition will be equally appropriate to all branches of science. Epidemiology has the practical purpose of discovering relations which offer the possibilities of disease prevention and for this purpose a causal association may usefully be defined as an association between categories of events or categories in which an alteration in the frequency or quality of one category is followed by a change in the other.[5(pp17–18)]

We'll return to the matter of associations among variables later in the chapter. For now, let's examine some of the types of causal frameworks that have been employed in epidemiology. **Table 6-3** presents examples of two major types of causality.

Deterministic Causality

A **deterministic model** (from the philosophy of **determinism**) of causality claims that a cause is invariably followed by an effect. Some examples of deterministic models can be derived from physics.[6] If you have taken a course in physics, you may be acquainted with Ohm's law, which is expressed by the following formula: ($I = V/R$). In this formula, the flow of current (I) is a function of the voltage (V) applied to a conductor divided by the resistance (R) of the conductor. If V is doubled, then I will double.

TABLE 6-3 Two Types of Causality with Examples	
Type of Causality	Example
Deterministic causality	Necessary and sufficient causes Sufficient-component causes
Probabilistic causality	Stochastic causes

How is this discussion relevant to epidemiology? Deterministic models have been applied to the etiology of diseases. In the epidemiologic context, a cause (independent variable) is often an exposure, and an effect is a health outcome (dependent variable). According to deterministic models of disease, the causes can be classified as to whether they are necessary or sufficient. A **necessary cause** is "[a] factor whose presence is required for the occurrence of the effect."[7] A **sufficient cause** is a cause that is sufficient by itself to produce the effect.

The concept of a necessary cause of a disease shares a common heritage with the discoveries of Pasteur and Koch, who both argued that infectious diseases have a single necessary cause, for example, a microbial agent.[8] Refer to **Figure 6-4** for an illustration of combinations

of necessary and sufficient causes. Given that we have variable X (a cause, e.g., exposure) and Y (an effect, e.g., health outcome), the four combinations of necessary and sufficient are the following:

- Necessary and sufficient
  - Definition: "Both X and Y are always present together, and nothing but X is needed to cause Y…"[9(p46)]
  - Example: This is an uncommon situation in epidemiology and one that is difficult to demonstrate.
- Sufficient but not necessary
  - Definition: "X may or may not be present when Y is present, because Y has other causes and can occur without X."[9(p46)] In other words, X is one of the causes of the disease, but there are other causes.
  - Example: Workers who have levels of exposures to a carcinogenic (cancer-causing) chemical can develop cancer. However, excessive exposure to radiation from a nuclear electric generating plant can also induce cancer.
- Necessary but not sufficient
  - Definition: "X must be present when Y is present, but Y is not always present when X is."[9(p46)] This formulation means that X is necessary for causation of Y, but X by itself does not cause Y.
  - Example: Consider seasonal influenza. The influenza virus is a necessary requirement for a flu infection; the flu virus will have interacted with people who develop an active case of the flu. Nevertheless, not everyone who is exposed to the virus will develop the flu; the reason is that development of an infection is influenced by one's general health status, the manner of one's exposure, and other factors such as one's immunity. Tuberculosis is another example of disease in which the agent (TB bacteria) is a necessary but not a sufficient cause of infection.
- Neither necessary nor sufficient
  - Definition: "… X may or may not be present when Y is present. Under these conditions, however, if X is present with Y, some additional factor must be present. Here X is a contributory cause of Y."[9(p46)]
  - Example: This form of causality is most applicable to chronic diseases (e.g., coronary heart disease) that have multiple contributing causes, none of which causes the disease by itself.

Sufficient-Component Cause Model

Epidemiologist Kenneth Rothman expounded on the **sufficient-component cause model**, also known as the *causal*

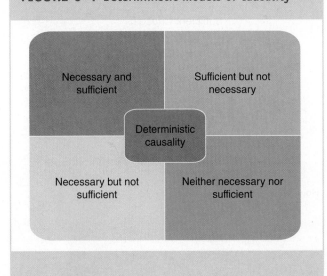

FIGURE 6-4 Deterministic models of causality

Necessary and sufficient

Sufficient but not necessary

Deterministic causality

Necessary but not sufficient

Neither necessary nor sufficient

pie model.[10] As the name implies, this model is constituted from a group of component causes, which can be diagrammed as a pie. One of the component causes in the pie is a necessary cause; the remaining component causes are not necessary causes. Together, the group of component causes makes up a sufficient cause complex. Recall in the previous section the combination labeled a necessary but not sufficient cause. According to the sufficient-component cause model, this necessary cause is accompanied by an additional set of component causes. The necessary cause in conjunction with the component causes forms a sufficient cause complex. Rothman indicated that, hypothetically speaking, more than one sufficient cause complex can be implicated in the etiology of a disease. However, for a particular disease (for example, an infectious disease) the necessary cause must be present in every causal complex. This somewhat confusing statement will become clearer when you consider an example.

Sufficient-component cause models are mapped in **Figure 6-5**, which uses the example of tuberculosis (TB). The causal bacterium for tuberculosis is the tubercle bacillus, which is a necessary cause of TB. This means that in order for one to develop tuberculosis, one must become infected with the bacterium. However, exposure to the tubercle bacillus is not a sufficient cause for contracting tuberculosis. A number of component causes (such as personal and environmental factors) operate in addition to exposure to the bacillus in order to cause TB; these additional component causes are not necessary causes. Figure 6-5 illustrates two hypothetical component cause complexes for TB. You can observe in the figure that for a person to develop TB, the bacterium is a necessary condition. One component cause complex might include crowding, sanitation, nutrition, and immune status. Another complex might include infection with HIV and homelessness. Exposure to the tubercle bacillus would be a necessary component of both complexes.

Probability Models and Probabilistic (Stochastic) Causality

Probability (probabilistic) models are the second major group of models used to describe disease etiology.[6] Another name for a probabilistic model is a stochastic model. A **stochastic process** is one "… that incorporates some element of randomness."[7] Probabilistic causation describes the probability of an effect (e.g., adverse health outcome) in mathematical terms,[11] given a particular dose (level of exposure). According to stochastic modeling, a cause is associated with the increased probability that an effect will happen. An example of stochastic causation applies to radiation exposure and carcinogenesis. Exposure to radiation from radioactive nuclear materials is related to the probability that the exposed person will develop radiation-induced cancer. Greater amounts of

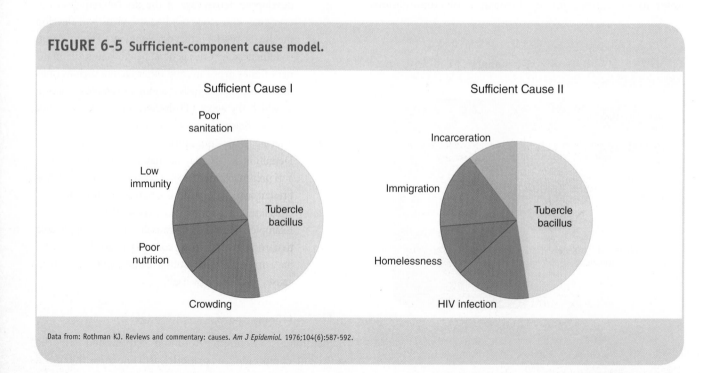

FIGURE 6-5 Sufficient-component cause model.

Sufficient Cause I

Poor sanitation
Low immunity
Poor nutrition
Crowding
Tubercle bacillus

Sufficient Cause II

Incarceration
Immigration
Homelessness
HIV infection
Tubercle bacillus

Data from: Rothman KJ. Reviews and commentary: causes. *Am J Epidemiol.* 1976;104(6):587-592.

exposure increase the probability of cancer induction. Phenomena such as carcinogenesis (and the etiology of many chronic diseases) are among the most interesting to epidemiologists. However, research has demonstrated that these conditions are not as predictable as specified by deterministic models. Hence, probabilistic causal models have gained favor among some epidemiologists who are investigating the etiology of chronic diseases.

EPIDEMIOLOGIC RESEARCH AND THE SEARCH FOR ASSOCIATIONS

One of the most important uses of epidemiology is to search for the etiology of diseases. The overriding question that epidemiologists ask is whether a particular exposure is causally associated with a given outcome. Esteemed epidemiologists, Brian MacMahon and Thomas Pugh, wrote, "In epidemiology, as in other sciences, progress in this search results from a series of cycles in which investigators (1) examine existing facts and hypotheses, (2) formulate a new or more specific hypothesis, and (3) obtain additional facts to test the acceptability of the new hypothesis. A fresh cycle then commences, the new facts, and possibly the new hypothesis, being added to the available knowledge."[5(p29)] An illustration of the cycle of epidemiologic research is shown in **Figure 6-6**.

Here is an explanation of the terms used in the figure. Epidemiologic research is guided by theories and explanatory models. In epidemiology, **theories** are general accounts of causal relationships between exposures and outcomes. There is a close connection between theories and explanatory models; an example of an explanatory model is the web of causation discussed later in the chapter. As new information is gathered in epidemiologic studies, theories and models need to be modified to take account of these new data.

Epidemiologic research studies are initiated with research questions, which are linked to the development of hypotheses. A **hypothesis** is defined as "[a]ny conjecture cast in a form that will allow it to be tested and, possibly, refuted."[7] One of the most commonly used hypotheses in research is called a negative declaration, or null hypothesis. A **null hypothesis** is a hypothesis of no difference in a population parameter among the groups being compared. For example, suppose an investigator wanted to study the association between smoking and lung cancer. The investigator could hypothesize that there is no difference in occurrence of lung cancer between smokers and nonsmokers. If an epidemiologic study found that there was a difference, then the null hypothesis would be rejected. Otherwise, the null hypothesis would fail to be rejected.

You might raise the question, "Where do hypotheses come from?" John Stuart Mill, in his writings on inductive reasoning, defined several methods for deriving hypotheses. These include the method of difference and the method of concomitant variation. The **method of difference** refers to a situation in which all of the factors in two or more domains are the same except for a single factor. The frequency of a disease that varies across the two settings is hypothesized to result from variation in a single causative factor. The method of difference is similar to a classic experimental design that in epidemiology is illustrated by clinical trials used to evaluate new medications and clinical procedures.

What is the linkage between the method of difference and hypotheses? An astute epidemiologist might observe that rates of coronary heart disease vary between sedentary and nonsedentary workers in a factory; he or she might hypothesize that the differences in coronary heart disease rates are due to differences in physical activity levels.

The **method of concomitant variation** refers to a type of association in which the frequency of an outcome increases with the frequency of exposure to a factor. One might hypothesize that this factor is associated with that outcome. An example from epidemiologic research is the dose-response relationship between the number of cigarettes smoked and mortality from lung cancer: The greater the number of cigarettes smoked, the higher the mortality levels from lung cancer.

Two additional terms shown in Figure 6-6 are *variables* and *operationalization*. Following the identification

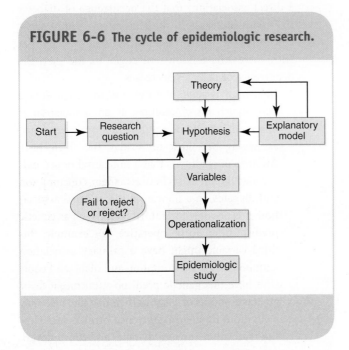

FIGURE 6-6 The cycle of epidemiologic research.

of hypotheses, the researcher needs to specify the variables that will be appropriate for the research project. In a previous chapter, the term *variable* was defined as "[a]ny quantity that can have different values across individuals or other study units."[7] After these variables have been specified, the measures to be used need to be identified. **Operationalization** refers to the process of defining measurement procedures for the variables used in a study. For example, in a study of the association between tobacco use and lung disease, the variables might be designated as number of cigarettes smoked and occurrence of asthma. The operationalization of these two variables might require a questionnaire to measure the amount of smoking and a review of the medical records to search for diagnoses of asthma. Using measures of association, the researcher could determine how strongly smoking is related to asthma. On the basis of the findings of the study, the researcher could obtain information that would help to update hypotheses, theories, and explanatory models, or that could be used for public health interventions.

TYPES OF ASSOCIATIONS FOUND AMONG VARIABLES

Previously, the author stated that one of the concerns of analytic epidemiology is to examine associations among exposure variables and health outcome variables. Variables that are associated with one another can be positively or negatively related. In a positive association, as the value of one variable increases so does the value of the other variable. In a negative (inverse) association, when the value of one variable increases, the value of the other variable decreases.

Let's refer generically to variable X (exposure factor) and variable Y (outcome). Consult **Figure 6-7** for an illustration of relationships between X and Y. Here are some possible relationships between X and Y:

- No association (X is unrelated to Y.)
- Associated (X is related to Y.)
  - **Noncausal** (X does not cause Y.)
  - **Causal** (X causes Y.)
    - Direct
    - Indirect

Take the hypothetical example of non–insulin-dependent (type 2) diabetes, which appears to be occurring at earlier and earlier ages in the United States. Suppose that in a hypothetical situation an epidemiologist wanted to study whether dietary consumption of sugar (exposure variable) is related to diabetes (health outcome). There are several possible types of

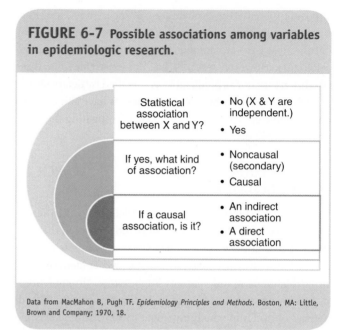

FIGURE 6-7 Possible associations among variables in epidemiologic research.

Data from MacMahon B, Pugh TF. *Epidemiology Principles and Methods*. Boston, MA: Little, Brown and Company; 1970, 18.

associations between these two variables (i.e., high levels of sugar consumption and diabetes).

- *No association between dietary sugar and diabetes.* The term "no association" means that the occurrence of diabetes is **statistically independent** of the amount of sugar consumed in the diet.
- *Dietary sugar intake and diabetes are associated.* A positive association would indicate (in the example of a direct association) that the occurrence of diabetes rises with increases in the amount of dietary sugar consumed. A negative association would show that with increasing amounts of sugar in the diet, the occurrence of diabetes decreases.
  - *Noncausal association between dietary sugar intake and occurrence of diabetes.* If an association is observed, it could be a purely random event (such as having bad luck on Friday the thirteenth). Another possibility is that a noncausal or secondary association exists between sugar consumption and diabetes. In a noncausal (secondary) association, it is possible for a third factor such as genetic predisposition to be operative. For example, this third variable might have a primary association with both sugar consumption and diabetes. People who have this genetic predisposition might favor greater amounts of sugar in their diet and also may have more frequent occurrence of diabetes. Thus the association between diabetes and consumption

Polio and "Spongy Tar"

Polio is a disease that can cause devastating paralysis in a small percentage of cases. Before virologists determined that the poliovirus was the cause of polio, some researchers alleged that polio was caused by exposure to spongy tar. The evidence for this assertion was an increase in the number of children's polio infections when the tar in playgrounds became spongy. In some areas, the tar in children's playgrounds was removed in order to prevent polio. Later, researchers discovered that polio infections increased when the weather became hotter; at the same time the tar in playgrounds softened during heat spells. Consequently, the relationship between polio and spongy tar was spurious and noncausal.

Data from *The Los Angeles Times*, October 11, 2015. Editorial: The misuse of research.

of a diet that is high in sugar is secondary to one's genetic predisposition and is a **noncausal association**. Refer to the above text box for another example of a noncausal association.

○ *Causal association between dietary intake of sugar and diabetes.* One form of relationship between these two variables might be an **indirect causal association**. As an example, excessive sugar consumption might be related to obesity, which in turn is related to diabetes. Thus obesity is an intermediate step between sugar consumption and diabetes. Another possibility is a direct association between the two factors. A **direct causal association** would mean that consumption of large amounts of sugar is directly related to the occurrence of diabetes, without the involvement of an intermediate step.

The foregoing examples demonstrate possible associations among exposures and health outcomes. Next, we need to take into account the framework for asserting that a causal relationship exists between factor X and factor Y. Before a causal association can be assumed, several criteria for causal relationships need to be evaluated and the associations need to be examined for possible errors.

THE CRITERIA OF CAUSALITY

In order for there to be a **causal association** between an exposure and a health outcome, several criteria, known as the **criteria of causality**, must be substantiated. Suppose that an epidemiologist has demonstrated an association between watching television commercials and binge drinking. As noted previously, an association can be either noncausal or causal. If noncausal, the association could be merely a one-time observation, due to chance and random factors, or due to errors in the methods and procedures used. On the other hand, there could be a causal association. What considerations are involved in a causal association?

The issue of causality has been explored extensively in the relationship between smoking and lung cancer. The 1964 U.S. Surgeon General's report *Smoking and Health* (see **Figure 6-8**) declared that smoking caused lung cancer. What was the rationale behind this pronouncement, which at the time was controversial? To reach this conclusion, the report's authors stated that the evaluation of a causal association does not depend solely on evidence from a probabilistic statement derived from statistics, but is instead a matter of judgment that depends on several criteria.[12] Subsequently, Sir Austin Bradford Hill developed an expanded list of causal criteria that augmented those presented in *Smoking and Health*. These criteria may be applied to the evaluation of the possible causal association between many types of exposures and health outcomes.

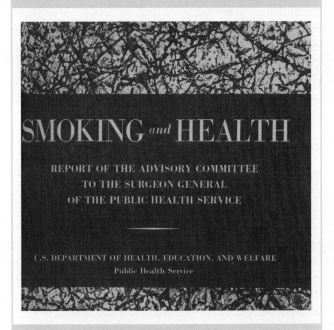

FIGURE 6-8 The cover page from the 1964 U.S. Surgeon General's report, *Smoking and Health*.

The determination of causal relationships between exposures and outcomes remains a difficult issue for epidemiology, which relies primarily on observational studies. One reason for the difficulty is that assessment of exposures is imprecise in many epidemiologic studies, as is the delineation of the mechanisms that connect exposures with outcomes.

One of the fields that have explored the relationship between exposures and disease is environmental health, as well as the closely related field of occupational health. Hill, a noted researcher, pointed out that in the realm of occupational health, extreme conditions in the physical environment or exposure to known toxic chemicals is expected to be invariably injurious.[13] More commonly, the situation prevails in which weaker associations have been observed between certain aspects of the environment and the occurrence of health events. An example of heavy occupational contact would be the development of lung diseases among people exposed to dusts (e.g., miners who work in dusty, unventilated mines). Hill raised the question of how one moves from such an observed association to the verdict of causation, e.g., exposure to coal dust causes a lung disease such as coal miners' pneumoconiosis. A second example is the perplexing question of the extent to which studies reveal a causal association between a specific environmental exposure and a particular form of cancer.[14]

Hill proposed a situation in which there is a clear association between two variables and in which statistical tests have suggested that this association is not due to chance. Under what circumstances would the association be causal? For example, data have revealed that smoking is associated with lung cancer in humans and that chance can be ruled out as being responsible for this observed association. Hill developed nine **causal criteria** that need to be taken into account in the assessment of a causal association between factor X and disease Y. We will next consider these criteria, which are listed in **Table 6-4.**

Strength

Strong associations are one of the criteria that give support to a causal relationship between a factor (exposure) and a disease. According to Hill, an example of a strong association comes from the observations of London surgeon Sir Percival Pott during the late 1700s. Pott noted that scrotal cancer was an occupational hazard among chimney sweeps. Hill pointed out the very large increase in scrotal cancer (by a factor of 200 times) among chimney sweeps in comparison to workers who were not occupationally exposed to tars and mineral oils.[13]

Another example of a strong association is the steeply elevated lung cancer mortality rates among heavy cigarette smokers in comparison to nonsmokers (20 to 30 times higher). Hill also cautioned that we should not be too ready to dismiss the

TABLE 6-4 Sir Austin Bradford Hill's Criteria of Causality

1. Strength
2. Consistency
3. Specificity
4. Temporality
5. Biological gradient
6. Plausibility
7. Coherence
8. Experiment
9. Analogy

Data from Hill AB. The environment and disease: association or causation? *Proc R Soc Med.* 1965; 58:295–300.

possibility of causal associations when the association is small, for there are many situations in which a causal association exists. One example would be exposure to an infectious agent (meningococcus) that produces relatively few clinical cases of meningococcal meningitis, a bacterial disease with symptoms that include headache, stiff neck, nausea, and vomiting.

Consistency

According to Hill, a consistent association is one that has been observed repeatedly "… by different persons, in different places, circumstances and times…"[13(p296)] An example of consistency comes from research on the relationship between smoking and lung cancer, a relationship that was found repeatedly in many retrospective and prospective studies.

Specificity

A specific association is one that is constrained to a particular disease–exposure relationship. In a specific association, a given disease results from a given exposure and not from other types of exposures. Hill gave the example of an association that "… is limited to specific workers and to particular sites and types of disease and there is no association between the work and other modes of dying…"[13(p297)] Returning to the smoking–lung cancer example, one may argue that the association is not specific, because "… the death rate among smokers is higher than the death rate of non-smokers from many causes of death…"[13(p297)] Nevertheless, Hill argued that one-to-one causation is unusual, because many diseases have more than one causal factor.

Temporality

This criterion specifies that we must observe the cause before the effect; Hill states that we cannot put the cart before the horse. For example, if we assert that air pollution causes lung cancer, we first must exclude persons who have lung cancer from our study; then we must follow those who are exposed to air pollution to determine whether lung cancer develops.

Biological Gradient

A biological gradient is known also as a dose-response curve, which shows a linear trend in the association between exposure and disease. An example is the dose-response association between the number of cigarettes smoked and the lung cancer death rate.

Plausibility

This criterion requires that an association be biologically plausible from the standpoint of contemporary biological knowledge. The association between exposure to tars and oils and the development of scrotal cancer among chimney sweeps is plausible in view of current knowledge about carcinogenesis. However, this knowledge was not available when Pott made his observations during the eighteenth century.

Coherence

This criterion suggests that "… the cause-and-effect interpretation of our data should not seriously conflict with the generally known facts of the natural history and biology of the disease…"[13(p298)] Examples related to cigarette smoking and lung cancer come from the rise in the number of lung cancer deaths associated with an increase in smoking, as well as lung cancer mortality differences between men (who smoke more and have higher lung cancer mortality rates) and women (who smoke less and have lower rates).

Experiment

Evidence from experiments (e.g., public health interventions) can help to support the existence of a causal relationship. Such experiments are conducted when research findings have shown an association between an exposure and a health outcome. If one changes the exposure during an experiment, then the disease or other health outcome should be altered. For example, if a smoking cessation intervention is successful, lung cancer deaths should decline among the participants in the intervention. This observation would suggest a causal association between the exposure and the disease. According to Hill, evidence from experiments is among the strongest forms of support for a causal hypothesis.

Analogy

The final criterion relates to the correspondence between known associations and one that is being evaluated for causality. The examples Hill cites are thalidomide and rubella. Thalidomide, administered in the early 1960s as an antinausea drug for use during pregnancy, was associated subsequently with severe birth defects. Rubella (German measles), if contracted during pregnancy, has been linked to birth defects, stillbirths, and miscarriages. Given that such associations already have been demonstrated, "… we would surely be ready to accept slighter but similar evidence with another drug or another viral disease in pregnancy."[13(p299)]

So where does epidemiology stand with respect to the evaluation of causal and noncausal associations? Any one of the criteria taken alone is not sufficient to demonstrate a causal relationship. The entire set of criteria must be evaluated. Generally speaking, the more criteria that are satisfied, the more convincing is the evidence in support of a causal association. The 1964 report *Smoking and Health* stated that cigarette smoking caused lung cancer in men because the relationship satisfied the majority of the criteria for causality.

You can think of the assertion of causality as being similar to a trial in court. The jury must ponder each of the bits of evidence, weigh them against the legal criteria (causal criteria) of guilt or innocence, and declare a verdict. (Refer to **Figure 6-9**, which shows a scale of justice.) Sometimes,

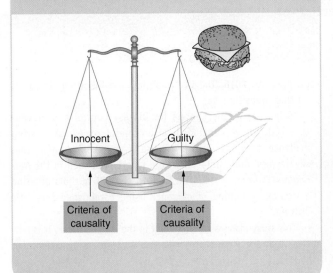

FIGURE 6-9 The declaration of a causal association involves a process that is similar to a jury weighing the evidence in a trial. Are foods (e.g., hamburgers) that are high in saturated fat "guilty" or "innocent" as causes of disease?

not all of the evidence will support a conclusion of guilt. However, a preponderance of the evidence must support a guilty verdict.

Applying the criteria of causality to the relationship between an exposure and a disease, we could say that "innocent" means that there is no causal association; "guilty" means that there is a causal association. In the case of the American diet, high-fat foods such as hamburgers are extremely popular and are consumed frequently. Heart disease is the leading cause of death in the United States; levels of obesity are increasing dramatically in the population. Evidence suggests that many high-fat foods contain large amounts of saturated fats, which have been implicated in heart disease and other adverse health outcomes. Consequently, the weight of the evidence (from the set of causal criteria) indicates that the scale has tipped toward a "guilty" verdict. Therefore, many authorities on nutrition and health recommend that consumption of large quantities of saturated fats should be minimized. Refer to the end of the chapter for an applicable example: Young Epidemiology Scholars Exercise "Alpine Fizz and Male Infertility: A Mock Trial."

Applying the Causal Criteria to a Contemporary Example: Zika Virus Disease and Microcephaly

For some time, the relationship between a female's infection with the Zika virus during pregnancy and microcephaly in the newborn was open to speculation. During April 2016, the Centers for Disease Control and Prevention (CDC) concluded "… that Zika virus is a cause of microcephaly and other severe brain defects"[15] Infection with the Zika virus increases the risk of adverse health outcomes; not all infected pregnant females will give birth to infants who have

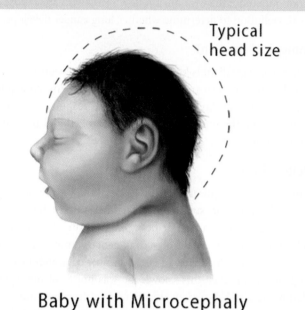

FIGURE 6-10 Baby with microcephaly.

Typical head size

Baby with Microcephaly

Reproduced from: Centers for Disease Control and Prevention. Facts about microcephaly. Available at: http://www.cdc.gov/ncbddd/birthdefects/microcephaly.html. Accessed August 14, 2016.

adverse health effects. See **Figure 6-10** for an illustration of microcephaly. Officials from CDC conducted a detailed review of empirical evidence regarding this relationship and applied Hill's criteria of causality to arrive at their conclusion. **Exhibit 6-1** reprints the details of CDC review.[16]

EXHIBIT 6-1 CDC Concludes that Zika Causes Microcephaly and Other Birth Defects

On April 13, 2016, The CDC published the following statement on their website:

"Scientists at the Centers for Disease Control and Prevention (CDC) have concluded, after careful review of existing evidence, that Zika virus is a cause of microcephaly and other severe fetal brain defects. In the report published in the *New England Journal of Medicine* [NEJM], the CDC authors describe a rigorous weighing of evidence using established scientific criteria.

'This study marks a turning point in the Zika outbreak. It is now clear that the virus causes microcephaly. We are also launching

further studies to determine whether children who have microcephaly born to mothers infected by the Zika virus is the tip of the iceberg of what we could see in damaging effects on the brain and other developmental problems,' said Tom Frieden, M.D., M.P.H., director of the CDC. 'We've now confirmed what mounting evidence has suggested, affirming our early guidance to pregnant women and their partners to take steps to avoid Zika infection and to health care professionals who are talking to patients every day. We are working to do everything possible to protect the American public.'

The report [in NEJM] notes that no single piece of evidence provides conclusive proof that Zika virus infection is a cause of

EXHIBIT 6-1 CDC Concludes that Zika Causes Microcephaly and Other Birth Defects (continued)

microcephaly and other fetal brain defects. Rather, increasing evidence from a number of recently published studies and a careful evaluation using established scientific criteria supports the authors' conclusions.

The finding that Zika virus infection can cause microcephaly and other severe fetal brain defects means that a woman who is infected with Zika during pregnancy has an increased risk of having a baby with these health problems ....[Not] all women who have Zika virus infection during pregnancy will have babies with problems ....[S]ome infected women have delivered babies that appear to be healthy."[†]

The noteworthy JAMA review illustrated the application of Sir Austin Bradford Hill's nine causal criteria to the relationship between the Zika virus and microcephaly and the need to weigh several causal criteria in order to reach the conclusion of a causal association regarding this relationship. The report posited that seven of Hill's criteria had been met; one (biologic gradient) was not applicable, and one (experiment) had not been met. The criteria that were met were the following:[*]

- Strength of association—"strong associations" (a risk ratio of about 50) were found between infection with the virus and subsequent microcephaly in French Polynesia; evidence from Brazil also supported a strong association.
- Consistency—consistent epidemiologic findings of an association in Brazil and French Polynesia have been observed.
- Specificity—an unusual form microcephaly appeared to be linked to Zika virus.
- Temporality—infection with the virus preceded the development of microcephaly.
- Plausibility—the effects are "similar to those seen after prenatal infection with some other viral teratogens."
- Coherence—animal models suggest that the virus is neurotropic (can affect nervous tissue).
- Analogy—animal studies have demonstrated that other flaviviruses (Zika is a flavivirus) can produce brain abnormalities and stillbirths.

*Modified from Rasmussen SA, Jamieson DJ, Honein MA, Petersen LR. Zika virus and birth defects—reviewing the evidence for causality. *N Engl J Med*. 2016;374(20):5 Centers for Disease Control and Prevention; April 13, 2016. CDC concludes Zika causes microcephaly and other brain defects. Available at: http://www.cdc.gov/media/releases/2016/s0413-zika-microcephaly.html. Accessed November 17, 2016.

Multivariate Causality

Currently, scientists believe that a preponderance of the etiologies of diseases (particularly chronic diseases) involve more than one causal factor. This type of causality is called **multivariate (multifactorial, multiple) causality**. For example, the etiology of chronic diseases as well as infectious diseases usually involves multiple types of exposures and other risk factors. In the case of the chronic disease lung cancer, these factors might include specific exposures (such as smoking), family history, lifestyle characteristics, and environmental influences. There are several models that portray multiple causality; we will present two of them—the epidemiologic triangle with the example of infectious diseases and the web of causation.

The epidemiologic triangle, which has been employed to explain the causation of infectious diseases, is composed of three major factors: agent, host, and environment. Each one of these major factors can be thought of as encompassing a

group of subfactors. In illustration, host factors can include such characteristics as age, immunity, and personal hygiene. Examples of environmental factors linked to infectious diseases are general sanitation, climate, and the presence of reservoirs of disease agents. According to the triangle, the agent, host, and environment operate jointly in the causation of infectious diseases (and other conditions).

Now let's turn to the web of causation, which portrays disease and a complex of variables (almost like a spider web). As shown in **Figure 6-11**, the etiology of coronary heart disease (CHD) involves a complex interplay of exposures and risk factors. Note that the figure does not exhaust the list of possible factors related to CHD. The web of causation agrees with the view that CHD, as is true of chronic diseases in general, has complicated etiology. No single exposure, by itself, has been demonstrated to be a cause of CHD.

FIGURE 6-11 The web of causation for coronary heart disease—a hypothetical model.

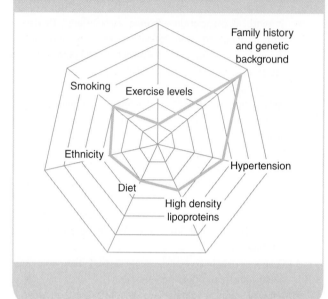

DEFINING THE ROLE OF CHANCE IN ASSOCIATIONS

Epidemiologists employ statistical procedures to assess the degree to which chance may have accounted for observed associations. The term **statistical significance** refers to the assertion that the observed association is not likely to have occurred as a result of chance. For an observed association to be valid, it cannot be due to chance.

As noted, an association can be merely a coincidental event: Suppose that it is Friday the thirteenth and that, on the way to class, you walk under a ladder and then a black cat crosses your path. Next, you go to class and receive the results of the midterm you took last week; you received an "F" on the exam. Later in the day you find out that you have been laid off from your job. When you approach your car to commute home, you discover that the door has been dented. There was an unfortunate and chance connection among the unlucky events on Friday the thirteenth after you walked under the ladder and saw the black cat run in front of you.

The field of inferential statistics explores the degree to which chance affects the conclusions that can be inferred from data. **Inference** is "[t]he process of evolving from observations and axioms to generalizations."[7] One of the goals of inference is to draw conclusions about a parent population from sample-based data. A **sample** is a subset of the data that have been collected from a population. An example of

inference would be to estimate the average age of all students in a university by randomly selecting a sample of students and calculating the average age of the sample.

Suppose we want to estimate the prevalence of multiple sclerosis in a population by using a sample. We collect a random sample from the population and determine how many individuals have multiple sclerosis. The value for the population is referred to as a **parameter** and the corresponding value for the sample is a **statistic**. The value of the statistic is used to estimate the parameter. Suppose we know from other research findings that the prevalence of multiple sclerosis is 2.0%. In our own research, the estimate (statistic) is calculated as 2.2%; this value is called a **point estimate**, which is a single value chosen to represent the population parameter. As a general rule, estimates gathered from samples do not exactly equal the population parameter because of sampling error.

As an alternative to a point estimate, an epidemiologist might use a **confidence interval estimate**, which is a range of values that with a certain degree of probability contain the population parameter. The degree of probability is called the **p-value**, an assessment that indicates the probability that the observed findings could have occurred by chance alone. Confidence interval (CI) estimates are shown in **Figure 6-12**,

FIGURE 6-12 Twenty hypothetical confidence interval estimates of population parameters.

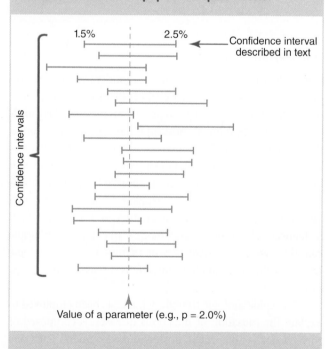

which represents the intervals as error bars. In the figure, the population proportion is denoted by the symbol p. (This is not the same as p-value.) The author will provide a hypothetical example of a CI estimate without performing the calculations.

To illustrate, an epidemiologist might want to be 95% certain that the confidence interval contains the population parameter. For example, suppose that the CI estimate of the prevalence of multiple sclerosis ranges from 1.5% to 2.5%, where p = 2.0%. In this hypothetical example, we could assert that we are 95% certain that the prevalence of multiple sclerosis in the population is from 1.5% to 2.5%. This CI is shown in the figure along with 19 additional hypothetical confidence intervals that have been constructed for 19 other samples, each having a different CI. Observe that one of the intervals does not include p. When the confidence interval is 95%, we would expect that 5% of the CIs will not contain p, the value of the parameter.

One of the factors that affect statistical significance is the size of the sample involved in the statistical test. Larger samples are more likely to produce significant results than smaller samples. In statistics, **power** is "… the ability of a study to demonstrate an association or effect if one exists."[7] Among the factors related to power are sample size and how large an effect is observed. The size of the effect is related to the strength of the association that has been observed. When the effect is small and the sample size is large, the association may be statistically significant. Conversely, if the effect is large and the sample size is small, the association may not be significant merely because of the small sample size that was employed.

A final comment about statistical significance: If an observed association is statistically significant, it is not necessarily **clinically significant**. Suppose an epidemiologist finds that a new drug produces a significant reduction in blood pressure level in the overall population, but the reduction is only slight. This significant result could have been influenced by including a large sample in the research. This slight reduction in blood pressure may not be clinically significant for an individual patient. The drug may not reduce the patient's morbidity or extend his or her life expectancy by any meaningful amount. In addition, some patients may experience side effects caused by the drug. As a result, use of the new drug may not be warranted.

Now, let's return to the examples that launched this chapter. Some media sources present research findings about the beneficial or deleterious effects of certain exposures on our health. Diet (consumption of organic foods, supplements, coffee, and alcoholic beverages) is a popular topic. These findings from empirical research need to be scrutinized according to the principles of causal inference and occurrence of chance associations. The author hopes that the information presented in this chapter will assist you in evaluating the findings of epidemiologic research.

CONCLUSION

This chapter explored the topics of epidemiologic associations, criteria of causality, and the effect of chance on observed relationships among variables. An association refers to a connection or linkage between or among two or more variables. An association among variables can be either noncausal or causal. Requiring the application of several causal criteria, causality is a complex topic. The greater the number of causal criteria that are satisfied by an observed association, the greater is the likelihood that a causal relationship exists. In addition to examining the criteria of causality, an epidemiologist must also rule out chance, which may account for observed associations. Statistical procedures enable one to estimate the role of chance.

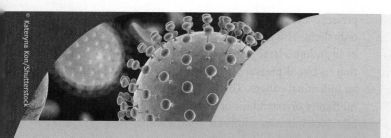

Study Questions and Exercises

1. Trace the landmarks in the history of disease causation from supernatural explanations to the germ theory of disease. Define each landmark, for example, contagion and miasmas, giving an example of each one.

2. How was the theory of miasmas reflected in sanitary reforms in Victorian Britain?

3. Define the terms *deterministic model* and *stochastic process*. Compare deterministic and stochastic models of disease causality, and provide examples of each type.

4. Distinguish between a cause that is sufficient but not necessary and one that is necessary but not sufficient. Be sure to give examples.

5. Describe the sufficient-component cause model and, using your own ideas, give an example.

6. In your opinion, how do theories and hypotheses guide the process of epidemiologic research?

7. Describe three types of associations (chance, noncausal, and causal) that are possible among exposures and health outcomes. Using your own experiences, give an example of each one.

8. Define what is meant by a causal association according to Hill's criteria. From your own experiences, give an example of how the three criteria of strength, consistency, and temporality might be satisfied with respect to the relationship between consumption of trans fats and heart disease. Note that trans fats are a type of liquid fat made solid through hydrogenation. Your answer might include a discussion of the health effects of eating French fries.

9. Statistics are an important aspect of evaluating associations.
   a. What is the difference between a parameter and a statistic?
   b. Distinguish between a point estimate and a confidence interval estimate.
   c. How does power apply to statistical testing?
   d. How is clinical significance different from statistical significance?

10. Conduct a search on the Internet for examples of possible chance associations reported in the media. Using your own ideas, give another example of a chance association between an exposure (e.g., diet or lifestyle) and a health outcome.

11. After reviewing Exhibit 6-1, restate how the first five of Hill's criteria were applied to the relationship between the Zika virus and microcephaly. Which criterion was not met? In your opinion, how important is it that that this one criterion was not met?

Young Epidemiology Scholars (YES) Exercises

The Young Epidemiology Scholars: Competitions website provides links to teaching units and exercises that support instruction in epidemiology. The YES program, discontinued in 2011, was administered by the College Board and supported by the Robert Wood Johnson Foundation. The exercises continue to be available at the following website: http://yes-competition.org/yes/teaching-units/title.html. The following exercises relate to topics discussed in this chapter and can be found on the YES competitions website.

Studying about causality

1. Huang FI, Baumgarten M. Alpine Fizz and Male Infertility: A Mock Trial

Studying associations

1. Kaelin M, Baumgarten M. An Association: TV and Aggressive Acts

2. Bayona M, Olsen C. Measures in Epidemiology

REFERENCES

1. Karamandou M, Panayiotakopoulos G, Tsoucalas G, et al. From miasmas to germs: a historical approach to theories of infectious disease transmission. *Infez Med*. 2012;20(1):58–62.
2. Science Museum, London. Miasma theory. Available at: http://www.sciencemuseum.org.uk/broughttolife/techniques/miasmatheory. Accessed August 9, 2016.
3. Brown M. From foetid air to filth: the cultural transformation of British epidemiological thought, ca. 1780–1848. *Bull Hist Med*. 2008;82:515–544.
4. Halliday S. Death and miasma in Victorian London: an obstinate belief. *BMJ*. 2001;323:1469–1471.
5. MacMahon B, Pugh TF. *Epidemiology Principles and Methods*. Boston, MA: Little, Brown and Company; 1970.
6. Clayton D, Mills M. *Statistical Models in Epidemiology*. New York, NY: Oxford University Press; 1993.
7. Porta M. *A Dictionary of Epidemiology*. 6th ed. New York, NY: Oxford University Press; 2014.
8. Vineis P. Causation in epidemiology. *Soz-Präventivmed*. 2003;48:80–87.
9. Susser M. *Causal Thinking in the Health Sciences*. New York, NY: Oxford University Press; 1973.
10. Rothman KJ. Reviews and commentary: causes. *Am J Epidemiol*. 1976;104(6):587–592.
11. Parascandola M, Weed DL. Causation in epidemiology. *J Epidemiol Commun Health*. 2001;55:905–912.
12. U.S. Public Health Service. *Smoking and Health*. Report of the Advisory Committee to the Surgeon General of the Public Health Service. U.S. Department of Health, Education, and Welfare, Public Health Service, Centers for Disease Control and Prevention, PHS Publication No. 1103. Washington, DC: U.S. Government Printing Office; 1964.
13. Hill AB. The environment and disease: association or causation? *Proc R Soc Med*. 1965;58:295–300.
14. DeBaun MR, Gurney JG. Environmental exposure and cancer in children. A conceptual framework for the pediatrician. *Pediatr Clin North Am*. 2001;48:1215–1221.
15. Centers for Disease Control and Prevention; April 13, 2016. CDC concludes Zika causes microcephaly and other brain defects. Available at: http://www.cdc.gov/media/releases/2016/s0413-zika-microcephaly.html. Accessed August 16, 2016.
16. Rasmussen SA, Jamieson DJ, Honein MA, Petersen LR. Zika virus and birth defects—reviewing the evidence for causality. *N Engl J Med*. 2016;374(20):1–7.

CHAPTER 7

Analytic Epidemiology: Types of Study Designs

By the end of this chapter you will be able to:

- List three ways in which study designs differ from one another.
- Describe case-control, ecologic, and cohort studies.
- Calculate an odds ratio, relative risk, and attributable risk.
- State appropriate uses of randomized controlled trials and quasi-experimental designs.
- Define sources of bias in epidemiologic study designs

CHAPTER OUTLINE

INTRODUCTION

Why is analytic epidemiology important to society? One reason is that analytic studies lead to the prevention of disease. The Framingham Study (a community cohort study mentioned elsewhere) was historically important because it contributed to our understanding of risk factors associated with coronary heart disease; modification of these risk factors has brought about reductions in morbidity and mortality from coronary heart disease. Another contribution of analytic epidemiology is the creation of quantitative evaluations of intervention programs (quasi-experimental designs), such as those directed at reduction of the incidence of sexually transmitted diseases. Without such evaluations, it would not be possible to determine whether intervention programs are efficacious or justified socially or economically. Finally, analytic epidemiology (implemented as clinical trials) aids in determining whether new drugs, immunizations, and medical procedures are safe and work as intended. Refer to **Table 7-1** for a list of important terms covered in this chapter.

OVERVIEW OF STUDY DESIGNS

Analytic epidemiologic studies are concerned with the etiology (causes) of diseases and other health outcomes. In comparison, descriptive epidemiology classifies a disease or other health outcome according to the categories of person, place, and time. Taking the perspective of analytic epidemiology, this chapter elaborates on the concept of association between exposures and health outcomes. This concept will be applied to the major categories of analytic designs—case-control, cohort, and ecologic study designs—as well as to intervention studies, all of which are covered in the present chapter.

TABLE 7-1 List of Important Terms Used in This Chapter

Observational Study Designs			Experimental Study Designs (Intervention Studies)	
Ecologic study	Case-control study	Cohort study	Clinical trial	Community trial
Ecologic comparison study	Matched case-control study	Cohort study (population based; exposure based; prospective; retrospective)	Crossover design	Stanford Five-City Project
Ecologic correlation	Odds ratio	Population risk difference	Prophylactic trial/ therapeutic trial	Program evaluation
Ecologic fallacy	Retrospective approach	Relative risk/ attributable risk	Randomized controlled trial	Quasi-experimental study

Other Terms Related to Epidemiologic Study Design		
Bias	Hawthorne effect	Protective factor
Confounding	Healthy worker effect	Randomization
Double-blind study	Internal validity	Recall bias
External validity	Intervention study	Selection bias
Family recall bias	Longitudinal design	Single-blind study

Figure 7-1 provides an organizational chart for study designs, subdividing them into the two major branches (descriptive and analytic). Here is some information about analytic epidemiology: Within the panel labeled analytic studies, the two subcategories are observational and intervention (experimental) studies. Observational studies include ecologic studies, case-control studies, and cohort studies. Three types of cohort studies are prospective, retrospective, and historical prospective. The two types of intervention studies (experimental studies) are clinical trials and community interventions. These terms will be defined later in the chapter.

Analytic studies, whether observational or experimental, explore associations between exposures and outcomes. Observational studies, which typify much epidemiologic research, are those in which the investigator does not have control over the exposure factor. Additionally, the investigator is unable to assign subjects randomly to the conditions of an observational study. Random assignment of subjects to study groups provides a degree of control over confounding. When the results of a study have been distorted by extraneous factors, confounding is said to have taken place. (More information on confounding is presented later in this chapter.)

In comparison with observational studies, experimental designs enable the investigator to control who is exposed to a factor of interest (for example, a new medication) and to randomly assign the participants into the groups used in the study. Random assignment of subjects is used in pure experimental designs. A quasi-experimental study is one in which

FIGURE 7-1 Two categories of epidemiologic studies.

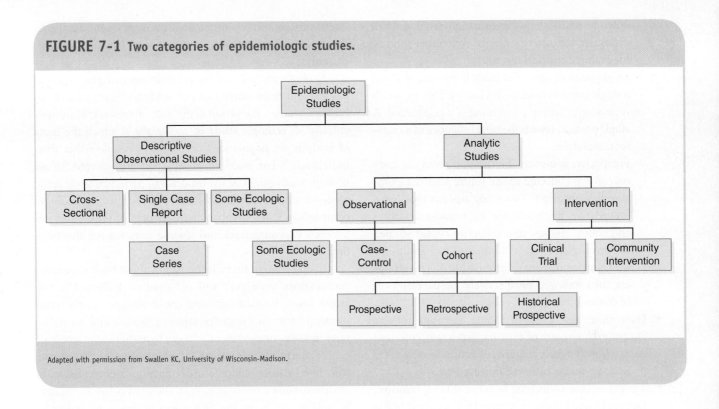

Adapted with permission from Swallen KC, University of Wisconsin-Madison.

the investigator is able to control the exposure of individuals or units to the factor but is unable to assign participants randomly to the conditions of the study.

A number of factors distinguish the study designs shown in Figure 7-1 from one another. (Refer to the text box.) These factors include who manipulates the exposure factor, either under the control of the investigator (in an experimental study) or not under the control of the investigator (in an observational study), the number of observations made, directionality of exposure, data collection methods, timing of data collection, unit of observation, and availability of subjects. An explanation of these terms is as follows:

- Number of observations made
  - In some cases, observations of subjects may be made only once. This is the approach of cross-sectional studies, many ecologic studies, and most case-control studies.
  - In other cases, two or more examinations may be made. This is the approach of cohort studies and experimental studies.
- Directionality of exposure: The directionality of exposure measurement relative to disease varies according to the type of study design used.
  - Retrospective approach: The term **retrospective** means obtaining information about exposures that occurred in the past. This method is used in case-control studies. The investigator starts with subjects who already have a disease and queries them about previous exposures that may have led to the

Seven factors that characterize study designs

1. Who manipulates the exposure factor?
   - Observational study: Exposure is not manipulated by the epidemiologist.
   - Experimental: Exposure is manipulated by the epidemiologist.
2. How many observations are made?
3. What is the directionality of exposure?
4. What are the methods of data collection?
5. What is the timing of data collection?
6. What is the unit of observation?
7. How available are the study subjects?

Adapted from Friis RH, Sellers TA. *Epidemiology for Public Health Practice*. 5th ed. Burlington, MA: Jones & Bartlett Learning; 2014:280–281.

outcome under study. Note that information about exposures can also be collected from other sources, for example, medical records.

- Single point in time: The study is referenced about a single point in time, as in a survey. This approach is similar to taking a snapshot of a population. A single point in time is the time reference of a cross-sectional study.
- Prospective approach: Information about the study outcome is collected in the future after the exposure has occurred. Two study designs that use a prospective approach are experimental studies and cohort studies. In prospective cohort studies, the investigator starts with disease-free groups for which exposures are determined first. The groups are then followed prospectively for development of disease.

- Data collection methods: Some methods require almost exclusive use of existing, previously collected data, whereas others require collection of new data.
  - Ecologic studies often use existing data.
- Timing of data collection: In some studies, information is obtained about exposures that occurred in the past. If long periods of time have elapsed between measurement of exposure and occurrence of disease, questions might be raised about the quality and applicability of the data. This information may be unreliable for various reasons including subjects' failure to remember past exposures. In other studies, subjects may be followed prospectively (i.e., into the future) over a period of time. Information about the outcome variable may be lost should subjects drop out during the course of the study.
- Unit of observation: The unit of observation can be the individual or an entire group. Most epidemiologic study designs employ the individual as the unit of observation; one type, known as an ecologic study design, uses the group as the unit of observation.
- Availability of subjects: Certain classes of subjects may not be available for epidemiologic research for several reasons, including ethical issues.

ECOLOGIC STUDIES

You are probably most familiar with studies in which the subjects are single individuals; this approach typifies most epidemiologic research. For example, information is collected from individual respondents by giving them a questionnaire, taking other measurements, and analyzing the data. In this situation, the individual is called the unit of analysis.

Ecologic studies are different from most familiar research designs and from other types of epidemiologic research. In ecologic studies, the group is the unit of analysis. More specifically, an **ecologic study** is "... a study in which the units of analysis are populations or groups of people rather than individuals."[1] For example, groups that are selected for an ecologic study might be the residents of particular geographic areas—nations, states, census tracts, or counties. An **ecologic comparison study** involves an assessment of the association between exposure rates and disease rates during the same time period.

In an ecologic study, information about both exposures (explanatory variables) and outcomes is collected at the group level. To illustrate, one could explore "... the relationship between the distribution of income and mortality rates in states or provinces."[1] In the hypothetical example of cancer mortality, researchers might hypothesize that people who live in lower-income areas have greater exposure to environmental carcinogens than those who live in higher-income areas, producing differences in cancer mortality.

Figure 7-2 illustrates an **ecologic correlation**, an association between two variables measured at the group level.

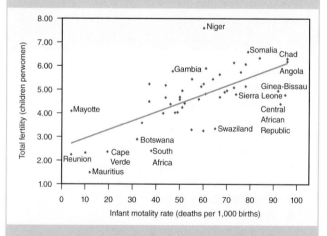

FIGURE 7-2 Relationship between total fertility and infant mortality, selected African countries: 2010–2015.

Notes: 48 African countries plus Mayotte and Reunion (departments of France) and excluding North Africa; R2 = 0.46.

Data from United Nations, Department of Economic and Social Affairs, Population Division (2015). *World Population Prospects: The 2015 Revision, Methodology of the United Nations Population Estimates and Projections*, Working Paper No. ESA/P/WP.242.

In the figure, infant mortality rates and average number of children per women are calculated for some African countries, which are the units of analysis. The graph portrays the strong positive linear relationship between fertility and infant mortality in sub-Saharan Africa. Countries that have high infant mortality rates (e.g., Sierra Leone) tend to have high birth rates.[2]

One of the reasons for conducting an ecologic study is that individual measurements might not be available, but group-level data can be obtained. Often the data used have already been collected and are stored in data archives. These group measurements are called aggregate measures, and they provide an overall measurement for the level (e.g., group or population) being studied. Often, ecologic studies are helpful in revealing the context of health—how demographic characteristics and the social environment contribute to morbidity and mortality.

Table 7-2 demonstrates some of the outcome variables, units of analysis, and explanatory variables (similar to exposure variables) used in ecologic studies. One of the common outcome variables of ecologic studies is mortality, either all-cause or cause-specific mortality (e.g., mortality from breast cancer or heart disease). In addition, outcome variables could include various types of morbidity; an example is occupational injuries. Other possible outcomes (not shown in the table) are rates of infectious diseases, congenital malformations, and chronic conditions.

Three examples of units of analysis are shown in Table 7-2: Spanish municipalities, U.S. counties, and regions in a Canadian province. Many other units of analysis at the group level are theoretically possible. Explanatory variables are those studied as correlates of outcome variables. The examples of explanatory variables shown are sex, socioeconomic level, age, income inequality, race, physician prevalence, unemployment, population density, and residential stability.

Here are the major findings of the studies shown in the table: Pollán et al.[3] reported an association between mortality and socioeconomic level among older women in Spain; Shi et al.[4] showed that availability of primary care physicians was related to a reduction in mortality; Breslin et al.[5] found that Ontario regions with stable populations had reduced levels of occupational injuries.

TABLE 7-2 Examples of Ecologic Studies

Author	Outcome Variable	Unit of Analysis	Representative Explanatory Variables
Pollán et al., 2007[a]	Breast cancer mortality	Municipalities in Spain, e.g., Madrid	Women; age group (≥ 50 and < 50); socioeconomic level; % population ≥ 65
Findings: Higher levels of socioeconomic status were associated with higher levels of breast cancer mortality among women age 50 years and older.			
Shi et al., 2005[b]	All-cause mortality; heart disease mortality; cancer mortality	U.S. counties	Income inequality; primary care physicians per 10,000 population; % black; % unemployed
Findings: Mortality was from 2% to 3% lower in counties that had more available primary care resources than counties with fewer resources.			
Breslin et al., 2007[c]	Occupational injuries	Regions in Ontario, Canada	Population density; residential stability; unemployment
Findings: Regional attributes such as low residential turnover were related to low injury rates.			

[a]Pollán M, Ramis R, Aragonés N, et al. Municipal distribution of breast cancer mortality among women in Spain. *BMC Cancer*. 2007;7(78). Available at: http://www.biomedcentral.com/1471-2407/7/78. Accessed July 12, 2016.
[b]Shi L, Macinko J, Starfield B, et al. Primary care, social inequalities, and all-cause, heart disease, and cancer mortality in US counties, 1990. *Am J Public Health*. 2005;95:674–680.
[c]Breslin FC, Smith P, Dunn JR. An ecological study of regional variation in work injuries among young workers. *BMC Public Health*. 2007;7(91). Available at: http://www.biomedcentral.com/1471-2458/7/91. Accessed July 11, 2016.

In addition to the examples shown in Table 7-2, what are some other examples of ecologic studies? Ecologic analyses have been applied to the study of air pollution by examining the correlation of air pollution with adverse health effects such as mortality. Instead of correlating individual exposures to air pollution with mortality, researchers measure the association between average levels of air pollution within a census tract (or other geographic subdivision) with the average mortality in that census tract. This type of study investigates whether mortality is higher in more polluted census tracts than in less polluted census tracts. Refer to the text box for definitions of the term *census tract* and related terms (statistical entities) used by the U.S. Census Bureau.

A major deficiency of the ecologic technique for the study of air pollution (and for virtually all ecologic studies), however, stems from uncontrolled factors. Examples relevant to air pollution include individual levels of smoking and smoking habits, occupational exposure to respiratory hazards and air pollution, differences in social class and other demographic factors, genetic background, and length of residence in the area.[6] Nonetheless, ecologic studies may open the next generation of investigations; the interesting observations gathered in ecologic studies may provide the impetus for more carefully designed studies. The next wave of studies that build on ecologic studies then may attempt to take advantage of more rigorous analytic study designs.

Ecologic studies have examined the association between water quality and both stroke and coronary diseases. A group of studies have demonstrated that hardness of the domestic water supply is associated inversely with risk of cerebrovascular mortality and cardiovascular diseases. However, a Japanese investigation did not support a relationship between water hardness and cerebrovascular diseases. In the latter ecologic study, the unit of analysis was municipalities (population subdivisions in Japan that consisted of from 6,000 to 3,000,000 inhabitants). In analyzing the 1995 death rates from strokes in relation to the values of water hardness, the researchers did not find statistically significant associations across municipalities.[7]

Other ecologic studies have examined the possible association between use of agricultural pesticides and childhood cancer incidence. For example, a total of 7,143 incident cases of invasive cancer diagnosed among children younger than age 15 years were reported to the California Cancer Registry during the years 1988–1994. In this ecologic study, the unit of analysis was census blocks, with average annual pesticide exposure estimated per square mile. The study

Some statistical entities used by the U.S. Census Bureau

- Census tract: A small, relatively permanent statistical subdivision of a county delineated by a local committee of census data users for the purpose of presenting data. Census tracts nest within counties, and their boundaries normally follow visible features, but may follow legal geography boundaries and other nonvisible features in some instances. Census tracts ideally contain about 4,000 people and 1,600 housing units.
- Census block: A statistical area bounded by visible features, such as streets, roads, streams, and railroad tracks, and by nonvisible boundaries, such as selected property lines and city, township, school district, and county boundaries. A block is the smallest geographic unit for which the Census Bureau tabulates decennial census data. Many blocks correspond to individual city blocks bounded by streets, but blocks, especially in rural areas, may include many square miles and may have some boundaries that are not streets.
- Metropolitan statistical area: A geographic entity delineated by the Office of Management and Budget for use by federal statistical agencies. Metropolitan statistical areas consist of the county or counties (or equivalent entities) associated with at least one urbanized area of at least 50,000 population, plus adjacent counties having a high degree of social and economic integration with the core as measured through commuting ties.

showed no overall association between pesticide exposure determined by this method and childhood cancer incidence rates. However, a significant increase in childhood leukemia rates was linked to census block groups that had the highest use of a type of pesticide known as propargite.[8]

Ecologic Fallacy

Information obtained from group-level data may not accurately reflect the relationship between exposure and outcomes at the individual level. The term **ecologic (or ecological) fallacy** is defined as "[a]n erroneous inference that may occur because an association observed between variables on an aggregate level does not necessarily represent or reflect the association that exists at an individual level;…"[1]

Here is an example: Epidemiologist and noted professor Raj Bhopal writes

> Imagine a study of the rate of coronary heart disease in the capital cities of the world relating the rate to average income. Within [sic] the cities studied, coronary heart disease will be higher in the richer cities than in the poorer ones. This finding would fit the general view that coronary heart disease is a disease of affluence. We might predict from such a finding that rich people in the individual cities too have more risk of CHD than poor people. In fact, in contemporary times, in the industrialized world the opposite is the case: within cities such as London, Washington DC, and Stockholm, poor people have higher CHD rates than rich ones. The forces that cause high rates of disease at a population level are different from those at an individual level.[9(p322)]

The advantages and disadvantages of ecologic studies can be summarized as follows:

- Advantages
  - May provide information about the context of health.
  - Can be performed when individual-level measurements are not available.
  - Can be conducted rapidly and with minimal resources.
- Disadvantages
  - Ecologic fallacy
  - Imprecise measurement of exposure

CASE-CONTROL STUDIES

A **case-control study** is one in which subjects are defined on the basis of the presence or absence of an outcome of interest. (Refer to **Figure 7-3**.) The cases are those individuals who have the outcome or disease of interest, whereas the controls do not. Because having a specific outcome such as a disease is the criterion for being included in the case group, a case-control study can examine only a single outcome or a limited set of outcomes. A **matched case-control study** is one in which the cases and controls have been matched according to one or more criteria such as sex, age, race, or other variables. The reasons for matching are discussed in the section on confounding.

Case-control studies use a retrospective approach to collect information about exposure to a factor, in which the exposure occurred in the past. One method to determine past

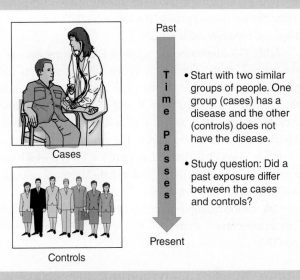

FIGURE 7-3 Diagram of a case-control study.

Modified from Cahn MA, Auston I, Selden CR, Pomerantz KL. *Introduction to HSR*, May 23, 1998. National Information Center on Health Services Research and Health Care Technology (NICHSR), National Library of Medicine; 1998. Available at: http://www.nlm.nih.gov/nichsr /pres/mla98/cahn/sld034.htm. Accessed July 30, 2008.

exposure is for the investigator to interview cases and controls regarding their exposure history. An advantage of case-control studies is that they can examine many potential exposures, such as exposure to toxic chemicals, use of medications, or adverse lifestyle characteristics. In some variations of the case-control approach, it may be possible to conduct direct measurements of the environment for various types of exposures.

Researchers have a variety of sources available for the selection of cases and controls. For example, investigators may use patients from hospitals, specialized clinics, or medical practices; also, they may select cases from disease registries (i.e., cancer registries). Sometimes, advertisements in the media solicit cases. For use as controls, investigators may identify patients from hospitals or clinics—patients who have different health problems than the cases. In other instances, controls may be friends or relatives of the cases or be people from the community.

Odds Ratio: Measure of Association Used in Case-Control Studies

The **odds ratio (OR)** is a measure of the association between frequency of exposure and frequency of outcome used in case-control studies. The OR is called an indirect measure of risk because incidence rates have not been used; instead, the risk of an outcome associated with an exposure is estimated by calculating the odds of exposure among the cases and controls. The OR is the ratio of odds in favor of exposure among the disease group (the cases) to the odds in favor of exposure among the no-disease group (the controls). This odds ratio is called the exposure odds ratio.[1]

Table 7-3 illustrates the method for labeling cells in a case-control study. The columns are labeled as cases and controls. Cells that contain the cases are A and C; the cells that contain the controls are B and D. The total number of cases and controls are A + C and B + D, respectively. Exposure status (reading across the rows) is identified as yes or no. The OR is defined as (A/C) ÷ (B/D), which can be expressed as (AD)/(BC). (Multiply the diagonal cells and divide them.)

Calculation example: Suppose we have the following data from a case-control study: A = 9, B = 4, C = 95, and D = 88. The OR is calculated as follows:

$$OR = \frac{AD}{BC} = \frac{(9)(88)}{(4)(95)} = 2.08$$

Interpretation: An odds ratio of more than 1.0 suggests a positive association between the exposure and disease or other outcome (provided that the results are statistically significant—not a chance association). In this sample calculation, the OR is 2.1, suggesting that the odds of the disease are about two times higher among the exposed persons than among the nonexposed persons. In some instances, an OR of less than 1.0 indicates that the exposure might be a protective factor. A **protective factor** is a circumstance or substance that provides a beneficial environment and makes a positive contribution to health. (Hypothetical example of a protective factor: We want to find out if heavy exercise is associated with early mortality among heart attack patients. One possibility is that exercise might strain the heart and cause the patient to die. In a case-control study, the OR should be greater than 1.0. Instead we find that the OR is less than 1.0, because mortality is lower among heart attack patients who exercise in comparison with nonexercisers. We conclude that exercise is a protective factor for heart disease mortality among heart attack patients.) When the OR is equivalent to 1.0, there is no association between exposure and outcome.

Case-control studies commonly are used in environmental epidemiologic research. For example, environmental health researchers have been concerned about the possible health effects of exposure to electromagnetic fields. A case-control study among female residents of Long Island, New York examined the possible association between exposure to electromagnetic fields (EMFs) and breast cancer.[10] Eligible subjects were those who were younger than age 75 years and had lived in the study area for 15 years or longer. Cases (*n* = 576) consisted of women diagnosed with *in situ* (early stage cancer in its original site) or invasive breast cancer. Controls (*n* = 585) were selected from the same community by random digit dialing procedures. (Random digit dialing is a computerized procedure for selecting telephone numbers at random within defined geographic areas; selected respondents are called and asked to participate in telephone interviews.) Several types of measurement of EMFs were taken in the subjects' homes and by mapping overhead power lines. The investigators reported that the odds ratio between EMF exposure and breast cancer was not statistically significantly different from 1.0; thus, the results suggested that there was no association between breast cancer and residential EMF exposure.

The advantages and disadvantages of case-control studies are as follows:

- Advantages
  - Can be used to study low-prevalence conditions.
  - Relatively quick and easy to complete.
  - Usually inexpensive.
  - Involve smaller numbers of subjects.
- Disadvantages
  - Measurement of exposure may be inaccurate.
  - Representativeness of cases and controls may be unknown.
  - Provide indirect estimates of risk.
  - The temporal relationship between exposure factor and outcome cannot always be ascertained.

In comparison with cross-sectional study designs, case-control studies may provide more complete exposure data,

TABLE 7-3 Fourfold Table that Demonstrates a Case-Control Study

	Disease Status	
Exposure status	Yes (Cases)	No (Controls)
Yes	A	B
No	C	D
Total	A + C	B + D

especially when the exposure information is collected from the friends and relatives of cases who died of a particular cause. Nevertheless, some unmeasured exposure variables as well as methodological biases (a term discussed later in this chapter) may remain in case-control studies. For example, in studies of health and air pollution, exposure levels are difficult to quantify precisely. Also, it may be difficult to measure unknown and unobserved factors, including smoking habits and occupational exposures to air pollution, which affect the lungs.[6]

Case-control studies are often inexpensive, yield results rapidly, and involve small sample sizes. They are useful for studying low-prevalence conditions—a specific disease or outcome is the basis for selection of the cases. Disadvantages of the case-control approach include the fact that risk is estimated indirectly by using the odds ratio; in addition, relationships between exposures and health outcomes may not have been measured accurately.

COHORT STUDIES

A **cohort study** tracks the incidence of a specific disease (or other outcome) over time. Variations of cohort studies include prospective cohort studies (longitudinal studies), retrospective cohort studies, population-based cohort studies, and exposure-based cohort studies. A cohort is defined as a population group, or subset thereof (distinguished by a common characteristic), that is followed over a period of time. Three examples of cohorts are:

- Birth or age cohort (e.g., the baby boom generation; generations X or Y; millennials)
- Work cohort (people in a particular type of employment studied for occupational exposures)
- School/educational cohort (people who graduated during a particular year)

As an introduction to cohort studies, the author notes that two major categories of cohort studies are population-based cohort studies and exposure-based cohort studies. As the name implies, a **population-based cohort study** leverages information from a total population or a representative sample of a population. An example of a population-based cohort study is the Framingham, Massachusetts study of coronary heart disease initiated in 1948. An **exposure-based cohort study** compares cohorts with or without different exposures. A simple example is a cohort study with two exposure groups (exposed and not exposed).

In a **prospective cohort study** design, subjects are classified according to their exposure to a factor of interest and are then observed over time to document the occurrence of new cases (incidence) of disease or other health events. (Refer to **Figure 7-4**.) At the inception or baseline of a prospective cohort study, participants must be certified as being free from the outcome of interest. For this reason cohort studies are not helpful for researching diseases that are uncommon in the population; during the course of the cohort study, only a few cases of the disease may occur. Cohort studies are a type of prospective or **longitudinal design**, meaning that subjects are followed over an extended period of time. Using cohort studies, epidemiologists are able to evaluate many different outcomes (such as causes of death or development of chronic diseases) but few exposures.[6] The reason is that the exposure is the criterion used to select subjects into a cohort study; for this reason, researchers are unable to examine more than one or two exposures in a single study.

A variation of a cohort study design uses a retrospective assessment of exposure. A **retrospective cohort study** is one that makes use of historical data to determine exposure level at some baseline in the past; follow-up for subsequent occurrences of disease between baseline and the present is performed. An alternative to a purely retrospective cohort study is a historical prospective cohort study, which combines retrospective and prospective approaches.

An example of a retrospective cohort study would be one that examined mortality among an occupational cohort such as shipyard workers who were employed at a specific

FIGURE 7-4 Diagram of a prospective cohort study.

Healthy people who have had an exposure

Time Passes

Healthy people and sick people

Baseline

Follow-up

Study question:
How many new cases of illness occur?

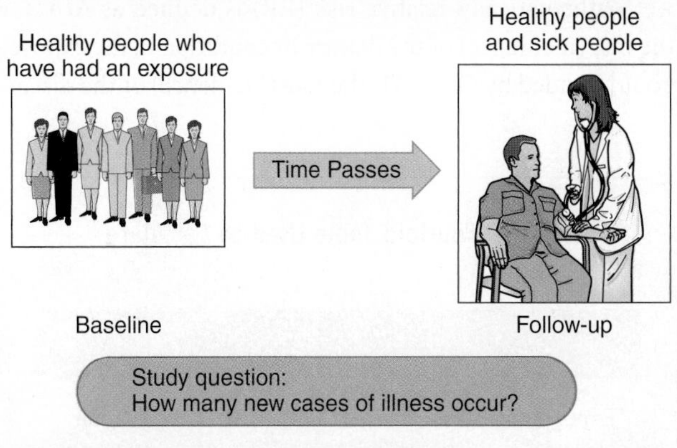

Modified from Cahn MA, Auston I, Selden CR, Pomerantz KL. *Introduction to HSR*, May 23, 1998. National Information Center on Health Services Research and Health Care Technology (NICHSR), National Library of Medicine; 1998. Available at: http://www.nlm.nih.gov/nichsr /pres/mla98/cahn/sld036.htm. Accessed July 30, 2008.

naval yard during a defined time interval (e.g., World War II). A retrospective cohort study is different from a case-control study because an entire cohort of exposed individuals is examined. In contrast, a case-control study makes use of a limited number of cases and controls who usually do not represent an entire cohort of individuals such as a group of people employed by a specific company.

Measure of Association Used in Cohort Studies

The measure of association used in cohort studies is called **relative risk (RR)**, the ratio of the incidence rate of a disease or health outcome in an exposed group to the incidence rate of the disease or condition in a nonexposed group. As noted previously, an incidence rate may be interpreted as the risk of occurrence of an outcome that is associated with a particular exposure. The RR provides a ratio of two risks—the risk associated with an exposure in comparison with the risk associated with nonexposure.

Relative risk = Incidence rate in the exposed ÷ Incidence rate in the nonexposed

The method for formatting the data from a cohort study and calculating a relative risk is shown in **Table 7-4**. Across the rows is the exposure status of the participants: either yes or no. The disease status of the participants is indicated in the columns and also is classified as either yes or no. The total number of subjects in the exposure group is A + B; the corresponding total for the nonexposed group is C + D.

Mathematically, relative risk (RR) is defined as A/A + B [the rate (incidence) of the disease or condition in the exposed group] divided by C/C + D [the rate (incidence) of the disease

or condition in the nonexposed group]. The formula for relative risk is:

$$RR = \frac{\dfrac{A}{A+B}}{\dfrac{C}{C+D}}$$

Calculation example: Suppose that we are researching whether exposure to solvents is associated with risk of liver cancer. Refer to the data shown in **Table 7-5**. From a cohort study of industrial workers, we find that three people who worked with solvents developed liver cancer (cell A of table) and 104 did not (cell B). Two cases of liver cancer occurred among nonexposed workers (cell C) in the same type of industry. The remaining 601 nonexposed workers (cell D) did not develop liver cancer.

Incidence rate in the exposed group = 3/107 = 0.02804 (rounded)

Incidence rate in the nonexposed group = 2/603 = 0.003317 (rounded)

The RR is:

$$RR = \frac{\dfrac{3}{3+104}}{\dfrac{2}{2+601}} = \frac{0.02804}{0.003317} = 8.45$$

We may interpret relative risk in a manner that is similar to that of the odds ratio. A relative risk of 1.0 implies that the risk (rate) of disease among the exposed is not different from the risk of disease among the nonexposed. A relative risk greater than 2.0 implies that the risk is more than twice as high among the exposed as among the nonexposed. In other words, there is a positive association between exposure and the outcome under study. In the calculation example, the risk of developing liver cancer is eight times

TABLE 7-4 Fourfold Table Used to Calculate a Relative Risk

	Disease Status		
Exposure status	Yes	No	Total
Yes	A	B	A + B
No	C	D	C + D

TABLE 7-5 Data Table for Liver Cancer Example

	Liver Cancer		
Exposure to solvents	Yes	No	Total
Yes	3	104	107
No	2	601	603

greater among workers who were exposed to solvents than among those who were not exposed to solvents.

Sometimes a relative risk calculation yields a value that is less than 1.0. If the relative risk is less than 1.0 (and statistically significant), the risk is lower among the exposed group; for example, a relative risk of 0.5 indicates that the exposure of interest is associated with half the risk of disease. This level of risk, i.e., less than 1.0, sometimes is called a protective effect.

Accurate disease determination is necessary to optimize measures of relative risk; disease misclassification affects estimates of relative risk. The type of disease and method of diagnosis affect the accuracy of diagnosis.[6] In illustration, death certificates are used frequently as a source of information about the diagnosis of a disease. Information from death certificates regarding cancer as the underlying cause of death is believed to be more accurate than the information for other diagnoses such as those for nonmalignant conditions. Nevertheless, the accuracy of diagnoses of cancer as a cause of death varies according to the particular form of cancer.

Difference in Rates (Risks)

The two measures of risk difference discussed in this section are attributable risk and population risk difference. Remember that the relative risk is the ratio of the incidence rate of an outcome in the exposed group to the incidence rate for that outcome in the nonexposed group; for a two-exposure group (exposed and nonexposed) cohort study, this comparison is made by dividing the two incidence rates. An alternative to relative risk is attributable risk, which is a type of difference measure of association.

Attributable risk, in a cohort study, refers to the difference between the incidence rate of a disease in the exposed group and the incidence rate in the nonexposed group. Returning to the calculation example shown in Table 7-5, the incidence rate (expressed as rate per 1,000) in the exposed group was 28.04 (rounded off) and the incidence rate (expressed as rate per 1,000) in the nonexposed group was 3.32 (rounded off). The attributable risk is the difference between these two incidence rates (28.04 per 1,000 − 3.32 per 1,000) and equals 24.72 per 1,000. This is the incidence rate associated with exposure to the solvent.

A second measure that assesses differences in rates is the population risk difference, which provides an indication of the benefit to the population derived by modifying a risk factor. The **population risk difference** is defined as the difference between the rate of disease in the nonexposed segment of the population and the overall rate in the population.

Population risk difference =
Incidence in the total population − Incidence in the nonexposed segment

Calculation example: What is the incidence of disease in the population attributed to smoking? Assume that the annual lung cancer incidence for men in the total population is 79.4 per 100,000 men; the incidence of lung cancer among nonsmoking men is 28.0 per 100,000 men. The population risk difference is (79.4 − 28.0), or 51.4 per 100,000 men. Among men, the incidence of lung cancer due to smoking is 51.4 cases per 100,000.

Uses of Cohort Studies

Cohort studies are applied widely in epidemiology. For example, they have been used to examine the effects of environmental and work-related exposures to potentially toxic agents. One concern of cohort studies has been exposure of female workers to occupationally related reproductive hazards and adverse pregnancy outcomes.[11]

A second example is an Australian study that examined the health impacts of occupational exposure to pesticides.[12] The investigators selected an exposure cohort of 1,999 male outdoor workers who were employed by the New South Wales Board of Tick Control between 1935 and 1995; these individuals were involved with an insecticide application program and had worked with a variety of insecticides. A control cohort consisted of 1,984 men who worked as outdoor field officers at any time since 1935 and were not known to have been exposed on the job to insecticides. The investigators carefully evaluated exposures and health outcomes such as mortality from various chronic diseases and cancer. They reported an association between exposure to pesticides and adverse health effects, particularly for asthma, diabetes, and some forms of cancer including pancreatic cancer.

In summary, the advantages and disadvantages of cohort studies are as follows:

- Advantages
  - Permit direct observation of risk.
  - Exposure factor is well defined.
  - Can study exposures that are uncommon in the population.
  - The temporal relationship between factor and outcome is known.
- Disadvantages
  - Expensive and time consuming.
  - Complicated and difficult to carry out.
  - Subjects may be lost to follow-up during the course of the study.
  - Exposures can be misclassified.

Regarding advantages, cohort studies provide information about incidence rates of disease and other health outcomes and thus provide direct assessment of risk. Exposure factors are defined at the inception of the study and are used as the basis for selection into the study. Cohort studies can examine exposures that are uncommon in the population, such as those that might be experienced by occupational groups that work with toxic chemicals and other hazardous substances. Finally, temporality between exposure variables and outcome is known; for example, in prospective cohort studies, assessment of exposures occurs before assessment of outcomes.

The disadvantages of cohort studies include the fact that they are expensive and may require several years before useful results can be obtained. Methodologically, they are difficult to carry out; frequently, the epidemiologist must account for large numbers of subjects, maintain extensive records, and follow subjects closely. Because cohort studies take place over a long period of time, subjects may be lost to follow-up because of dropping out, moving, or dying. Lastly, it is important to ascertain whether exposures have been correctly identified in cohort studies; one scenario in which misclassification of exposures can occur is in retrospective cohort studies because accurate exposure records may no longer be available.

EXPERIMENTAL STUDIES

In epidemiology, experimental studies are implemented as intervention studies. An **intervention study** is "[a]n investigation involving intentional change in some aspect of the status of the subjects, e.g., introduction of a preventive or therapeutic regimen or an intervention designed to test a hypothesized relationship;..."[1] This section covers the topics of clinical trials and two types of experimental study designs: randomized controlled trials and quasi-experiments.

Clinical Trials

A **clinical trial** refers to "[a] research activity that involves the administration of a test regimen to humans to evaluate its efficacy or its effectiveness and safety."[1] The term *clinical trial* has several meanings that can range from the early trials conducted in history without the benefit of control or comparison groups to randomized controlled trials. Early clinical trials, such as those used to treat battlefield wounds or cure the nutritional disease scurvy, did not use control groups. Another example of an early forerunner of a clinical trial was Edward Jenner's development of his smallpox vaccine; Jenner did not have a control group.

Some applications of clinical trials are to test the efficacy of new medications and vaccines and evaluate medical treatment regimens and health education programs. A **prophylactic trial** is designed to test preventive measures; **therapeutic trials** evaluate new treatment methods.

Clinical trials are conducted in three, and sometimes more, phases. Imagine a clinical trial for a new vaccine. The first phase might involve initial human testing for safety. The second phase could evaluate the immune responses of a limited group of vaccine recipients. The third phase would be a large-scale study involving randomization of participants to test and control conditions. **Randomization** is defined as a process whereby chance determines the subjects' likelihood of assignment to either an intervention group or a control group. Each subject has an equal probability of being assigned to either group.

Clinical trials have evolved over time into increasingly expensive, complex, and time-consuming undertakings. Multicenter trials (collaborations among groups of medical facilities) have been adopted as a means of creating larger sample sizes. These efforts have spurred the need for improved communication among investigators and have challenged data analysis capacity by creating vast data sets. One of the solutions for addressing modern advances in clinical trials is increasing the use of the Internet as a platform for conducting clinical trials. This innovation may help to speed results and lower costs.[13]

Randomized Controlled Trial

A **randomized controlled trial (RCT)** is defined as "[a] clinical-epidemiological experiment in which subjects are randomly allocated into groups, usually called *test* and *control* groups, to receive or not to receive a preventive or a therapeutic procedure or intervention. The results are assessed by comparison of rates of disease, death, recovery, or other appropriate outcome in the study control groups."[1] A diagram of a randomized controlled trial (RCT) is shown in **Figure 7-5**. In comparison with observational studies, a randomized controlled trial is considered the most scientifically rigorous study design and to have the highest level of validity for making etiologic inferences; an RCT can control for many of the factors that affect study designs, including assignment of exposures and biases in assessment of study outcomes. RCTs are limited to a narrow range of applications; they are not as helpful for studying the etiology of diseases as are observational designs. For obvious ethical reasons, it is not possible for an investigator to run experiments that determine whether an exposure causes disease in human subjects.

FIGURE 7-5 Diagram of a randomized controlled trial.

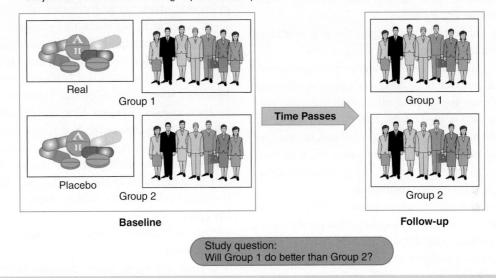

- The researcher takes a larger group of people and uses *random assignment* to divide them into two smaller groups.
- Group 1 gets a real medicine.
- Group 2 gets a *placebo*.
- Subjects are *blinded* as to their group membership.

Real

Group 1

Placebo

Group 2

Baseline

Time Passes

Group 1

Group 2

Follow-up

Study question:
Will Group 1 do better than Group 2?

Modified from Cahn MA, Auston I, Selden CR, Pomerantz KL. *Introduction to HSR*, May 23, 1998. National Information Center on Health Services Research and Health Care Technology (NICHSR), National Library of Medicine. 1998. Available at: http://www.nlm.nih.gov/nichsr/pres/mla98/cahn/sld036.htm. Accessed July 30, 2008.

An example of the difficulty in using RCTs arises in the study of environmental health hazards. For several reasons, the use of experimental methods in environmental epidemiology is difficult to achieve. In fact, the majority of research on health outcomes associated with the environment use observational methods.[14] Epidemiologist Kenneth Rothman points out that:

> Randomized assignment of individuals into groups with different environmental exposures generally is impractical, if not unethical; community intervention trials for environmental exposures have been conducted, although seldom (if ever) with random assignment. Furthermore, the benefits of randomization are heavily diluted when the number of randomly assigned units is small, as when communities rather than individuals are randomized. Thus, environmental epidemiology consists nearly exclusively of non-experimental epidemiology. Ideally, such studies use individuals as the unit of measurement; but

often environmental data are available only for groups of individuals, and investigators turn to so-called ecologic studies to learn what they can.[15(p20)]

Randomized controlled trials follow a carefully executed research protocol with a treatment group (test group) and a control group. Research participants are allocated randomly to either one of these two conditions. An RCT bears similarities to experimental designs that you might have studied in experimental psychology, other behavioral science courses, or biology. In an experimental design, an investigator manipulates a study factor. Participants are assigned randomly to the study groups.

As noted in the foregoing definition, RCTs can have more than one treatment group and control group. In a **crossover design**, participants may be switched between or among treatment groups; an example is the transfer of members of treatment group A (e.g., test group) to treatment group B (e.g., placebo group—defined in the following section), or vice versa. An RCT combines the features of a traditional experimental design with several unique characteristics described in the following sections. Refer again to Figure 7-4 for an illustration of an RCT. Here are the components of an RCT:

- Selection of a study sample: Participants in an RCT could be volunteers or patients who have a particular disease. Rigorous inclusion and exclusion criteria are used in the selection of participants.
- Assignment of participants to study conditions: Random assignment is used.
  - The treatment group receives the new treatment, procedure, or drug.
  - The control group receives an alternative, commonly used treatment or procedure or a placebo, which is a medically inactive medication or pill (e.g., sugar pill). In a study of medical procedures, the control group might receive the usual standard of care. In a study of behavioral change, the control group might be given a self-instructional booklet. (The treatment group might receive group counseling.)
- Blinding or masking to prevent biases: When the participants or the investigators know the conditions of the study (i.e., treatment and control groups) to which participants have been assigned, multiple biases can be introduced.
  - **Single-blind study**: The subjects are unaware of whether they are participating in the treatment or control conditions.
  - **Double-blind study**: Neither the participants nor the investigators are aware of who has been assigned to the treatment or control conditions.
- Measurement of outcomes: Outcomes must be measured in a comparable manner in the treatment and control conditions. Outcomes of RCTs can include behavioral changes such as smoking cessation, increases in exercise levels, and reduction of behaviors that increase the risk of sexually transmitted diseases. An outcome of a clinical trial is called a clinical endpoint (examples are rates of disease, recovery, or death).

Quasi-Experimental Designs

A **community intervention (community trial)** is an intervention designed for the purpose of educational and behavioral changes at the population level. In most situations, community interventions use quasi-experimental designs. A **quasi-experimental study** is a type of research in which the investigator manipulates the study factor but does not assign individual subjects randomly to the exposed and nonexposed groups. Some quasi-experimental designs assign study units

(e.g., communities, counties, schools) randomly to the study conditions. In addition, some quasi-experimental designs may not use a control group or may use fewer study subjects (or other units) that are randomized into the study conditions than in a randomized controlled trial. The operation of community trials is expensive, complex, and time consuming. An important component of community interventions is **program evaluation**, the determination of whether the program meets stated goals and is justified economically.

A specific example of a community trial was a test of the efficacy of fluoridation of drinking water in preventing tooth decay.[16] During the 1940s and 1950s, two comparable cities in New York state—Newburgh and Kingston—were contrasted for the occurrence of tooth decay and related dental problems among children. Newburgh had received fluoride for about one decade and Kingston had received none. In Newburgh, the frequency of such problems decreased by about one-half in comparison to the period before fluoridation. Over the same period, those dental problems increased slightly in Kingston.[16] This study is an example of a quasi-experiment because the "subjects" (cities) were assigned arbitrarily and not randomly.

There are many other examples of community trials. One is the **Stanford Five-City Project**, which sought to reduce the risk of cardiovascular diseases. This trial was a media-based campaign directed at Monterey and Salinas, California. Control cities were Modesto and San Luis Obispo, with Santa Maria selected as an additional comparison city.[17] Another example is the Community Intervention Trial for Smoking Cessation (COMMIT), which began in 1989. This intervention trial involved 11 matched pairs of communities throughout the United States. The trial aimed to promote long-term smoking cessation.[18]

CHALLENGES TO THE VALIDITY OF STUDY DESIGNS

In addition to the type of study design chosen, several other factors affect the confidence that one may have in the results of a study. These factors are as follows:

- External validity: **External validity** refers to one's ability to generalize from the results of the study to an external population. Some studies may select subjects by taking a sample of convenience (a "grab bag" sample) or by using random samples of a population. Random samples are generally more representative of the parent population from which they are selected and thus are more likely to demonstrate external validity than are samples of convenience.

Nevertheless, random samples may depart from (be unrepresentative of) their parent populations. Sampling error is a type of error that arises when values (statistics) obtained for a sample differ from the values (parameters) of the parent population.

- Internal validity: Care must be taken in the manner in which a study is carried out. **Internal validity** refers to the degree to which the study has used methodologically sound procedures. For example, in an experimental design, subjects need to be assigned randomly to the conditions of the study. Appropriate and reliable measurements need to be taken. Departures from acceptable procedures such as those related to assignment of subjects and measurement as well as other errors in the methods used in the research may detract from the quality of inferences that can be made.

- Biases in outcome measurement: Several types of bias can affect the results of a study. These are discussed in the section that follows.

Bias in Epidemiologic Studies

Epidemiologic studies may be impacted by **bias**, which is defined as "[s]ystematic deviation of results or inferences from truth. Processes leading to such deviation. An error in the conception and design of a study—or in the collection, analysis, interpretation, reporting, publication, or review of data—leading to results or conclusions that are systematically (as opposed to randomly) different from truth."[1] There are many types of bias; particularly meaningful for epidemiology are those that impact study procedures. Examples of such bias are related to how the study was designed, the method of data collection, interpretation and review of findings, and procedures used in data analysis. For example, in measurements of exposures and outcomes, faulty measurement devices may introduce biases into study designs.

One of these biases is the **Hawthorne effect**, which refers to participants' behavioral changes as a result of their knowledge of being in a study. Three other types of bias are recall bias, selection bias, and confounding. The first is particularly relevant to case-control studies. **Recall bias** refers to the fact that cases (subjects who participate in the study) may remember an exposure more clearly than controls.[14] For example, **family recall bias** is a type of recall bias that occurs when cases are more likely to remember the details of their family history than are controls. The consequence of recall bias can be an overestimation of an association between an exposure and a health outcome.

Selection bias is defined as "[b]ias in the estimated association or effect of an exposure on an outcome that arises the from procedures used to select individuals into the study…"[1] An example of selection bias is the healthy worker effect, which may reduce the validity of exposure data. Occupational epidemiologist Richard Monson wrote that the **healthy worker effect** refers to the "observation that employed populations tend to have a lower mortality experience than the general population."[19(p114)] The healthy worker effect may have an impact on occupational mortality studies in several ways. People whose life expectancy is shortened by disease are less likely to be employed than healthy people. One consequence of this phenomenon would be a reduced (or attenuated) measure of effect (e.g., odds ratio or relative risk) for an exposure that increases morbidity or mortality. That is, because the general population includes both employed and unemployed individuals, the mortality rate of that population may be somewhat elevated in comparison with a population in which everyone is healthy enough to work. As a result, any excess mortality associated with a given occupational exposure is more difficult to detect when the healthy worker effect is operative. The healthy worker effect is likely to be stronger for nonmalignant causes of mortality, which usually produce worker attrition during an earlier career phase, than for malignant causes of mortality, which typically have longer latency periods and occur later in life. In addition, healthier workers may have greater total exposure to occupational hazards than those who leave the work force at an earlier age because of illness.

Confounding is another example of a type of study bias. **Confounding** denotes "… the distortion of a measure of the effect of an exposure on an outcome due to the association of the exposure with other factors that influence the occurrence of the outcome."[1] Confounding means that the effect of an exposure has been distorted because an extraneous factor has entered into the exposure–disease association. Confounding factors are those that are associated with disease risk (exposure factors) and produce a different distribution of outcomes in the exposure groups than in the comparison groups. An example of a potential confounder is age. Here is a possible scenario: An epidemiologist might have studied the relationship between exposure and disease in an exposed group and a nonexposed group; the exposed group might have higher rates of morbidity and mortality than the nonexposed group. If the study participants in the exposed group are older than those in the nonexposed group, the age difference could have caused the rates of disease to be higher in the exposed group. (Keep in mind that age is associated with morbidity.) The existence of confounding factors such as age might lead to invalid conclusions regarding exposure–outcome associations.

In addition to age as a confounder, a second example is the confounding effect of smoking. Exposure of workers to occupational dusts is associated with the development of lung diseases such as lung cancer. One of the types of dust encountered in the workplace is silica, e.g., from sand used in sandblasting. Suppose we find that workers exposed to silica have a higher mortality rate for lung cancer than is found in the general population. A possible conclusion is that the workers do, indeed, have a higher risk of lung cancer. However, the issue of confounding also should be considered: It is conceivable that employees exposed to silica dusts have higher smoking rates than the general population, which might be used as a comparison population. When smoking rates are taken into account, the strength of the association between silica exposure and lung cancer is reduced, suggesting that smoking is a confounder that needs to be considered in the association.[20]

How can bias due to confounding be controlled? One should attempt to make certain that the effects of potential confounders are controlled by using study groups that are comparable with respect to such confounders. Possible approaches would be to match study groups on age and sex (a procedure called matching) or to use statistical procedures such as multivariate analyses (not discussed here).

CONCLUSION

Epidemiologic study designs encompass descriptive and analytic approaches. One of the most common epidemiologic approaches, whether descriptive or analytic, is an observational study design. Examples of observational analytic study designs covered in this chapter were ecologic studies, case-control studies, and cohort studies. Ecologic studies are distinguished by the use of the group as the unit of analysis; the other study designs use individual subjects as the unit of analysis.

Differing from the observational approach are experimental designs (intervention studies). By definition, the investigator controls who is and who is not exposed to the study factor in an intervention study. Experimental designs include clinical trials and quasi-experimental designs. Clinical trials are used to test new medications, vaccines, and medical procedures. Clinical trials are implemented as randomized controlled trials (RCTs), which are rigorously designed experiments. Among the applications of quasi-experimental designs is the assessment of the effects of public health interventions. One must be aware of the strengths, weaknesses, and appropriate uses of each type of study design. Also, one must examine carefully possible biases, such as confounding, that can affect the validity of epidemiologic research.

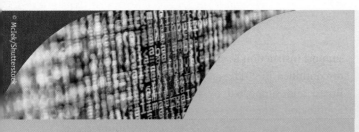

Study Questions and Exercises

1. Describe the two major approaches (observational and experimental) used in analytic studies. What circumstances would merit use of either of these approaches?

2. List the seven factors that characterize study designs and explain each one.

3. Define each of the following terms used by the U.S. Census Bureau:
   a. Census tract
   b. Census block
   c. Metropolitan statistical area

4. State one of the most important ways in which ecologic studies differ from other observational study designs used in epidemiology. What is meant by the ecologic fallacy? Using your own ideas, suggest a possible design for an ecologic study; how might the study design be affected by the ecologic fallacy?

5. Define the term *case-control study*. Describe how to calculate an odds ratio.

6. Define the term *cohort study*. What measure of association is used in a cohort study?

7. Interpret the following values for an odds ratio (OR) and a relative risk (RR):
   a. OR = 1.0; OR = 0.5; OR = 2.0
   b. RR = 1.0; RR = 0.5; RR = 2.0

8. Compare and contrast randomized controlled trials and quasi-experimental designs.

9. Identify the type of study design that is described by each of the following statements:
   a. The association between average unemployment levels and mortality from coronary heart disease was studied in counties in New York State.
   b. A group of women who had been diagnosed with breast cancer was compared with a group of cancer-free women; participants were asked whether they used oral contraceptives in the past.
   c. A group of recent college graduates (exercisers and nonexercisers) were followed over a period of 20 years in order to track the incidence of coronary heart disease.
   d. A pharmaceutical company wanted to test a new medicine for control of blood sugar. Study participants were assigned randomly to either a new medication group or a group that used an older medication. The investigator and the participants were blinded as to enrollment in the study conditions.

10. Define the terms *attributable risk* and *population risk difference*. What types of information do these measures provide?

11. Construct a grid that compares the advantages and disadvantages of the following study designs: ecologic, case-control, and cohort.

12. Define what is meant by bias in epidemiologic studies. Give examples of four types of bias.

13. In a hypothetical case-control study of female participants regarding exposure to EMFs and breast cancer, the following data were obtained: (Refer to Table 7-3 for labeling of cells.)

    A = 11, B = 108, C = 5, D = 436. Calculate the odds ratio for the association between exposure to EMFs and breast cancer. Interpret the results. (Answer for calculation: 8.9)

14. A hypothetical cohort study of pesticide exposure and cancer followed exposed pesticide workers and a comparison group of non-exposed employees of the same company over a 30-year period. Researchers found that the incidence of cancer among exposed workers was 55.3 per 1,000. In the comparison cohort not exposed to pesticides, the incidence of cancer was 15.7 per 1,000. Calculate the relative and attributable risks of exposure to pesticides and development of cancer. (Answer: RR = 3.5; AR = 39.7 per 1,000 exposed workers)

Young Epidemiology Scholars (YES) Exercises

The Young Epidemiology Scholars: Competitions website provides links to teaching units and exercises that support instruction in epidemiology. The YES program, discontinued in 2011, was administered by the College Board and supported by the Robert Wood Johnson Foundation. The exercises continue to be available at the following website: http://yes-competition.org/yes/teaching-units/title.html. The following exercises relate to topics discussed in this chapter and can be found on the YES competitions website.

1. Kaelin MA, Bayona M. Case-Control Study
2. Kaelin MA, Bayona M. Attributable Risk Applications in Epidemiology
3. Bayona M, Olsen C. Observational Studies and Bias in Epidemiology
4. Bayona M, Olsen C. Measures in Epidemiology
5. Huang FI, Stolley P. Testing Ephedra: Using Epidemiologic Studies to Teach the Scientific Method

REFERENCES

1. Porta M, ed. *A Dictionary of Epidemiology*. 6th ed. New York, NY: Oxford University Press; 2014.
2. Tabutin D, Schoumaker B. The demography of sub-Saharan Africa from the 1950s to the 2000s. *Population-E*. 2004;59(3–4):457–556.
3. Pollán M, Ramis R, Aragonés N, et al. Municipal distribution of breast cancer mortality among women in Spain. *BMC Cancer*. 2007;7(78). Available at: http://www.biomedcentral.com/1471-2407/7/78. Accessed July 12, 2016.
4. Shi L, Macinko J, Starfield B, et al. Primary care, social inequalities, and all-cause, heart disease, and cancer mortality in US counties, 1990. *Am J Public Health*. 2005;95:674–680.
5. Breslin FC, Smith P, Dunn JR. An ecological study of regional variation in work injuries among young workers. *BMC Public Health*. 2007;7(91). Available at: http://www.biomedcentral.com/1471-2458/7/91. Accessed July 11, 2016.
6. Blair A, Hayes RB, Stewart PA, Zahm SH. Occupational epidemiologic study design and application. *Occup Med*. 1996;11:403–419.
7. Miyake Y, Iki M. Ecologic study of water hardness and cerebrovascular mortality in Japan. *Arch Environ Health*. 2003;58:163–166.
8. Reynolds P, Von Behren J, Gunier RB, et al. Childhood cancer and agricultural pesticide use: an ecologic study in California. *Environ Health Perspect*. 2002;110:319–324.
9. Bhopal R. *Concepts of Epidemiology: Integrating the Ideas, Theories, Principles and Methods of Epidemiology*. 2nd ed. New York, NY: Oxford University Press; 2008.
10. Schoenfeld ER, O'Leary ES, Henderson K, et al. Electromagnetic fields and breast cancer on Long Island: a case-control study. *Am J Epidemiol*. 2003;158:47–58.
11. Taskinen HK. Epidemiological studies in monitoring reproductive effects. *Environ Health Perspect*. 1993;101(Suppl 3):279–283.
12. Beard J, Sladden T, Morgan G, et al. Health impacts of pesticide exposure in a cohort of outdoor workers. *Environ Health Perspect*. 2003;111:724–730.
13. Paul J, Seib R, Prescott T. The Internet and clinical trials: background, online resources, examples and issues. *J Med Internet Res*. 2005;7(1):e5.
14. Prentice RL, Thomas D. Methodologic research needs in environmental epidemiology: data analysis. *Environ Health Perspect*. 1993;101(Suppl 4):39–48.
15. Rothman KJ. Methodologic frontiers in environmental epidemiology. *Environ Health Perspect*. 1993;101(Suppl 4):19–21.
16. Morgenstern H, Thomas D. Principles of study design in environmental epidemiology. *Environ Health Perspect*. 1993;101(Suppl 4):23–38.
17. Fortmann SP, Flora JA, Winkleby MA, et al. Community intervention trials: reflections on the Stanford Five-City Project experience. *Am J Epidemiol*. 1995;142:579–580.
18. COMMIT Research Group. Community Intervention Trial for Smoking Cessation (COMMIT): summary of design and intervention. *J Natl Cancer Inst*. 1991;83:1620–1628.
19. Monson RR. *Occupational Epidemiology*. 2nd ed. Boca Raton, FL: CRC Press; 1990.
20. Steenland K, Greenland S. Monte Carlo sensitivity analysis and Bayesian analysis of smoking as an unmeasured confounder in a study of silica and lung cancer. *Am J Epidemiol*. 2004;160:384–392.

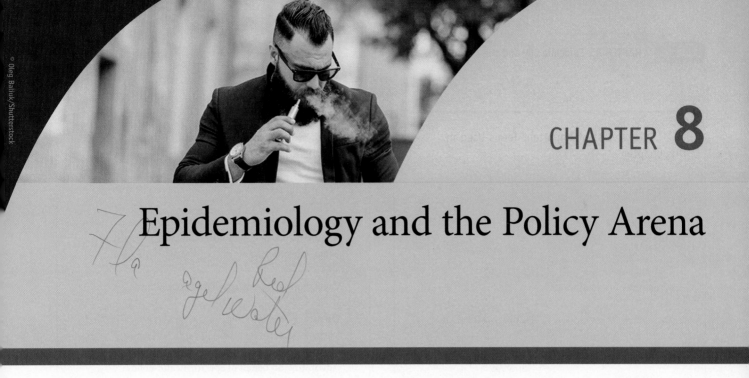

CHAPTER **8**

Epidemiology and the Policy Arena

Fla egeliester

LEARNING OBJECTIVES

By the end of this chapter you will be able to:

- State how policy development relates to the core functions of public health.
- Define the terms *policy* and *health policy*.
- Describe the steps of risk assessment, giving an example of each step.
- Compare two examples of policies that derive from epidemiologic research.
- Give three examples of ethics guidelines for epidemiology.

CHAPTER OUTLINE

INTRODUCTION

One of the most noteworthy and perhaps least recognized uses of epidemiology is the application of epidemiologic methods to the policy arena. Increasingly, epidemiologists

have been concerned with policy development. At first glance, this application would appear to differ from epidemiologists' usual focus on the design of studies, data collection, and analysis of exposure–disease relationships. However, you will learn that epidemiologic methods are transferrable to the policy domain. Implementation and enforcement of public health policies can require the expenditure of substantial monetary, personnel, and other resources.

This chapter relates epidemiologic methods to the broad issue of policy formulation. You will learn about the terminology of policy development and examples of major public health policies that have been informed through the application of epidemiologic methods. Increasing involvement of epidemiologists in policy development is justified by the recognition that many significant public health policies are established or abandoned in the absence of specific empirical evidence. Epidemiologists have the expertise to acquire the data needed for policy development and partner with policy makers to formulate cost-effective programs. Policy issues illustrate a situation where "the rubber hits the road" for applied epidemiology. Refer to **Table 8-1** for a list of important terms covered in this chapter.

EPIDEMIOLOGISTS' ROLES IN POLICY DEVELOPMENT

What are the roles of epidemiologists regarding policy development? They can provide the quantitative evidence for justifying needed policies. In addition, the input of

TABLE 8-1 List of Important Terms Used in This Chapter

Bisphenol A	Hazard identification
Core functions of public health	Healthy People
Cost-effectiveness (cost-benefit) analysis	Health policy
Cost-effectiveness ratio	Health in All Policies
Decision analysis	National Prevention Strategy
Dose-response assessment	Policy
Essential public health services	Policy cycle
Ethics	Risk assessment
Ethics guidelines	Risk characterization
Evidence-based public health	Risk management
Exposure assessment	*Trans* fats
Hazard	Tuskegee Study

TABLE 8-2 How Can Epidemiologists Contribute to Public Health Policy?

Performing research and sharing the results with others
Joining policy-making bodies that have expertise in public health issues
Contributing expertise to legal proceedings
Offering expert testimony to the various policy-making arms of government–from local to national
Advocating on behalf of specific health policy initiatives.

Data from Brownson RC. Epidemiology and health policy. In: Brownson RC, Petitti DB. *Applied Epidemiology: Theory to Practice*. 2nd ed. New York: Oxford University Press; 2006, 270.

epidemiologists can be helpful in demonstrating the effectiveness of policies once they have been adopted. These roles are accomplished in several ways.

The findings of epidemiologic research can result in the development of health policies and applicable laws. To illustrate, epidemiologists' discovery that asbestos exposure was associated with lung disease led to bans in the use of asbestos in consumer products.

Professional epidemiologists are called upon to give expert testimony regarding the potential health effects of exposures to environmental hazards; also, they serve on panels of scientific experts. **Table 8-2** gives additional examples of the roles of epidemiologists in health policy.

Epidemiologists take an objective stance with respect to data collection. Empirical data gathered in epidemiologic studies can provide quantitative and qualitative evidence for the efficacy of health policies. For example, policies that prohibit smoking in eating and alcohol-serving establishments initially met resistance because of their possible impact on the economy. Subsequent empirical evidence suggested that the economic impact of smokefree laws was minimal and that the positive health effects of such laws were likely to be substantial. In this case, the data supported the policy.

Epidemiologists operate in a rational domain by sequencing through gathering of data, contributing to interpretation of findings, and arriving at a consensus based on scientific principles.[1] All too often, health policies are implemented (or fail to be implemented) as a result of political pressures. In some cases, valuable and needed health policies may be abandoned in response to political backlash or the demands of a self-interested, vociferous minority. Policy making is inherently a messy political process; the governmental political domain is *terra incognita* for most epidemiologists.

Epidemiologists who aspire to function in the policy arena need to be mindful of the vastly different worlds of scientific objectivity and the realities of policy development. James Tallon, a leader in the field of healthcare policy, has written "[r]esearchers are from Mars; policy makers are from Venus."[2(p344)] As he noted, the realities of the policy maker and researcher are quite different, "similar to oil and water." Tallon states

> … [at the state level] legislators work within a broader context of state government, which includes governors, executive agencies, executive staffs, budget divisions, and the like. They also work within a context of interest groups, of media attention, and of course of a broader public who are, in a final analysis for legislators, their constituents…. But researchers can make their work relevant to state health policy if they are willing to focus on how to operate in that world. Most of us think of our research as our findings, our observations, our analysis. Let me take a step back and remind researchers that

they also do two other things—they frame the question and they create the context in which the question is analyzed.[2(p344)]

POLICY AND THE 10 ESSENTIAL PUBLIC HEALTH SERVICES

This section discusses policy from the standpoint of the three core functions of public health and the 10 Essential Public Health Services. In 1994, the Core Public Health Functions Steering Committee developed the framework for the essential services. The steering committee included members from well-known public health groups plus agencies that were part of the U.S. Public Health Service. **Figure 8-1** presents these core functions in a wheel, showing their alignment with the 10 essential public health services. The three **core functions of public health**

FIGURE 8-1 Essential public health services.

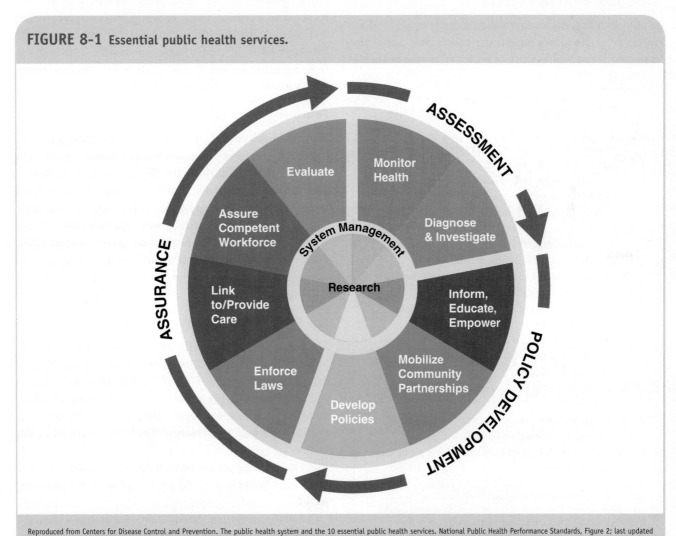

are assurance, assessment, and policy development. Note that policy development is one of the three categories of the core functions of public health. Subsumed under the three core functions are the 10 **essential public health services**. The wheel is helpful in showing the interrelationships among the core functions and essential services, which are listed in **Table 8-3**.

Refer for a moment to Table 8-3. From our previous discussion of the uses of epidemiology, you are aware of how epidemiology can aid with item 1 (identify community health problems) and item 2 (diagnose health problems and health hazards). Epidemiology also can contribute to item 9 (evaluate personal and population-based health services). These three items are necessary antecedents of policy development, which involves mobilization of community partnerships and education of people about health issues.

WHAT IS A HEALTH POLICY?

Before providing more information on the epidemiologic aspects of policy development, the author will define the terms *policy* and *health policy*. A **policy** is "a plan or course

TABLE 8-3   The 10 Essential Public Health Services

1. Monitor health status to identify and solve community health problems.
2. Diagnose and investigate health problems and health hazards in the community.
3. Inform, educate, and empower people about health issues.
4. Mobilize community partnerships and action to identify and solve health problems.
5. Develop policies and plans that support individual and community health efforts.
6. Enforce laws and regulations that protect health and ensure safety.
7. Link people to needed personal health services and assure the provision of health care when otherwise unavailable.
8. Assure competent public and personal healthcare workforce.
9. Evaluate effectiveness, accessibility, and quality of personal and population-based health services.
10. Research for new insights and innovative solutions to health problems.

Reproduced from Centers for Disease Control and Prevention. The public health system and the 10 essential public health services. National Public Health Performance Standards; last updated May 29, 2014. Available at: http://www.cdc.gov/nphpsp/essentialservices.html. Accessed June 16, 2016.

of action, as of a government, political party, or business, intended to influence and determine decisions, actions, and other matters."[3]

A **health policy** is one that pertains to the health arena, for example, in dentistry, medicine, public health, or regarding provision of healthcare services. "Health policies, in the form of laws, regulations, organizational practices, and funding priorities, have a substantial impact on the health and well-being of the population. Policies influence nearly every aspect of daily life, ranging from seat belt use in cars, to where smoking is allowed, to access to health care."[4(p260)] Public health policies apply to such aspects of health as water quality, food safety, health promotion, and environmental protection.

Policies are not equivalent to laws, which either require or proscribe certain behaviors. Nevertheless, health policies are linked with the development of laws such as those involved in licensing (e.g., licensing medical practitioners and medications), setting standards (e.g., specifying the allowable levels of contaminants in food), controlling risk (e.g., requiring the use of child safety seats), and monitoring (e.g., surveillance of infectious diseases).

Policy Implementation

How is a health policy implemented? An overarching mission of government health agencies, such as health departments, is to protect the public from the effects of infectious diseases. This mission is translated into health policies. Government agencies implement these policies by enacting laws and regulations that apply to specific domains. Examples are laws that require the immunization of children against communicable diseases, maintenance of hygienic sanitary conditions in restaurants, and protection of the public water supply from contamination.

The Policy Cycle and Policy Creation

The **policy cycle** refers to the distinct phases involved in the policy-making process[5] (See **Figure 8-2**). The policy cycle comprises several stages: (1) problem definition, formulation, and reformulation; (2) agenda setting; (3) policy establishment (i.e., adoption and legislation); (4) policy implementation; and (5) policy assessment. These are described in this section.

The terms subsumed under the policy cycle are explained more fully in **Table 8-4** and are described in the following section.

Problem definition, formulation, and reformulation: the processes of defining the problem for which the policy actors believe that policies are necessary. This early stage—problem

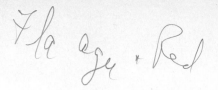

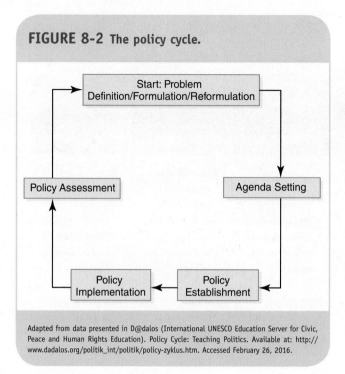

FIGURE 8-2 The policy cycle.

Adapted from data presented in D@dalos (International UNESCO Education Server for Civic, Peace and Human Rights Education). Policy Cycle: Teaching Politics. Available at: http://www.dadalos.org/politik_int/politik/policy-zyklus.htm. Accessed February 26, 2016.

definition and development of alternative solutions—often is regarded as the most crucial phase of the policy development process. The problems chosen should be significant for public health and have realistic and practical solutions. Poorly defined problems are unlikely to lead to successful policy implementation. Note that Figure 8-2 (The policy cycle)

shows that, following a process of review, problem definitions may need to be reformulated and the steps in the policy cycle repeated.

Agenda setting: establishing priorities, deciding at what time to deal with a public health problem or issue, and determining who will deal with the problem. Policy makers need to establish priorities in order to reconcile budgetary constraints, resource restrictions, and the complexity of public health problems against the need to develop those policies that are most feasible, realistic, and workable. A successful approach in developing priorities for public health policies is to involve the community and stakeholders. However, agenda setting is hampered by limited information on health risks and lack of coordination among government agencies.

One of the difficulties in establishing priorities stems from the lack of information on risks.[6] Consider the development of policies related to control of environmental health hazards. (Environmental health is a topic with an extensive track record of policy development.) For example, the public may be concerned about the presence of suspected carcinogenic chemicals used in plastic containers for storing food. Suppose that the carcinogenic properties of plastic containers (or whether, in fact, they are indeed carcinogenic) have not been established definitively. Nor is it known how much exposure to the chemical is needed in order to produce an adverse health effect. Given the dearth of information about the level of risk posed by the chemical, one would have difficulties in establishing an appropriate policy for manufacture

TABLE 8-4 Components of the Policy Cycle

	Problem Definition, Formulation, and Reformulation	Agenda Setting	Policy Establishment	Policy Implementation	Assessment/ Evaluation
What happens?	Define problems and alternatives	Set priorities; involve stakeholders	Formally adopt public policy; legitimization	Put the policy into practice	Assess or evaluate effectiveness
Who performs the function?	Formal and informal policy actors	Formal and informal policy actors	Formal decision makers	Government agencies	Arm of government responsible for assessment

(continues)

TABLE 8-4 Components of the Policy Cycle (continued)

	Problem Definition, Formulation, and Reformulation	Agenda Setting	Policy Establishment	Policy Implementation	Assessment/ Evaluation
What factors influence policy?	Research and science; interest groups; public opinion; social and economic factors	Research and science; interest groups; public opinion; social and economic factors	Research and science; interest groups; public opinion; social and economic factors	Research and science; interest groups; public opinion; social and economic factors	Research and science; interest groups; public opinion; social and economic factors
What problems are encountered?	Poorly defined problems	Lack of information on risk; lack of coordination	Inability to coordinate and assess research information	Lack of government support	Lack of sound scientific data

Definitions:

Policy actors: individuals who are involved in policy formulation; these include members of the legislature, citizens, lobbyists, and representatives of advocacy groups.

Stakeholders: individuals, organizations, and members of government who are affected by policy decisions.

Legitimization: the process of making policies legitimate, meaning to be acceptable to the norms of society.

Interest group: "Non-profit and usually voluntary organization whose members have a common cause for which they seek to influence public policy, without seeking political control"[7] (e.g., business groups, trade unions, religious groups, and professional associations).

Adapted from Friis RH. *Essentials of Environmental Health.* 2nd ed. Burlington, MA: Jones & Bartlett Learning; 2012:71.

and use of the plastic containers that incorporate the chemical. When the nature of the risks associated with an environmental hazard or toxin is uncertain, planners are left in a quandary about what aspects of the exposure require policy interventions. In illustration, this level of uncertainty has surrounded the safety of BPA, a chemical ingredient used in plastic containers for food storage. (Currently, BPA may be added to plastics used to manufacture food storage containers. Its use in baby bottles, sippy cups, and infant formula packaging is not permitted.)

Another barrier to agenda setting is lack of coordination among government agencies.[8] A criticism levied against the U.S. Congress, which is a crucial policy-formulating body for the government of the United States, is its inability to set priorities because of fragmentation of authority among numerous committees and subcommittees that are involved with environmental policy.

Policy establishment: the formal adoption of policies, programs, and procedures that are designed to protect society from public health hazards. Once again, in the environmental

health arena, a factor that impedes policy establishment is the unavailability of empirical information on the scope of risks associated with environmental hazards. According to Bailus Walker, former president of the American Public Health Association, "Limitations on our ability to coordinate, assess, and disseminate research information hampers efforts to translate policy into programs and services designed to reduce environmental risk."[7(p190)]

Policy implementation: the phase of the policy cycle that "… focuses on achieving the objectives set forth in the policy decision."[7(p186)] Often this phase of the policy cycle is neglected in favor of the earlier phases of policy development. Barriers to policy implementation can arise from the actions of lobbying groups to influence the government administration in power. In the case of the United States, political considerations can lead to weakened policies.

The political and social contexts may stimulate or impede the creation and implementation of public health policies. As Tallon noted, government officials work within the political context and must be able to negotiate this domain if they are to be successful. The impetus for policy development often arises from advocacy groups and lobbyists. Also, special interest groups can mount effective campaigns to block policy initiatives.

In order to overcome barriers to policy implementation, policy developers may include incentives for the adoption of policies. An illustration is the availability of economic incentives to increase energy efficiency. Some states and the federal government have offered rebates for the purchase of energy-saving devices: solar electric panels, solar hot water heating systems, energy-efficient appliances, and fuel-efficient automobiles.

Policy assessment/evaluation: determining whether the policy has met defined objectives and related goals. The final stage in the policy cycle, this process may be accomplished by applying the methods of epidemiology as well as other tools, such as those from economics. The result is a body of quantitative information that can reveal the degree to which the policy has met stated objectives.

Environmental policies illustrate the linkage between assessment and objectives. In order to facilitate their assessment, environmental policies may incorporate *environmental objectives*, which "are statements of policy… intended to be assessed using information from a monitoring program. An

environmental monitoring program has to be adequate in its quality and quantity of data so that the environmental objectives can be assessed."[9(p144)] An example of an environmental objective is the statement that the amount of particulate matter in an urban area (e.g., Mexico City) will be reduced by 10% during the next 5 years.

Another example of a statement of objectives can be found on the Healthy People website (www.healthypeople.gov). The national collaborative effort known as **Healthy People** articulates science-derived objectives for advancing the health of Americans.[10] These objectives are meant to be accomplished within 10-year cycles. *Healthy People 2010* set forth objectives for the decade beginning in 2000. The Healthy People agenda is intended for use both by individuals and numerous, groups, agencies, and organizations in the United States.

Healthy People 2020 continues along similar lines as the preceding document. This version specifies 1,200 objectives in 42 public health topic areas.[11] Twenty-six leading health indicators address high-priority areas such as reduction of tobacco use and increasing physical activity. Regarding tobacco use, the indicator is the age-adjusted percentage of adults who smoke cigarettes. As of March 2014, the percentage of smokers had declined, marking progress regarding this indicator. **Figure 8-3** presents information regarding the status of the 26 indicators.

FIGURE 8-3 Status of the 26 *Healthy People 2020* leading health indicators, March 2014.

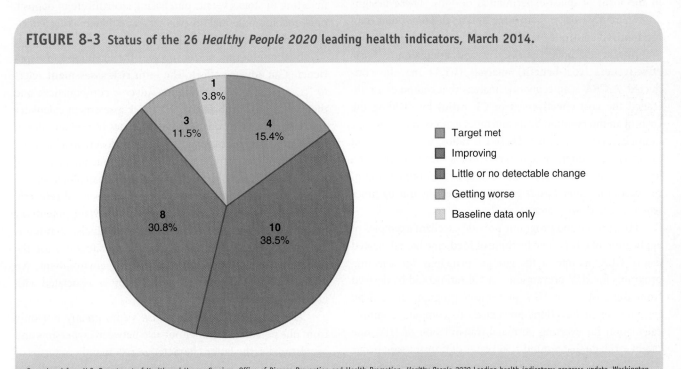

Evidence-Based Policy

Policy assessment and evaluation are a function of the quality of evidence that is available to policy makers. **Evidence-based public health** refers to the adoption of policies, laws, and programs that are supported by empirical data. "Evidence reduces uncertainty in decision making. Evidence is about reality, about what is true and not true."[12(p357)]

Pertinent to the discussion of evidence is the evidence-based medicine movement, which has been attributed to the late Archie Cochrane. The noted physician argued that medical care often used procedures that lacked empirical data with respect to their safety and efficacy.[13] Cochrane advocated the use of clinical trials for substantiating the efficacy of medical practices.

Empirical data varies in quality; one of the most reliable forms of evidence comes from randomized controlled trials, one of the varieties of clinical trials. Epidemiologic studies can be arranged according to a hierarchy with respect to their validity for etiologic inference. Less valid are those studies that fall lower on the hierarchy (e.g., case studies, ecologic studies, and cross-sectional studies). However, it is not always feasible to attain the high standard of randomized controlled trials in providing justification for public health interventions that are reflections of policy implementation. Evaluation of most public health policies takes place in the form of quasi-experimental designs. These designs are inherently weaker from a methodologic standpoint than randomized controlled trials.

As part of policy assessment and evaluation, a **cost-effectiveness (cost-benefit) analysis (CEA)** may be conducted. A CEA is an economic analysis that computes a ratio (called the **cost-effectiveness** or **CE ratio**) by dividing the costs of an intervention by its outcomes expressed as units, for example, deaths averted.[14] These CE ratios, when compared for alternative programs and interventions, help to identify the least costly alternatives. A CEA facilitates the optimization of resources for public health programs, especially during times when resources are scarce.

HIV prevention programs provide excellent examples of application of CEAs. The Institute of Medicine has advocated use of CEAs as one of the guiding principles for selecting programs for HIV prevention.[15] A CE ratio could be derived from the cost of an HIV prevention program divided by the number of infections prevented. To compute a sample calculation for averting perinatal transmission of HIV, one might estimate that around 1,560 cases of transmission occur annually. The costs for screening and treatment of infected mothers might total $51 million. The CE ratio would be $32,700 per case prevented ($51,000,000/1,560). By applying this same methodology, the CE ratio of alternative programs for HIV prevention could be developed and then all of the CEs compared in order to determine which program is the most cost effective.

DECISION ANALYSIS BASED ON PERCEPTIONS OF RISKS AND BENEFITS

Decision analysis involves developing a set of possible choices and stating the likely outcomes linked with those choices, each of which may have associated risks and benefits. Ideally, policy makers will select alternatives that minimize health risks and maximize desirable health outcomes and other benefits. Let us briefly examine the concept of risk. Be aware of the fact that life is not free from risks that have the potential to harm our health and well-being. Even the most benign activities carry risk: while riding on a busy street, a bicyclist may be struck by a car. Once the author heard about a professor who had struggled during most of his professional life, eagerly anticipating retirement; eventually the long-awaited moment arrived. A short time after his retirement, the campus received the sad news that the professor had choked to death on his meal while viewing an intense sports event on television. In summary, many aspects of life involve weighing risks—e.g., buying versus renting a house, investing in stocks versus purchasing a certificate of deposit, or choosing a potential life partner—and then making a decision about what action to take.

In simple terms, a *risk* involves the likelihood of experiencing an adverse effect. The term **risk assessment** refers to "... a process for identifying adverse consequences and their associated probability."[16(p611)] Risk assessment calculates either qualitative or quantitative estimates of probabilities of undesirable outcomes, given a specific exposure to a hazard.[17] The process can include the input of various forms of data, for example from epidemiologic research, toxicologic assays, or environmental investigations. In environmental research, risk assessment strives to identify and alleviate potentially harmful situations that could injure individuals, communities, or ecosystems.[18] In many cases, these situations are the result of people's impact on the natural environment. An example is risks of adverse health outcomes associated with use of fossil fuels.

The meaning of the term *risk* varies greatly not only from one person to another but also between laypersons and professionals; the latter characterize risk mainly in terms of mortality.[19] In a psychometric study, Slovic reported that laypersons classified risk according to two major factors.

(Psychometrics is a field concerned with psychological measurements.) His methods enabled risks to be portrayed in a two-dimensional space so that their relative positions could be compared. The two factors that Slovic identified were the following:

> Factor 1, labeled "dread risk," is defined at its high (right-hand) end by perceived lack of control, dread, catastrophic potential, fatal consequences, and the inequitable distribution of risks and benefits....
> Factor 2, labeled "unknown risk," is defined at its high end by hazards judged to be unobservable, unknown, new, and delayed in their manifestation of harm.[19(p283)]

Refer to **Figure 8-4**, which maps the spatial relationships among a large number of risks. For example, nuclear reactor accidents fall in the space that defines uncontrollable dread factors that are of unknown risk. In other words, nuclear reactor accidents fall in the quadrant defined by both high levels of unknown risk and high levels of dread risk. Another example is home swimming pools, which pose risks that are not dreaded and are known to those exposed.

Risk assessment generally takes place in four steps: (1) hazard identification, (2) dose-response assessment, (3) exposure assessment, and (4) risk characterization.[20,21] Refer to **Figure 8-5** for an illustration. Let's examine each one of the foregoing terms in more detail.

Hazard Identification

Hazard identification applies generally to public health but is particularly well developed in environmental health research with toxic substances. **Hazard identification** (hazard assessment) "... examines the evidence that associates exposure to an agent with its toxicity and produces a qualitative judgment about the strength of that evidence, whether it is derived from human epidemiology or extrapolated from laboratory animal data."[21(p286)] Evidence regarding hazards linked to toxic substances may be derived from the study of health effects among exposed humans and animals. These health effects may range from dramatic outcomes, such as mortality or cancer, to lower-level conditions, such as developmental delays in children and reductions in immune status.[20]

A **hazard** is defined as the "inherent capability of an agent or a situation to have an adverse effect. A factor or exposure that may adversely affect health."[17] Hazards may originate from chemicals, biological agents, physical and mechanical energy and force, and psychosocial influences. Toxic agents such as organic toxins and chemicals are examples of potential sources of hazards. Physical hazards arise from ionizing radiation emitted by medical x-ray devices or from naturally occurring background radiation. Other hazards originate from non-ionizing radiation—sunlight, infrared and ultraviolet light, and electromagnetic radiation from power lines and radio transmissions. In urban and work environments, mechanical energy is associated with high noise levels that can be hazardous for hearing and psychological well-being. Psychosocial hazards include work-related stresses, combat fatigue, and recall of posttraumatic events.

Dose-Response Assessment

Dose-response assessment is the measurement of "... the relationship between the amount of exposure and the occurrence of the unwanted health effects."[20(p38)] Dose-response assessment is one of the activities of toxicology, the science of poisons. In their research, some toxicologists examine biologic responses to exposure to toxicants, which are toxic substances created by human activity or natural processes. According to Russell and Gruber, "Dose-response assessment examines the quantitative relation between the experimentally administered dose level of a toxicant and the incidence or severity or both of a response in test animals, and draws inferences for humans. The presumed human dosages and incidences in human populations may also be used in cases where epidemiological studies are available."[21(p286)]

Exposure Assessment

Exposure assessment is defined as the procedure that "... identifies populations exposed to the toxicant, describes their composition and size, and examines the roots, magnitudes, frequencies, and durations of such exposures."[21(p286)] High-quality data on exposure are necessary for making valid interpretations of a study's findings.[22] The quality of exposure assessment data determines the accuracy of risk assessments and therefore is a limiting factor in the risk assessment process.[23] However, the process of human exposure assessment is believed to be one of the weakest aspects of risk assessment in epidemiology, particularly when exposures occur at low levels.

When referring to a toxic substance, exposure assessment must take into account where the exposure occurs, how much exposure occurs, and how the substance is absorbed by the body. The process of human exposure assessment examines "... the manner in which pollutants come into actual contact with the human body—the concentration levels at the points of contact and the sources of these pollutants

FIGURE 8-4 Location of 81 hazards on factors 1 and 2 derived from the relationships among 15 risk characteristics.

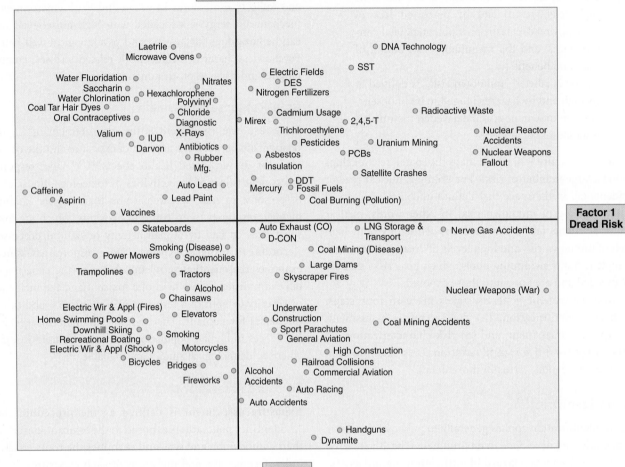

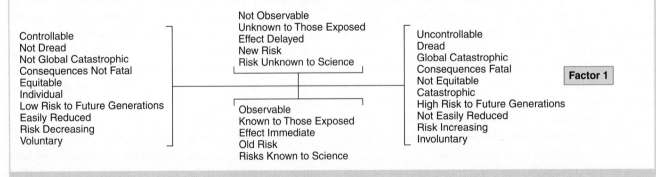

FIGURE 8-5 Steps in risk assessment.

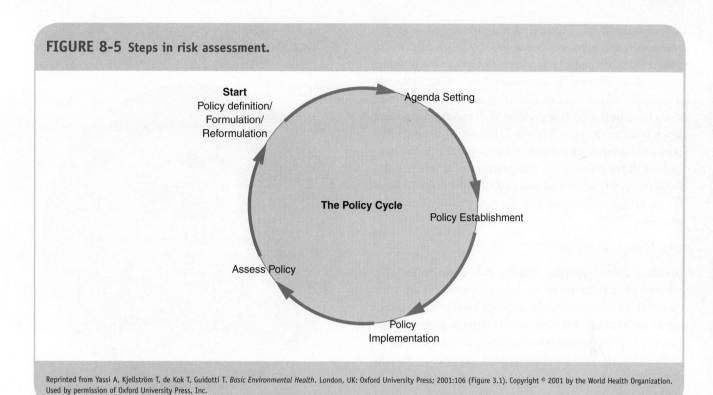

making contact. The key word here is 'contact'—the occurrence of two events at the same location and same time."[24(p449)] The methods by which human beings are exposed to toxic substances include encountering them in water, air, food, soil, and various consumer products and medications. Several methods of exposure assessment are used in toxicology, environmental epidemiology, and other environmental health disciplines. These include direct measures of the environment and personal exposure monitoring. Two examples covered in this section are reviews of archival materials to document exposures and use of biomarkers (biological markers) of exposure.

A review of company personnel records is one of the methods used in occupational health research for assessing exposures to work-related hazards. A simplified illustration is the examination of job classifications, which may record on-the-job exposures to hazardous substances; information regarding tenure of employment may suggest duration of these exposures.

If the records of former and retired workers have been retained by the company, a complete data set spanning long time periods may be available. This information could be obtained for retrospective cohort studies. Ideally, every previous and current worker exposed to the factor should be included in an occupational health study. Selection bias may

occur if some workers are excluded because their records have been purged from the company's database.[25] Data relevant to exposures that might be collected from employment records may include:

- Personal identifiers to permit record linkage to Social Security Administration files and retrieval of death certificates
- Demographic characteristics, length of employment, and work history with the company
- Information about potential confounding variables, such as the employee's medical history, smoking habits, lifestyle, and family history of disease

Another way to measure exposures is to measure biomarkers. Some environmental studies use biomarkers that may be correlated with exposures to potential carcinogens and other chemicals. These biomarkers involve changes in genetic structure that are thought to be the consequence of an exposure.

Risk Characterization

Risk characterization develops "... estimates of the number of excess unwarranted health events expected at different time intervals at each level of exposure."[20(p38)] Risk characterization follows the three foregoing steps by integrating the information from hazard identification, dose-response assessment, and exposure assessment.[26] The process of risk characterization yields "a synthesis and summary of information about a hazard that addresses the needs and interests of decision makers and of interested and affected parties. Risk characterization is a prelude to decision making and depends on an iterative, analytic-deliberative process."[27(p216)] "Risk characterization presents the policy maker with a synopsis of all the information that contributes to a conclusion about the nature of the risk and evaluates the magnitudes of the uncertainties involved and the major assumptions that were used."[21(p286)]

Risk Management

Oriented toward specific actions, **risk management** "... consists of actions taken to control exposures to toxic chemicals in the environment. Exposure standards, requirements for premarket testing, recalls of toxic products, and outright banning of very hazardous materials are among the actions that are used by governmental agencies to manage risk."[20(p37)]

EXAMPLES OF PUBLIC HEALTH POLICIES AND LAWS

This section presents information regarding major health policies and several public health–related laws. The Healthy People documents, covered earlier in the chapter, exemplify a groundbreaking body of health-related policies for the United States.

A second policy formulation, the **National Prevention Strategy**, is an effort to improve the nation's level of health and well-being through four strategic directions and seven targeted priorities.[28] **Figure 8-6** shows the strategic directions and targeted priorities. A sample strategic direction is promotion of healthy and safe community environments; targeted priorities include healthy eating, active living, and mental and emotional well-being. A group known as the National Prevention Council oversees national leadership for the National Prevention Strategy. The Affordable Care Act established the National Prevention Council, which is chaired by the U.S. Surgeon General. Data from ongoing data collection activities such as those by Healthy People are used for tracking progress toward key indicators.

Still another policy formulation is Health in All Policies, described in the next section. The philosophical underpinnings of Health in All Policies are unique for their emphasis on collaboration at multiple levels.

FIGURE 8-6 National Prevention Strategy.

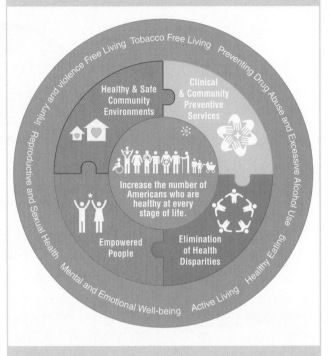

Reproduced from National Prevention Council, National Prevention Strategy, Washington, DC: U.S. Department of Health and Human Services, Office of the Surgeon General; 2011, 7.

Health in All Policies

"**Health in All Policies** is a collaborative approach to improving the health of all people by incorporating health considerations into decision making across sectors and policy areas."[29(p6)] (See **Figure 8-7**.) An example at the governmental level is incorporating health considerations into the design of neighborhoods. Design considerations that promote a healthy environment include availability of clean water and air, excellent housing quality, access to public parks, and neighborhood walkability. Another illustration of an application of Health in All Policies is in addressing the obesity epidemic in the United States. A strategy would be a multisectoral approach, which might include the coordinated efforts of educational institutions (health education), agriculture (production of nutritious foods), and the media (promotion of active lifestyles). Refer to **Table 8-5** for more information.

Public Health–Related Laws and Regulations

Some public health–related laws and regulations are presented in **Table 8-6**. One especially noteworthy example applies to laws for controlling exposure to cigarette smoke in alcohol-serving

FIGURE 8-7 What is Health in All Policies?

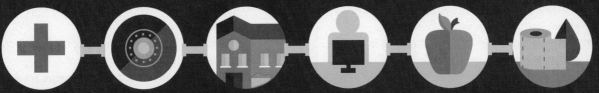

Good health requires policies that actively support health

It requires different sectors working together, for example:

HEALTH   TRANSPORT   HOUSING   WORK   NUTRITION   WATER & SANITATION

TO ENSURE ALL PEOPLE HAVE EQUAL OPPORTUNITIES TO ACHIEVE THE HIGHEST LEVEL OF HEALTH

Reproduced from United Nations. Available at: http://www.who.int/social_determinants/publications/health-policies-manual/HiAP_Infographic.pdf?ua=1. Accessed June 27, 2016.

TABLE 8-5 Health in All Policies

- Health in All Policies is a collaborative approach to improving the health of all people by incorporating health considerations into decision making across sectors and policy areas.
- Health is influenced by the social, physical, and economic environments, collectively referred to as the "social determinants of health."
- Health in All Policies, at its core, is an approach to addressing the social determinants of health that are the key drivers of health outcomes and health inequities.
- Health in All Policies supports improved health outcomes and health equity through collaboration between public health practitioners and those nontraditional partners who have influence over the social determinants of health.
- Health in All Policies approaches include five key elements: promoting health and equity, supporting intersectoral collaboration, creating cobenefits for multiple partners, engaging stakeholders, and creating structural or process change.
- Health in All Policies encompasses a wide spectrum of activities and can be implemented in many different ways.
- Health in All Policies initiatives build on an international and historical body of collaborative work.

Reprinted from Rudolph L, Caplan J, Ben-Moshe K, Dillon L. Health in All Policies: a guide for state and local governments. Washington, DC and Oakland, CA: American Public Health Association and Public Health Institute; 2013.

establishments, other public venues, and the workplace. Second, much effort has been expended to regulate the nutritional content and portion sizes of beverages and foods sold in chain restaurants. A final example relates to safeguarding the public from chemicals (e.g., bisphenol A) that can leach into food from storage containers.

TABLE 8-6 Public Health–Related Laws and Regulations

- Smokefree public venues, e.g., bars and restaurants
- Prohibition of smoking in automobiles when children are present
- Prohibition of texting and requiring the use of hands-free cellular telephones while driving
- Regulating the amount of particulate matter that can be emitted from motor vehicles
- Regulating the nutritional content of food sold in restaurants
- Removing high-fat and high-sugar content foods from vending machines in schools
- Requiring the use of helmets by motorcyclists and by children when riding bicycles
- Controlling toxic chemicals in foods

Smokefree Bars Laws

A significant public policy development concerns smokefree bars laws that were first adopted in California. The impetus for the implementation of smokefree laws was the growing body of information about the health hazards that second-hand cigarette exposure presented in the work setting. These hazards endangered the employees of alcohol-serving establishments, as well as customers. Epidemiologic studies were one of the sources of data that demonstrated the adverse health effects of smoking and exposure to secondhand cigarette smoke.

In 1998, the California state legislature passed a law (AB 3037) that prohibited smoking in all workplaces, including alcohol-serving establishments. The purpose of AB 3037 was to protect workers from the health effects associated with secondhand smoke. Initially, it was feared that the law would be opposed or ignored by the public and the business community and thus be doomed to failure. A survey of the residents of a large city (Long Beach) in California found strong approval of the prohibition of smoking in all indoor public places. Two-thirds and three-fourths of the respondents approved of the law in 1998 and 2000, respectively.[30]

Remarkable is the decline in the percentage of adult smokers over time following California's implementation of tobacco control policies; as of late 2013, the prevalence of smoking in California had fallen to slightly less than 12%. In 2016, new California laws eliminated electronic cigarettes from smokefree areas and increased the minimum age for purchasing tobacco products to age 21.

The strong endorsement of the smokefree bars law in California has had major public health and policy implications. Some of these policy implications are the following:

- Should smoking be restricted at public venues such as public beaches?
- Should tobacco taxes be increased further to fund smoking cessation programs and research?
- What are the economic effects of the law, e.g., how have businesses been impacted?
- Are smokefree policies being enforced?
- Are businesses complying?
- Does banning of cigarette smoking result in increases in the use of other forms of tobacco?
- Should films be prevented from showing smoking by societal role models such as glamorous movie stars?

National and Global Status of Smokefree Laws

Smokefree bars laws that were first adopted in California have spread across the United States. Eventually, countries in Europe and many other countries across the world have enacted smokefree laws. **Exhibit 8-1** presents a case study that reviews the status of smokefree bars laws.

Banning *Trans* Fats in Foods

Trans fats are manufactured though the process of hydrogenation, whereby hydrogen is added to vegetable oils. Hydrogenated oils increase the shelf life of products, hence their widespread use. They are added to many popular foods including baked goods and French fries. Epidemiologic evidence suggests that the use of *trans* fats (hydrogenated fats) is associated with coronary heart disease as well as stroke and diabetes. Consumption of *trans* fats can lead to increases in "bad cholesterol" and the build-up of arterial plaques. (Refer to **Figure 8-8**, which shows a low-fat baked potato versus high-fat French fries.)

With the adoption of a new law (AB 97) in 2008, California became the first state in the United States to ban the use of *trans* fats in restaurants. As of January 1, 2010, all restaurants in the state of California were prohibited from cooking with *trans* fats.[31] In 2015, the U.S. Food and Drug Administration required the removal of *trans* fats from processed foods.[32] The regulation is being phased in over a 3-year period.

Should the Use of Bisphenol A (BPA) Be Curtailed?

Bisphenol A (BPA) is a chemical ingredient used in the manufacture of plastics and resins. This chemical is used in food containers, on ATM receipts, and in many other applications. It is no longer used in baby bottles, sippy cups,

EXHIBIT 8-1 Case Study: Status of Smokefree Bars Laws, United States and Europe

United States

Since the adoption of California's smokefree bars law, other states and government agencies in the United States have adopted similar laws. For example:

- 30 U.S. states plus the District of Columbia, Puerto Rico, and the U.S. Virgin Islands, require two venues (bars and restaurants) to be 100% smokefree (as of July 2016).
- 25 states plus the District of Columbia, Puerto Rico, and the U.S. Virgin Islands, require three venues (bars and restaurants plus nonhospitality worksites) to be 100% smokefree.
- The U.S. government prohibits smoking on commercial aircraft; smoking is prohibited in airports and many other confined public areas.

Global Situation

Here are selected examples in Europe: Total bans on smoking in bars (2013 data) have been implemented by some member states of the European Union (EU), for example Ireland, Spain, and Norway. Bans on smoking in bars but with areas set aside for smokers exist in Belgium, France, Italy, and Sweden. Partial bans on smoking (special smoking zones and exemptions of some categories of bars) have been instituted in Denmark, Germany, and Netherlands. The United Kingdom, which plans to exit the EU, also has a total ban on smoking in bars. In addition, many other countries across the globe, for example, Turkey, have adopted smokefree laws or are considering such legislation.

Data from American Nonsmokers' Rights Foundation[33] and the European Commission.[34]

and infant formula packaging. Human beings are exposed to BPA through food and contact with BPA-containing products. National biomonitoring studies have suggested that more than 90% of the U.S. population have detectable levels of BPA in their urine. The policy issue with respect to BPA is whether this omnipresent chemical poses a significant health hazard and, consequently, whether its use should be curtailed.

According to the National Toxicology Program (NTP), the scientific evidence supports a conclusion of *some concern* for exposures to BPA in fetuses, infants, and children. The justification of the NTP's position comes from some laboratory animal studies, which suggest that BPA may affect the development of fetal and newborn animals. The NTP concluded that "… there is limited evidence of developmental changes occurring in some animal studies at doses that are experienced by humans. It is uncertain if similar changes would occur in humans, but the possibility of adverse health effects cannot be dismissed."[35(p2)]

Although the National Toxicology Program declared that there was some concern regarding exposures to BPA, the U.S. Food and Drug Administration stated that "… the available information continues to support the safety of BPA for the currently approved uses in food containers and packaging."[36]

ETHICS AND EPIDEMIOLOGY

Description of Ethics in Research

The final topic in this chapter relates to ethics and epidemiology. Ethical concerns have implications for policy issues regarding treatment of human subjects and the design of research protocols. The term **ethics** refers to "… *norms for*

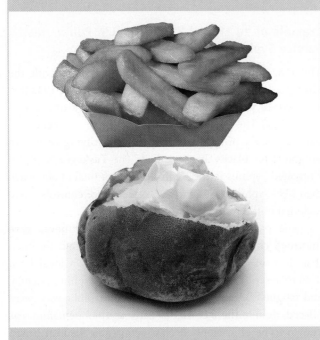

FIGURE 8-8 Baked potato or French fries?

Reproduced from National Institute on Aging. Taking in calories. Available at: https://www.nia.nih.gov/health/publication/whats-your-plate/taking-calories. Accessed July 21, 2016.

conduct that distinguish between... acceptable and unacceptable behavior."[37] David B. Resnik, bioethicist for the National Institute of Environmental Health Sciences, has written the following statement about ethics in research:

> When most people think of ethics (or morals), they think of rules for distinguishing between right and wrong, such as the Golden Rule ("Do unto others as you would have them do unto you"), a code of professional conduct like the Hippocratic Oath ("First of all, do no harm"), a religious creed like the Ten Commandments ("Thou Shalt not kill..."), or a wise aphorisms [sic] like the sayings of Confucius. This is the most common way of defining "ethics": *norms for conduct* that distinguish between acceptable and unacceptable behavior....
>
> Many different disciplines, institutions, and professions have norms for behavior that suit their particular aims and goals. These norms also help members of the discipline to coordinate their actions or activities and to establish the public's trust of the discipline. For instance, ethical norms govern conduct in medicine, law, engineering, and business. Ethical norms also serve the aims or goals of research and apply to people who conduct scientific research or other scholarly or creative activities. There is even a specialized discipline, research ethics, which studies these norms.
>
> There are several reasons why it is important to adhere to ethical norms in research. First, norms *promote the aims of research*, such as knowledge, truth, and avoidance of error. For example, prohibitions against fabricating, falsifying, or misrepresenting research data promote the truth and avoid error. Second, since research often involves a great deal of cooperation and coordination among many different people in different disciplines and institutions, ethical standards promote the *values that are essential to collaborative work*, such as trust, accountability, mutual respect, and fairness. For example, many ethical norms in research, such as guidelines for authorship, copyright and patenting policies, data sharing policies, and confidentiality rules in peer review, are designed to protect intellectual property interests while encouraging collaboration. Most

researchers want to receive credit for their contributions and do not want to have their ideas stolen or disclosed prematurely. Third, many of the ethical norms help to ensure that researchers can be held *accountable to the public*. For instance, federal policies on research misconduct, conflicts of interest, the human subjects protections, and animal care and use are necessary in order to make sure that researchers who are funded by public money can be held accountable to the public. Fourth, ethical norms in research also help to build *public support* for research. People [are] more likely to fund research project [sic] if they can trust the quality and integrity of research. Finally, many of the norms of research promote a variety of other important *moral and social values*, such as social responsibility, human rights, animal welfare, compliance with the law, and health and safety. Ethical lapses in research can significantly harm human and animal subjects, students, and the public. For example, a researcher who fabricates data in a clinical trial may harm or even kill patients, and a researcher who fails to abide by regulations and guidelines relating to radiation or biological safety may jeopardize his health and safety or the health and safety of staff and students.[37]

Example of an Ethical Violation: U.S. Public Health Service Syphilis Study at Tuskegee

The U.S. Public Health Service, in conjunction with the Tuskegee Institute, began a syphilis investigation in 1932 that spanned 40 years. (Refer to the text box for a description of syphilis.) The purpose of the study was to "... record the natural history of syphilis in hopes of justifying treatment programs for blacks. It was called 'The **Tuskegee Study** of Untreated Syphilis in the Negro Male.'"[38] A total of 600 black men (399 syphilis cases and 201 syphilis-free controls) were included in the study.

The participants in the Tuskegee Study never gave informed consent to take part. "Researchers told the men that they were being treated for 'bad blood,' a local term used to describe several ailments, including syphilis, anemia, and fatigue."[38] Appropriate treatment for syphilis was never offered, despite the fact that as early as 1947 penicillin was known to be efficacious. A class-action suit filed on behalf of the men in 1973 resulted in a $10 million settlement plus

A description of syphilis

A sexually transmitted disease associated with the bacterial agent *Treponema pallidum,* syphilis can have both acute (having sudden onset) and chronic (long-term) phases. The initial infection (primary lesion) produces a painless sore (called a chancre) that appears approximately 3 weeks after exposure. After the primary lesion seems to resolve, a secondary infection (e.g., a rash on the palms of the hands and soles of the feet) may appear in about 2 months. This secondary infection resolves several weeks or months later and then becomes a latent infection. Some infections will remain latent for life and others will progress to tertiary syphilis, resulting in diseases of the central nervous system, cardiovascular system (see **Figure 8-9**), or other organs of the body.[39] At present, syphilis is treatable with penicillin and other antibiotics. Before the advent of modern antibiotics, compounds that contained mercury or arsenic were used to treat syphilis. These treatments were not completely effective and often were harmful.

FIGURE 8-9 Stenosis (narrowing) of the coronary arteries due to cardiovascular syphilis.

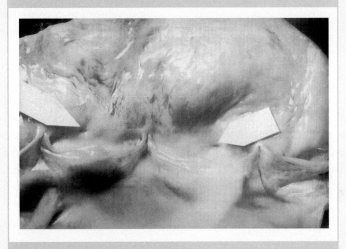

Courtesy of Susan Lindsley/CDC.

medical and health benefits. **Figure 8-10** shows a nurse conversing with some of the participants in the study.

Nowadays, universities maintain Human Subjects Review Boards to ensure that all research protocols that involve human beings and animals are reviewed to make certain that the procedures meet the requirements for informed consent among humans and other ethical standards. In addition, many professional organizations have adopted codes of professional ethics to prevent ethical lapses by their members. For example, epidemiologists operate according to a set of core values that guide practice in the field. The American College of Epidemiology (ACE) has developed a statement of **ethics guidelines**.[40] Five of the

guidelines have been abstracted from the ACE ethics statement (refer to text box).

CONCLUSION

The worlds and realities of the epidemiologist and policy maker are quite dissimilar. Epidemiologists strive to maintain objectivity; their focus is on designing studies, collecting information, and analyzing data. Policy makers must function in the world of politics and are subject to the influences of elected officials, constituents, and special interest groups. This chapter has stressed the importance of increasing the input of epidemiologists into the policy-making

FIGURE 8-10 Tuskegee syphilis study participants with Nurse Rivers.

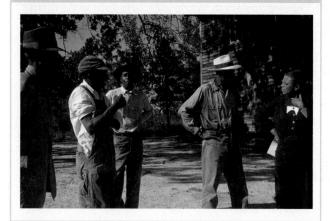

Courtesy of the National Archives Southeast Region, Atlanta.

Ethics guidelines for epidemiologists

- Minimizing risks and protecting the welfare of research subjects
- Obtaining the informed consent of participants
- Submitting proposed studies for ethical review
- Maintaining public trust
- [Meeting] obligations to communities

Data from American College of Epidemiology, Ethics guidelines. *Annals of Epidemiology*. 2000;10(8):487–497. Available at: http://www.acepidemiology.org/statement/ethics-guidelines. Accessed December 27, 2015.

process because of their expertise in study design. Another important role for epidemiologists is in policy assessment and evaluation, which require the establishment of clearly articulated objectives, the use of evidence-based approaches, and cost-effectiveness analysis. Policies often are developed as a consequence of risk assessment, which culminates in risk management. The method of risk assessment has been used extensively in the study and control of environmental health problems, for example, hazards associated with smoking and exposure to secondhand cigarette smoke. In response to the perceived hazards associated with these exposures, governments in the United States and abroad have developed smokefree bars laws. This chapter concluded with the policy-related issue of research ethics as they apply to epidemiology.

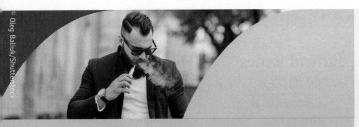

Study Questions and Exercises

1. Define the following terms:
   a. Cost-effectiveness analysis
   b. Evidence-based public health
   c. Healthy People

2. Discuss the roles of epidemiologists in the policy arena. How do the roles of epidemiologists differ from those of policy makers?

3. Explain the differences between health policies and health laws/health regulations.

4. Describe the stages of the policy cycle. Which one of these stages is the most important for epidemiology? Or, would you assign them equal importance?

5. What is meant by risk assessment? Describe the process of risk assessment for a potentially toxic chemical used in containers for food storage.

6. Suppose you live in a community that is being affected by a hazardous chemical from a factory located in the neighborhood. The local health department has conducted a formal risk assessment and has documented people's high levels of exposure to this chemical. Several cases of adverse health effects have been reported to the health department. Previous research has documented that this chemical is a potent neurotoxin. Children are particularly vulnerable to the effects of this chemical. In your own opinion, what steps might be taken for risk management with regard to this exposure?

7. Name five public health laws (and/or regulations) that have been implemented within the past few years.

8. Invite a public health official to your classroom and ask the individual to discuss public health policy issues that currently confront his or her organization.

9. How likely it is that ethical violation of research standards could happen in the United States? In your opinion, what is probability that an event such as in the Tuskegee incident could recur during the contemporary era?

10. Give two reasons why it is important for epidemiologic researchers to conform to high ethical standards. What are three examples of ethical standards in epidemiology?

11. In your own words, formulate relationships between epidemiology and the three core functions of public health? Describe roles for epidemiologists with respect to the 10 essential public health services; be sure to give three examples.

Young Epidemiology Scholars (YES) Exercises

The Young Epidemiology Scholars: Competitions website provides links to teaching units and exercises that support instruction in epidemiology. The YES program, discontinued in 2011, was administered by the College Board and supported by the Robert Wood Johnson Foundation. The exercises continue to be available at the following website: http://yes-competition.org/yes/teaching-units/title.html. The following exercises relate to topics discussed in this chapter and can be found on the YES competitions website.

Epidemiology and policy

1. Novick LF, Wojtowycz M, Morrow CB, Sutphen SM. Bicycle Helmet Effectiveness in Preventing Injury and Death
2. Huang FI, Stolley P. Epidemiology and Public Health Policy: Using the Smoking Ban in New York City Bars as a Case Study

Ethical issues

1. Kaelin MA, St. George DMM. Ethical Issues in Epidemiology
2. Huang FI, St. George DMM. Should the Population Be Screened for HIV?
3. McCrary F, St. George DMM. The Tuskegee Syphilis Study

REFERENCES

1. Sommer A. How public health policy is created: scientific process and political reality. *Am J Epidemiol.* 2001;154(12 Suppl):S4–S6.

2. Tallon J. Health policy roundtable—view from the state legislature: translating research into policy. *HSR: Health Services Research.* 2005;40(2):337–346.

3. *The American Heritage Dictionary of the English Language.* 5th ed. Boston, MA: Houghton Mifflin Harcourt; 2015

4. Brownson RC. Epidemiology and health policy. In: Brownson RC, Petitti DB. *Applied Epidemiology: Theory to Practice.* 2nd ed. New York, NY: Oxford University Press; 2006.

5. D@dalos (International UNESCO Education Server for Civic, Peace and Human Rights Education). Policy cycle: teaching politics. Available at: http://www.dadalos.org/politik_int/politik/policy-zyklus.htm. Accessed February 26, 2016.

6. Businessdictionary.com. Online Business Dictionary. Interest group. Available at: http://www. Businessdictionary.com/definition/interest-group.html. Accessed August 7, 2015.

7. Walker B Jr. Impediments to the implementation of environmental policy. *J Public Health Policy.* 1994;15:186–202.

8. Rabe BG. Legislative incapacity: the congressional role in environmental policy-making and the case of Superfund. *J Health Polit Policy Law.* 1990;15:571–589.

9. Goudey R, Laslett G. Statistics and environmental policy: case studies from long-term environmental monitoring data. *Novartis Found Symp.* 1999;220:144–157.

10. U.S. Department of Health and Human Services, Office of Disease Prevention and Health Promotion. About Healthy People. Available at: http://www.healthypeople.gov/2020/About-Healthy-People. Accessed August 6, 2015.

11. U.S. Department of Health and Human Services, Office of Disease Prevention and Health Promotion. *Healthy People 2020.* Leading health indicators: progress update. Available at: http://www.healthypeople.gov/sites/default/files/LHI-ProgressReport-ExecSum_0.pdf. Accessed August 8, 2015.

12. Raphael D. The question of evidence in health promotion. *Health Promot Int.* 2000;15:355–367.

13. Ashcroft RE. Current epistemological problems in evidence based medicine. *J Med Ethics.* 2004;30:131–135.

14. Centers for Disease Control and Prevention. HIV cost effectiveness. Available at: http://www.cdc.gov/hiv/prevention/ongoing/costeffectiveness/. Accessed August 6, 2015.

15. Ruiz MS, Gable AR. Kaplan EH, et al., eds. No time to lose: getting more from HIV prevention. Washington, DC: National Academy of Sciences; 2001.

16. McKone TE. The rise of exposure assessment among the risk sciences: an evaluation through case studies. *Inhal Toxicol.* 1999;11: 611–622.

17. Porta M, ed. *A Dictionary of Epidemiology.* 6th ed. New York, NY: Oxford University Press; 2014.

18. Amendola A, Wilkinson DR. Risk assessment and environmental policy making. *J Hazard Mater.* 2000;78:ix–xiv.

19. Slovic P. Perception of risk. *Science.* April 17, 1987;236(4799):280–285.

20. Landrigan PJ, Carlson JE. Environmental policy and children's health. *Future Child.* 1995;5(2):34–52.

21. Russell M, Gruber M. Risk assessment in environmental policy-making. *Science.* 1987;236:286–290.

22. Gardner MJ. Epidemiological studies of environmental exposure and specific diseases. *Arch Environ Health.* 1988;43:102–108.

23. Lippmann M, Thurston GD. Exposure assessment: input into risk assessment. *Arch Environ Health.* 1988;43:113–123.

24. Ott WR. Human exposure assessment: the birth of a new science. *J Expos Anal Environ Epidem.* 1995;5:449–472.

25. Monson RR. *Occupational Epidemiology.* Boca Raton, FL: CRC Press; 1990.

26. Duffus JH. Risk assessment terminology. *Chemistry Internat.* 2001;23(2):34–39.

27. Stern PC, Fineberg HV, eds. National Academy of Sciences' National Research Council, Committee on Risk Characterization. *Understanding Risk: Informing Decisions in a Democratic Society.* Washington, DC: National Academies Press; 1996.

28. U.S. Surgeon General. National Prevention Strategy. Available at: http://www.surgeongeneral.gov/priorities/prevention/strategy/national-prevention-strategy-fact-sheet.pdf. Accessed July 20, 2016.

29. Rudolph L, Caplan J, Ben-Moshe K, Dillon L. *Health in All Policies: a guide for state and local governments.* Washington, DC and Oakland, CA: American Public Health Association and Public Health Institute, 2013.

30. Friis RH, Safer AM. Analysis of responses of Long Beach, California residents to the smoke-free bars law. *Public Health.* 2005;119:1116–1121.

31. McGreevy P. State bans trans fats. [Editorial]. *Los Angeles Times.* July 26, 2008.

32. U.S. Food and Drug Administration. Final determination regarding partially hydrogenated oils (removing *trans* fat). Available at: http://www.fda.gov/Food/IngredientsPackagingLabeling/FoodAdditivesIngredients/ucm449162.htm. Accessed July 20, 2016.

33. American Nonsmokers' Rights Foundation. Overview list—how many smokefree laws. Available at: www.no-smoke.org. Accessed July 20, 2016.

34. European Commission. Report on the implementation of the Council recommendation of 30 November 2009 on smoke-free environments. Brussels, Belgium: European Commission; March 14, 2013.

35. National Institute of Environmental Health Sciences (NIEHS), National Institutes of Health, The National Toxicology Program (NTP). Bisphenol A (BPA). Research Triangle Park, NC: NIEHS, 2010.

36. U.S. Food and Drug Administration. Bisphenol A (BPA): use in food contact application. Available at: http://www.fda.gov/newsevents/publichealthfocus/ucm064437.htm. Accessed August 7, 2015.

37. Resnik DB. What is ethics in research and why is it important? Research Triangle Park, NC: National Institute of Environmental Health Sciences. Available at: http://www.niehs.nih.gov/research/resources/bioethics/whatis/. Accessed October 9, 2016.

38. Centers for Disease Control and Prevention. U.S. Public Health Service Syphilis Study at Tuskegee: the Tuskegee timeline. Available at: http://www.cdc.gov/tuskegee/timeline.htm. Accessed July 17, 2015.

39. Heymann DL, ed. *Control of Communicable Diseases Manual.* 20th ed. Washington, DC: American Public Health Association; 2015.

40. American College of Epidemiology. Ethics guidelines. Available at: http://www.acepidemiology.org/statement/ethics-guidelines. Accessed December 27, 2015.

Epidemiology and Screening for Disease

LEARNING OBJECTIVES

By the end of this chapter you will be able to:

- Synchronize screening for disease with a model for prevention of disease.
- Compare two types of screening programs.
- State the differences and relationships between reliability and validity.
- Calculate measures for evaluating screening tests for disease.
- Give three examples of specific screening programs.

CHAPTER OUTLINE

INTRODUCTION

This chapter covers the topic of screening for disease, an important method for reducing morbidity and mortality in the population. One of the preeminent components of public health, screening aligns with the natural history of disease and models of disease prevention. You will discover the unique characteristics of screening and how screening differs from other encounters with healthcare providers. In addition, you will learn about the types of screening, for example, mass screening and selective screening, and their applications. Key examples of screening methods and programs will be presented. A related topic will be measures used to evaluate the reliability and validity of screening tests. The term "gold standard" will be introduced; its applications for evaluating a screening test by using a four-fold table to classify screening results and calculate validity measures will be reviewed. Refer to **Table 9-1** for a list of important terms covered in this chapter. **Figure 9-1** details the lexicon of screening for disease.

OVERVIEW OF SCREENING

This section defines the term *screening*, provides examples of screening tests, and distinguishes between two types of screening programs—mass and selective screening. You will learn how screening for disease can be linked to surveillance programs as part of health promotion in various settings. Screening makes a vital contribution to the control of major chronic diseases such as cancer by helping to identify them as early as possible so that appropriate and timely interventions can be made. The procedure is used to exclude persons with certain health conditions from joining military service or participating in vigorous sports activities. Applicants for a driver license have their vision screened in order to protect the public. In addition to these examples, this section will present appropriate uses, controversies, and policy issues regarding the implementation of screening tests.

TABLE 9-1 List of Important Terms Used in This Chapter

Deoxyribonucleic acid (DNA)	Natural history of disease
BRCA gene	Prepathogenesis
Cholesterol	Pathogenesis
False negative	Overdiagnosis
False positive	Phenylketonuria (PKU)
Gold standard	Predictive value (+ and −)
Genetic screening	Reliability (precision)
Levels of prevention	Screening for disease
Primary	Selective screening
Secondary	Sensitivity
Tertiary	Specificity
Lipoprotein panel	True negative
Mammogram	True positive
Mass screening	Validity (accuracy)

Definition of Screening

Screening for disease is defined as "[t]he presumptive identification of unrecognized disease or defect by the application of tests, examinations, or other procedures which [sic] can be applied rapidly."[1] Some examples of screening tests are those that check for the presence of abnormalities in newborn infants, tests for sexually transmitted diseases, and screens for diabetes. Community health fairs and campus health fairs are voluntary programs that screen for diverse conditions, such as high blood pressure, high cholesterol levels, and tooth decay. Some local retail drug stores encourage their customers to have their blood pressure and cholesterol checked while shopping.

In comparison with other medical encounters, the uses of information from screening tests are unfamiliar to many people. Screening tests are applied to people who appear to be well (do not have active signs or symptoms of a disease) and who are probably not aware that they may have an undetected illness or risk factors for an illness. Usually one conceives of a clinical encounter as involving a visit to a doctor or other provider for treatment of a specific illness—the patient's chief complaint.

FIGURE 9-1 Screening for disease.

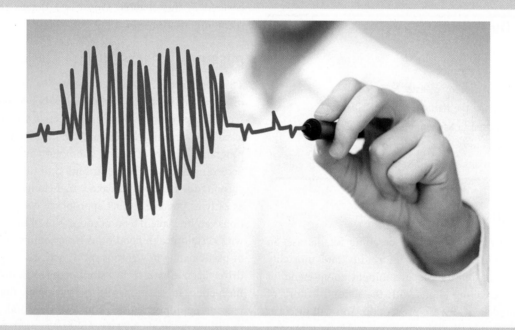

One caveat regarding screening is that positive results are preliminary information only; a diagnostic workup of any positive results of a screening test is required. For example, this confirmation might involve additional procedures, including clinical examinations and more extensive testing. Screening is not the same as diagnosis, although some screening tests are also used for diagnostic testing.

Often screening is performed in conjunction with disease surveillance.[2] In fact, these two activities may be considered as complementary. One of the applications of this complementary approach is in occupational health. Surveillance information can be combined with screening data in order to implement programs to reduce hazardous job-related exposures. The process of disease surveillance denotes the ongoing collecting of information about morbidity and mortality in a population. In comparison, screening programs help in detecting occupational diseases. Both of these data sources (screening and surveillance) are then pooled and analyzed in order to pinpoint high-risk occupations. The resulting information is invaluable in formulating interventions for limiting suspected adverse health outcomes identified by screening.

Beyond the realm of occupational health, surveillance and screening programs monitor high-risk groups, as in the cases of patients with sexually transmitted diseases and intravenous (IV) drug users who could transmit bloodborne infections.

The Types of Screening Tests: Mass Versus Selective Screening

Mass screening refers to the application of screening tests to total population groups, regardless of their risk status. One example of mass screening pertains to work settings: All new employees may be required to obtain tuberculin skin tests, chest x-rays, and urine drug screens. A second example is screening of all newborn infants for phenylketonuria (PKU). A final example is measuring the temperatures of all incoming passengers at an airport in order to identify those who might be importing a deadly communicable disease.

Selective screening is the type of screening applied to high-risk groups, such as those at risk for sexually transmitted diseases. Selective screening is likely to result in the greatest yield of true cases and to be the most economically productive form of screening. This type of screening is most efficient for detecting infectious diseases, chronic diseases, and other conditions among persons who have specific risk factors. For example, smoking, obesity, IV drug use, or engaging in unprotected sex place individuals at increased risk of adverse health outcomes. Such high-risk individuals are advised to receive screening tests.

Appropriate Situations for Use of Screening Tests

Considerations regarding the appropriate use of screening tests include whether the condition being screened is sufficiently important for the individual and the community. Also, the screening test should have a high cost-benefit ratio; this means that the condition needs to be sufficiently prevalent in the population to justify the cost of screening. In addition, the screening test should be applied mainly to conditions for which an effective treatment is available. Finally screening tests should be simple to perform and safe for participants.

Controversies Regarding Screening Tests

Two controversies regarding the use of screening tests are the following:

- False alarms (false positive results) are disconcerting for patients who receive them.
- Screening may result in overdiagnosis of potentially benign conditions.

A false alarm from a screening test causes undue concern for the patient when no significant disease process has occurred and anxiety is not warranted. A related point is that as screening tests improve in sensitivity and their use becomes more widespread, they are increasingly able to identify minute lesions or other signs of disease, and consequently, lead to the detection of abnormalities that have little clinical significance. This is the issue of **overdiagnosis**. In the instance of either false positive results or overdiagnosis, the patient may need to undergo painful, invasive (albeit unwarranted) medical testing and procedures.

Mammography (taking a mammogram) is the recommended screening procedure for breast cancer. A **mammogram** is an **x**-ray image of the human breast. Some experts believe that overdiagnosis is an issue for screening mammography. One opinion is that screening mammography provides limited benefits in terms of reduced mortality and its use should be restricted. Mammograms for breast cancer can lead to "…diagnosis of cancers that otherwise would never have bothered women."[3]

Consequently, several policy and related issues pertain to the appropriate use of screening tests. Simple policy questions (without simple answers!) are: How frequently should screening tests be administered? Who should be screened? What conditions should be screened? Under which circumstances should screening tests be used? and At what age should screening begin? For example, controversy surrounds the age at which routine screening for breast cancer should begin. Similarly, opinion is divided on the timing and application of screening tests for prostate cancer.

EXAMPLES OF SCREENING TESTS

This section provides examples of common screening tests. These illustrations are grouped according to the categories of tests for newborn infants, those relevant to children and adolescents, those focused on adults (including sex-specific tests), and genetic screening. Screening tests have been developed for an extensive list of conditions, from chronic diseases to infectious diseases including sexually transmitted diseases, hepatitis B in IV drug users, and hepatitis C—to name a few examples. Sex-specific screening tests for women include screening for cancers that affect females (breast and cervical cancer), osteoporosis, and sexually transmitted infections. Mental health screening is a component of routine medical practice.

This review is not exhaustive. However, in case you are not familiar with the specific types of screening, you will learn how screening goes hand in hand with preventive services and how screening can address the major causes of morbidity and mortality in the United States.

Screening Tests for Newborn Infants

Figure 9-2 highlights the crucial role of newborn screening in children's health promotion. Despite appearing healthy at birth, every newborn infant requires screening.[4] Conditions that affect the newborn are not readily observable and can cause irreversible brain impairment, organ damage, and possibly death. The purpose of screening tests for newborns is to search for potentially harmful metabolic, genetic, and developmental disorders.[5] Such conditions tend to be rare, but when identified early are treatable.

Newborn screening is conducted at the state level in the United States.[6] Universal access to testing is mandated by

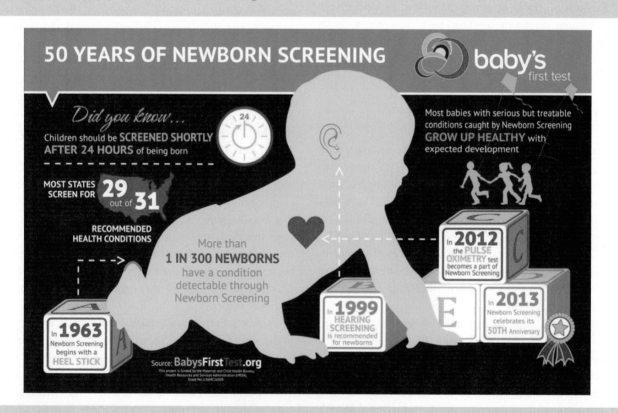

FIGURE 9-2 Fifty years of newborn screening.

Reprinted from Baby's First Test. About newborn screening. Available at: http://www.babysfirsttest.org/newborn-screening/about-newborn-screening. Accessed July 11, 2016.

all states and is made available regardless of ability to pay. A uniform panel of about 40 disorders to be included in the screening program has been developed. However, the states determine independently the exact makeup of their screening programs. As a result, states have varying requirements regarding the conditions that are screened. As of April 2011, all states screen for at least 26 of the disorders included in the panel.[7]

Recommended screening programs for newborns include hearing evaluations, screening for congenital heart defects (CHDs), and blood tests. Severe CHDs are known as critical CHDs.[8] These defects require surgical or other interventions during the infant's first year. Pulse oximetry screening, which measures blood oxygen levels, is the screening test for critical CHDs.

In addition to screens for hearing deficits and heart defects, blood samples are collected as part of newborn screening. Blood tests screen for a variety of conditions that may affect newborn infants; one of the universal tests (given in all states) is for **phenylketonuria (PKU)**. **Table 9-2** gives several examples of blood screening tests recommended for newborn screening. Note that the list is not exhaustive.

TABLE 9-2 Examples of Blood Screening Tests for Newborns

Name of Disorders Screened	Definition
Amino acid metabolism disorders Example: phenylketonuria (PKU)	PKU is a condition marked by the inability to metabolize the amino acid phenylalanine. PKU is a genetic disorder that is associated with intellectual disability.
Biotinidase deficiency	Inability of the body to recycle biotin, a B vitamin; a cause of motor disorders and seizures.
Congenital adrenal hyperplasia	An adrenal gland disorder that disrupts hormone production.
Congenital hypothyroidism	A hereditary disorder of the thyroid gland associated with insufficient production of thyroid hormone.
Cystic fibrosis	A condition in which very thick mucus forms in the body and restricts breathing and other functions.
Fatty acid metabolism disorders	A disorder in which the body is unable to change fat into energy.
Galactosemia	The body is unable to metabolize galactose, a simple sugar.
Glucose-6-phosphate dehydrogenase deficiency (G6PD)	Too little of the enzyme G6PD, which can cause hemolysis (destruction of red blood cells).
Organic acid metabolism disorders	Disorders that affect ability to metabolize food.
Infectious diseases	Examples: human immunodeficiency virus disease (HIV); toxoplasmosis
Hemoglobin disorders and traits Example: sickle cell disease (SCD)	SCD is a hereditary disorder in which red blood cells are C-shaped and can block blood flow as they circulate in the body.

Data from U.S. National Library of Medicine. MedlinePlus. Newborn screening tests. Available at: https://www.nlm.nih.gov/medlineplus/ency/article/007257.htm. Accessed July 11, 2016; and March of Dimes. Newborn screening tests for your baby. Available at: http://www.marchofdimes.org/baby/newborn-screening-tests-for-your-baby.aspx. Accessed July 18, 2016.

Children and Adolescents

Screening programs for children and adolescents are oriented toward their respective growth stages. During early childhood (from 9 months to 30 months), developmental screening helps to determine whether a child's behavioral and mental status reflect attainment of normal developmental milestones.[9] This procedure aids in the identification of developmental delays and disabilities, for example, autism and intellectual disabilities. Developmental screening encompasses observations of the child's behaviors and responses to questions during an examination. Additional examples of screening tests for children are vision and dental screening.

For adolescents who have specific risk factors, screening for hypertension, diabetes, and obesity may be appropriate. Other screens for adolescents might include those for behavioral risk factors such as tobacco use. Still another example is screening for chlamydia beginning around 15 years of age among girls who have become sexually active.

Adults

Screening programs for adults target the major chronic diseases and their risk factors. Some examples of screening programs are those for cancer, diabetes, and heart disease risk factors. Attention to these conditions is warranted as each one ranks among the major causes of mortality in the United States and contributes substantially to health care and societal costs. Early identification can extend lives and reduce needless suffering.

Cancer Screening

The first set of screening examples pertains to cancer—breast cancer, colorectal cancer, cervical cancer, and prostate cancer. Regarding breast cancer, screening mammography is the recommended procedure for screening for breast cancer. The U.S. Preventive Services Task Force advises that women between age 50 and 74 years obtain a mammogram every 2 years. Women between the ages of 40 through 49 should consult their own physicians about whether to be screened and make a decision based on personal circumstances. **Figure 9-3** shows a woman receiving a mammogram.

Three different screening tests are used for colon cancer,[10] the second leading cause of cancer death in the United States. One is a stool test for presence of blood in the stool. A second—a flexible sigmoidoscopy—searches for cancer and polyps in the lower third of the colon and the rectum. The third is the colonoscopy, which explores the rectum and the entire colon for lesions. A polyp is an abnormal growth that could become cancerous and thus should be excised. **Figure 9-4** illustrates a polyp located in the colon.

FIGURE 9-3 Screening mammography.

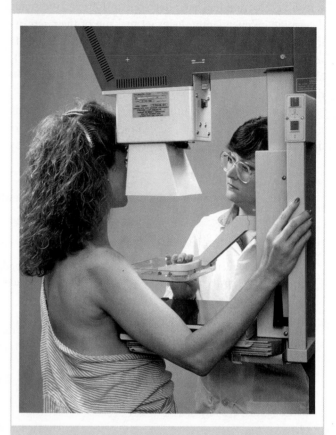

Reprinted from National Cancer Institute: Visuals Online. Mammography patient. Available at: https://visualsonline.cancer.gov/details.cfm?imageid=2483. Photo credit: Bill Branson.

Refer to **Table 9-3** for detailed information regarding screening tests for four prevalent types of cancer, including cervical cancer and prostate cancer, neither of which is discussed further in the text.

Diabetes

Among the forms of diabetes, type 2 diabetes has the highest prevalence.[11] The condition is characterized by abnormally high levels of blood glucose (hyperglycemia). Diabetes is associated with damage to organs of the body, for example, kidney disease, eye disease, and neurologic dysfunction. In 2012, approximately 21.3 million people in the United States had diabetes.[12] Projections suggest that by 2050 this figure will grow to one out of three adults. The economic costs of diabetes in 2012 were enormous—an estimated $245 billion. In view of the economic toll of this prevalent disease, public health officials have prioritized screening for diabetes. The screening test for type 2 diabetes is a blood test known as the fasting plasma glucose (FGP) test.

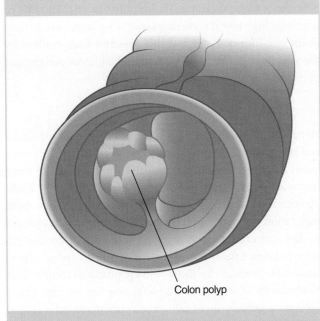

FIGURE 9-4 A polyp growing in the colon.

Colon polyp

Reprinted from Centers for Disease Control and Prevention. Colorectal cancer screening saves lives. CDC Publication #99-6948. Atlanta, GA: CDC; revised July 2009, p 2. Available at: www.cdc.gov/cancer/colorectal/pdf/SFL_brochure.pdf.

Cholesterol

Elevated blood cholesterol has been substantiated as a dominant risk factor for coronary heart disease and atherosclerosis.[13] **Cholesterol** is a waxy material that can be found throughout the body.[14] Excessive amounts of "bad" cholesterol (called low-density lipoproteins [LDL]) are known to block arteries and result in heart disease. **Figure 9-5** illustrates cholesterol circulating in the bloodstream. Circulating cholesterol can be deposited and build up in the arteries over time.

Cholesterol screening tests require fasting blood samples (patient is not allowed to eat for 9 to 12 hours beforehand).[15] Two versions of these screening tests are available. One measures total cholesterol present in the blood; a **lipoprotein panel** assesses total cholesterol as well as three types of blood lipids: LDL cholesterol, high-density lipoprotein (HDL) cholesterol ("good" cholesterol), and triglycerides. In most cases, cholesterol screening is recommended for men starting at age 35 and women at age 45, with 5-year follow-ups if normal results were obtained previously.

Coronary heart disease is the leading cause of death in the United States. Consequently, cholesterol screening is a public health priority. The Behavioral Risk Factor

TABLE 9-3 Examples of Cancer Screening Tests

Type of Cancer	Name of Test	Comments
Breast cancer	Screening mammography, an x-ray of the breast	The U.S. Preventive Services Task Force recommends that women between age 50 and 74 years obtain a mammogram every 2 years.
Cervical cancer	Pap test (Pap smear)	Recommended for all women between age 21 and 65 years of age.
Colorectal cancer	Fecal occult blood testing (FOBT)—stool test Flexible sigmoidoscopy Colonoscopy	Men and women between 50 and 70 years of age
Prostate cancer	Prostate-specific antigen (PSA) test Digital rectal exam	Previously recommended for men beginning at age 20. Some organizations caution against routine use of the PSA test.

FIGURE 9-5 Cholesterol circulating in the blood.

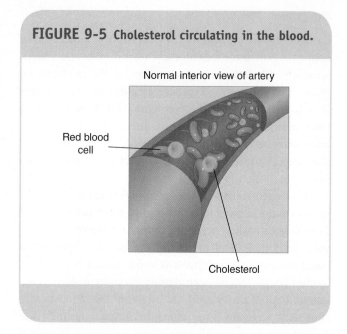

Normal interior view of artery

Red blood cell

Cholesterol

Surveillance System (BRFSS) collects data on the prevalence of cholesterol screening in the United States. The results of the BRFSS study demonstrate that two-thirds of adults who have high cholesterol do not have it under control.

Figure 9-6 shows statewide variations in the prevalence of screening for cholesterol. A desirable public health goal is to screen a high percentage (for example, more than 80%) of adults for high blood cholesterol over a 5-year period. In only about one-fifth of states had this objective been realized by the year 2011.[16] The remaining states had lower percentages of residents who had been screened.

Hypertension

Hypertension (high blood pressure) is a risk factor for stroke and heart disease. Approximately one-third of the U.S. population has hypertension; unfortunately, just one-half of these individuals have it under control.[17] (See **Figure 9-7**.) Early identification can help patients avoid complications from high blood pressure. Lifestyle modifications such as changes in diet and exercise levels aid in preventing or controlling hypertension. Effective medications for treatment of hypertension are available for those who are unable to control their condition by other means. The screening test for high blood pressure is measurement using a sphygmomanometer (blood pressure cuff), as demonstrated in **Figure 9-8**. This test is performed routinely as part of a medical encounter. Sometimes, blood pressure screening takes place in others venues such as community health fairs and senior centers.

FIGURE 9-6 Prevalence of cholesterol screening in the past 5 years, adults age 20 years and older (percentage)—United States, 2011.

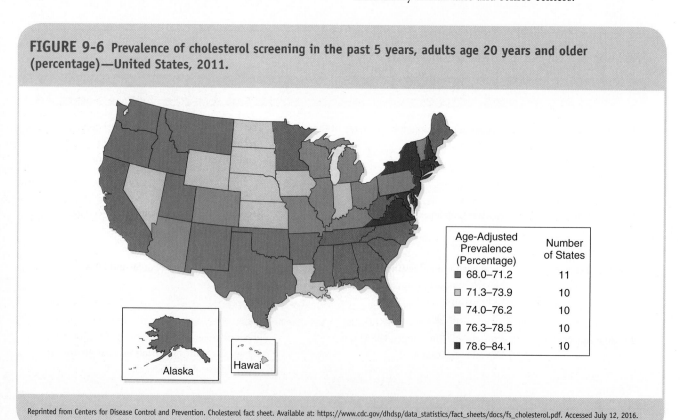

Age-Adjusted Prevalence (Percentage)	Number of States
■ 68.0–71.2	11
▢ 71.3–73.9	10
■ 74.0–76.2	10
■ 76.3–78.5	10
■ 78.6–84.1	10

Alaska

Hawaii

FIGURE 9-7 Hypertensive* population aware, treated, and controlled, age 18 to 74 years—United States, 1976–1980 to 2005–2008.

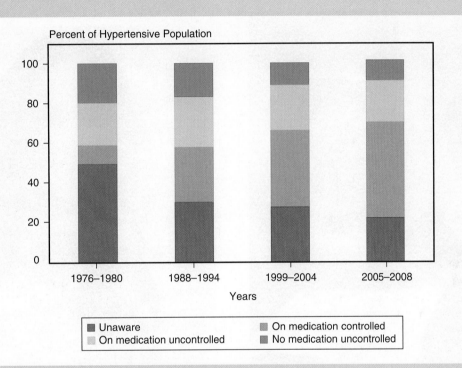

*Hypertension is defined as systolic blood pressure (BP) ≥ 140 mmHg, or diastolic BP ≥ 90 mmHg, or on medication.

Reprinted from National Heart, Lung, and Blood Institute. *Morbidity and Mortality: 2012 Chart Book on Cardiovascular, Lung, and Blood Diseases.* Bethesda, MD: NHLBI; 2012:56.

Human Immunodeficiency Virus (HIV)

HIV is the virus associated with the acquired immunodeficiency syndrome (AIDS). The prevalence of HIV in the United States is slightly more than one million; approximately 13% of persons with HIV infection are unaware that they have HIV.[18] Estimates suggest that undiagnosed HIV-infected individuals transmit about one-third of new HIV cases annually. Testing is recommended for all persons between age 13 and 64 years at least once; testing can be done in conjunction with routine health care. At-risk persons should be tested annually.[18] Initial screening is done with antibody tests or combination tests. Antibody tests (screens for antibodies against HIV) detect antibodies in blood or oral samples. Combination tests screen for the presence of HIV antibodies as well as antigens (parts of the HIV virus).

Genetic Screening

Genetic screening refers to "[t]he use of genetic, clinical, and epidemiological knowledge, reasoning, and techniques to detect genetic variants that have been demonstrated to place an individual at increased risk of a *specific disease*."[1] A *gene* is a particular segment of a DNA (deoxyribonucleic acid) molecule on a chromosome that determines the nature of an inherited trait in an individual. Genetic screening involves the use of genetic tests that are applied to populations, as in the example of screening for PKU. Samples taken for genetic tests may include blood, hair, amniotic fluid, skin, and other body tissues. Buccal smears (swabs of the inside surface of the cheek) may be collected.

Genetic testing can also be conducted with individuals. An example is preconception genetic testing of couples who would like to conceive a child. Future parents can determine whether they carry genes for inherited diseases including cystic fibrosis and Tay Sachs disease. Another application of genetic testing is the detection of the genetic mutations that increase risk of specific conditions. A genetic mutation is a change in deoxynucleic acid (DNA) that may adversely affect the organism. **DNA (deoxyribonucleic acid)**, which is found in the cells of humans and most other organisms, is a nucleic acid that carries genetic information.

FIGURE 9-8 Blood pressure screening.

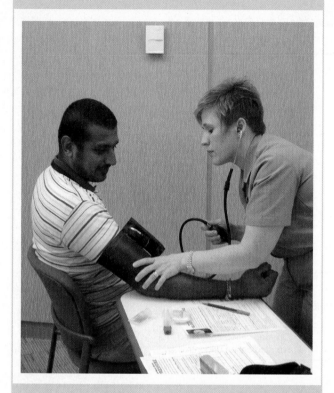

Reprinted from Centers for Disease Control and Prevention. Public Health Image Library. PHIL I.D. # 14869. Photo credit: Yvonne Green, RN, CNM, MSN.

FIGURE 9-9 Angelina Jolie, carrier of the *BRCA1* gene.

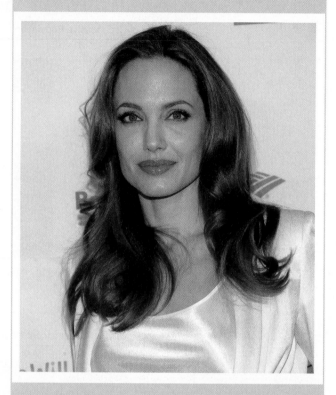

© Jason Kempin/Staff/Getty Images

A case in point is genetic tests for mutations in the **BRCA genes** (called *BRCA1* and *BRCA2*) that increase risk of breast and ovarian cancers. In a well-publicized happening (causing the "Angelina effect"), film star Angelina Jolie elected to undergo a double mastectomy because she carried the *BRCA1* gene.[19] The surgery was performed even though Ms. Jolie had not been diagnosed with breast cancer. (See **Figure 9-9**.) As a result of the so-called Angelina effect, providers worried that hordes of women who were positive for BRCA might flood into their offices demanding a mastectomy. Mastectomies for cancer-free women who are positive for the BRCA genetic mutations may not be the optimal course of medical action.

Depression

Depression, a prevalent mental disorder in the United States, causes significant morbidity and has large economic impacts. The condition afflicts many groups of adults including children, adolescents, college students, and persons active in the workforce. Among the tools for identifying depression is the Patient Health Questionnaire (PHQ-9), which has several applications, including screening for depression. The PHQ-9 contains nine

items that reflect symptoms of depression. A sample item is worded, "Over the past 2 weeks, how often have you been bothered by any of the following problems? [Item 1] Little interest or pleasure in doing things."[20] A Likert scale (ranging from "not at all" [0 points] to "nearly every day" [3 points]) allows respondents to rate the frequency with which they have experienced each symptom. A total score is then calculated from the set of nine items. The instrument has high sensitivity (88%) and high specificity (88%) for major depression.[21] The terms *sensitivity* and *specificity* will be defined later in the chapter.

SCREENING AND THE NATURAL HISTORY OF DISEASE

Screening is a method for secondary prevention of disease. The rationale for this terminology will become clear when we define the term *natural history of disease*. In this section the author will describe a public health model for prevention of disease, which coincides with the phases of the natural history of disease. You will learn about the linkage between prevention and the natural history of disease and see how screening fits in with the model of prevention.

Natural History of Disease

The **natural history of disease** refers to the time course of disease from its beginning to its final clinical endpoints. This time course encompasses the two time segments designated as the period of prepathogenesis and the period of pathogenesis. (Refer to **Figure 9-10.**) The terms that appear in the figure are defined in the following sections.

Prepathogenesis occurs during the time period in the natural history of disease before a disease agent (e.g., a bacterium) has interacted with a host (the person who develops the disease). The agent simply exists in the environment. For example, an infectious agent is residing in the soil, circulating among wild animals, or is coating an environmental surface.

Pathogenesis occurs after the agent has interacted with a host. This situation can happen when a susceptible host comes into contact with a disease agent, such as a virus or bacterium. As a simple example, when someone who has a cold comes to class with the sniffles and sore throat, other susceptible students may be exposed to the cold virus and become infected (start of pathogenesis). Later in pathogenesis, some infected students will develop active cold symptoms. During late pathogenesis, the symptoms will usually resolve and the student will recover fully.

Three **levels of prevention** From the public health point of view, the three types of prevention are primary, secondary, and tertiary. These coincide with the periods of prepathogenesis and pathogenesis.

Primary prevention involves the prevention of disease before it occurs; primary prevention targets the stage of prepathogenesis and embodies general health promotion and specific protections against diseases. Methods of primary prevention include the creation of a healthful environment, implementation of health education programs, and administration of immunizations against specific infectious diseases (called specific protection).

Secondary prevention takes place during the early phases of pathogenesis and includes activities that limit the progression of disease. Illustrations are programs described in this chapter for cancer screening and early detection of other chronic diseases.

Tertiary prevention is directed toward the later stages of pathogenesis and includes programs for restoring the patient's optimal functioning; examples are physical therapy for stroke victims and fitness programs for recovering heart attack patients.

MEASURES USED IN SCREENING
Reliability and Validity

Screening tests need to demonstrate reliability and validity in order to be useful. The term **reliability** (synonym: precision) refers to the ability of a measuring instrument to give consistent results on repeated trials. The term *repeated measurement reliability* pertains to the degree of consistency between or among repeated measurements of the same individual on more than one occasion.

In comparison with reliability, **validity** (synonym: accuracy), is the ability of the measuring instrument to give a true measure of the entity being measured. The "true measure" sometimes is called the **gold standard**, which refers to a definitive diagnosis that has been determined by biopsy, surgery, autopsy, or other method[22] and has been accepted as the standard.

Reliability and validity are interrelated terms; it is possible for a measure to be invalid and reliable, but not the converse. An example would be a bathroom weight scale that has been tampered with so that it does not give a correct weight measurement but consistently gives the same incorrect (invalid) measurement.

It is never possible for a measure that is unreliable to be valid, however. A valid measure must give a true measure of an attribute on repeated occasions; an unreliable measure would give different results each time a measurement is taken. Consider the analogy of a bullet hitting a target. For several rifle shots at a target, when the bullet hits the bullseye consistently, this outcome is analogous to validity (and also to

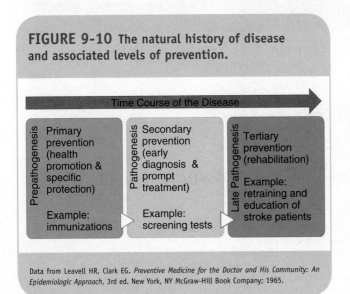

FIGURE 9-10 The natural history of disease and associated levels of prevention.

Data from Leavell HR, Clark EG. *Preventive Medicine for the Doctor and His Community: An Epidemiologic Approach*, 3rd ed. New York, NY McGraw-Hill Book Company; 1965.

a reliable, valid measure). A situation that would be analogous to an unreliable, invalid measure would be when the bullet hits several different places on the target (not the bullseye every time). Ideally, a screening test should be both reliable and valid. (See **Figure 9-11**.)

Measures of Validity of Screening Tests

In the context of screening, there are four measures of validity that must be considered: sensitivity, specificity, predictive value (+), and predictive value (−). A good screening test needs to be high in sensitivity, high in specificity, high in predictive value (+), and high in predictive value (−). **Table 9-4** represents a sample of individuals who have been examined with both a screening test for disease (rows) and a definitive diagnostic test or gold standard (columns). Thus, we are able to determine how well the screening test performed in identifying individuals with disease.

Sensitivity is the ability of the test to identify correctly all screened individuals who actually have the disease. In Table 9-4, a total of a + c individuals were determined to have the disease according to the gold standard. Sensitivity

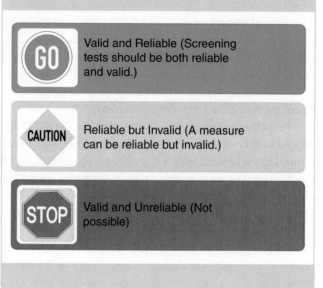

FIGURE 9-11 Reliability and validity of screening tests.

GO — Valid and Reliable (Screening tests should be both reliable and valid.)

CAUTION — Reliable but Invalid (A measure can be reliable but invalid.)

STOP — Valid and Unreliable (Not possible)

TABLE 9-4 Fourfold Table for Classification of Screening Test Results

Definitions: **True positives** are individuals who have both been screened positive and truly have the condition; **false positives** are individuals who have been screened positive but do not have the condition. **False negatives** are individuals who have been screened negative but truly have the condition; **true negatives** are individuals who have both been screened negative and do not have the condition.

		Condition According to Gold Standard			
		Present	Absent	Total	
Test result	Positive	a = True positives	b = False positives	a + b	Predictive value (+) $\frac{a}{a+b}$
	Negative	c = False negatives	d = True negatives	c + d	Predictive value (−) $\frac{d}{c+d}$
	Total	a + c	b + d	**Grand total a + b + c + d**	
		Sensitivity $\frac{a}{a+c}$	Specificity $\frac{d}{b+d}$		

is defined as the number of true positives divided by the sum of true positives and false negatives according to the formula a/(a + c). Suppose that in a sample of 1,000 individuals there were 120 who actually had the disease. If the screening test correctly identified all 120 cases, the sensitivity would be 100%. If the screening test was unable to identify all these individuals, then the sensitivity would be less than 100%.

Specificity is the ability of the test to identify only non-diseased individuals who actually do not have the disease. It is a proportion defined as the number of true negatives divided by the sum of false positives and true negatives as denoted by the formula d/(b+d). If a test is not specific, then individuals who do not actually have the disease will be referred for additional diagnostic testing.

Predictive value (+) is the proportion of individuals who are screened positive by the test and who actually have the disease. In Table 9-4, a total of a + b individuals were screened positive by the test. Predictive value (+) is the proportion screened positive who actually have the condition, according to the gold standard; this is the probability that an individual who is screened positive actually has the disease. The formula for predictive value (+) is a/(a+b).

Predictive value (−) is an analogous measure for those screened negative by the test; it is designated by the formula d/(c + d); this is the probability that an individual who is screened negative does not have the disease. Note that the only time these measures can be estimated is when the same group of individuals has been examined using both the screening test and the gold standard.

Additional interpretations of Table 9-4 are the following: false positive and false negative test results are vexing for both patients and healthcare providers. (See **Figure 9-12**.) A false positive result could unnecessarily raise the anxiety levels of people who are screened positive and subjected to invasive medical tests. On the other hand, a false negative test result would not detect disease in people who actually have the disease and require treatment. For example, if a screening test missed a case of breast cancer (false negative result), the disease could progress to a more severe form.

Sensitivity and Specificity: Calculation Example

Suppose that a pharmaceutical company wishes to evaluate the validity of a new measure for screening people who are suspected of having diabetes. (Refer to **Table 9-5**.) A total of 1,473 persons are screened for diabetes; 244 of them

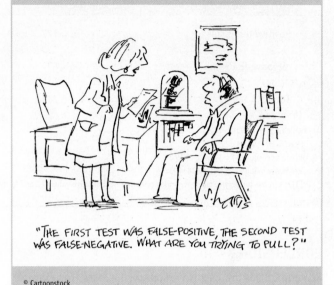

FIGURE 9-12 False positive and false negative test results.

"THE FIRST TEST WAS FALSE-POSITIVE, THE SECOND TEST WAS FALSE-NEGATIVE. WHAT ARE YOU TRYING TO PULL?"

© Cartoonstock

have been confirmed as diabetic according to the gold standard. Here are the results of the screening test: true positives (a = 177), false positives (b = 268), false negatives (c = 67), true negatives (d = 961). Table 9-5 shows the calculations for sensitivity, specificity, and predictive value (positive and negative). This test has moderate sensitivity and specificity, low predictive value (+), and fairly high predictive value (−).

Effect of Disease Prevalence on Predictive Value

Predictive value (+) and predictive value (−) are variable properties of screening tests that depend on the prevalence of a disease in the population. In comparison, sensitivity and specificity are called stable properties of a screening test. Consequently, sensitivity and specificity remain stable regardless of the prevalence of a disease in a population. More specifically, the predictive value (+) decreases as the prevalence of a condition decreases; however, the predictive value (−) increases at the same time. For this reason, if you apply a screening test in an instance in which the prevalence of a disease is low, any individual who is screened positive for the disease has a low probability of actually having the condition.

TABLE 9-5 Calculation Example

	Gold Standard (present)	Gold Standard (absent)	Total
Positive test result	a = 177	b = 268	445
Negative test result	c = 67	d = 961	1,028
Total	244	1,229	1,473

Sensitivity = 177/244 = 72.5%
Specificity = 961/1,229 = 78.2%
Predictive value (+) = 177/445 = 39.8%
Predictive value (−) = 961/1,028 = 93.5%
[This test has moderate sensitivity and specificity, low predictive value (+), and fairly high predictive value (−).]

CONCLUSION

Screening tests are used to search for diseases (for example, cancer) and risk factors for disease (for example, hypertension) among apparently "well" persons. A positive screening test needs to be followed up with a diagnostic workup. Mass screening tests are applied to populations without regard to risk factor status. Selective screening involves the use of screening tests among high-risk groups. Screening tests can cause false alarms, which can be disconcerting to those who have been mistakenly told that they had a positive test result. A multitude of screening tests are available for use with specific populations, such as newborns, children and adolescents, and adults. These tests contribute to effective public health practice by limiting morbidity and mortality from prevalent chronic diseases, infectious diseases, and genetic conditions. Screening, classified as secondary prevention of disease, requires the application of reliable and valid screening tests. Sensitivity and specificity are measures of the validity of screening tests. Two additional measures used to evaluate screening tests are predictive value (+) and predictive value (−). This chapter described formulas and calculations for the foregoing four measures.

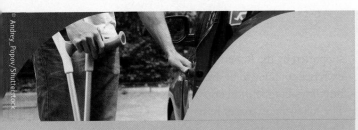

Study Questions and Exercises

1. Define the following groups of terms:
   a. Primary, secondary, and tertiary prevention
   b. Prepathogenesis and pathogenesis

2. How does screening for disease align with the three levels of prevention—primary, secondary, and tertiary?

3. Define the following terms that are related to screening tests:
   a. Reliability and validity
   b. Sensitivity and specificity
   c. Predictive value (+) and predictive value (−)

4. **Table 9-6** presents the results of a screening test. Calculate sensitivity, specificity, predictive value (+), and predictive value (−).

   Answers:

   Sensitivity = 55/66 × 100 = 83.3%

   Specificity = 145/150 × 100 = 96.7%

   Predictive value (+) = 55/60 × 100 = 91.7%

   Predictive value (−) = 145/156 × 100 = 92.9%

5. What are the most appropriate applications of mass screening and selective screening? Give one example each of a mass screening test and a selective screening test.

6. How could screening performed in conjunction with disease surveillance contribute to the alleviation of work-related hazardous exposures?

7. What is meant by overdiagnosis?

8. Conduct a web search for "whole body scans." They are CT scans of the entire body and are promoted as a method for early detection of abnormalities. Using your own ideas, construct a list of the advantages and disadvantages of whole body scans and reach a conclusion. To what extent are whole body scans related to the issue of overdiagnosis?

9. Why is newborn screening important for public health practice? Give examples of programs for newborn screening.

10. What is a method used for developmental screening? At what ages is developmental screening most relevant?

11. Describe methods of screening for each of the following conditions:
    a. Breast cancer
    b. Colon cancer
    c. Type 2 diabetes
    d. Elevated lipid levels
    e. Hypertension
    f. Infections with HIV

TABLE 9-6 Data for Question 4

	Gold Standard: disease present	Gold Standard: disease absent
Screening test positive	55	5
Screening test negative	11	145

Young Epidemiology Scholars (YES) Exercises

The Young Epidemiology Scholars: Competitions website provides links to teaching units and exercises that support instruction in epidemiology. The YES program, discontinued in 2011, was administered by the College Board and supported by the Robert Wood Johnson Foundation. The exercises continue to be available at the following website: http://yes-competition.org/yes/teaching-units/title.html. The following exercises relate to topics discussed in this chapter and can be found on the YES competitions website.

1. Huang, FI, St. George DMM. Should the Population Be Screened for HIV?

REFERENCES

1. Porta M, ed. *A Dictionary of Epidemiology*. 6th ed. New York, NY: Oxford University Press; 2014.

2. Wagner GR. Screening and surveillance of workers exposed to mineral dust. Geneva, Switzerland: World Health Organization; 1996.

3. Welch HG. When screening is bad for your health. [Editorial]. *Los Angeles Times*. July 19, 2015:A22.

4. Centers for Disease Control and Prevention. National Center on Birth Defects and Developmental Disabilities. Importance of newborn screening. Available at: http://www.cdc.gov/ncbddd/newbornscreening/. Accessed July 11, 2016.

5. U.S. National Library of Medicine. MedlinePlus. Newborn screening tests. Available at: https://www.nlm.nih.gov/medlineplus/ency/article/007257.htm. Accessed July 11, 2016.

6. Health Resources and Services Administration. Newborn screening: toward a uniform screening panel and system. Available at: https://www.hrsa.gov/advisorycommittees/mchbadvisory/heritabledisorders/uniform screening.pdf. Accessed July 11, 2016.

7. Centers for Disease Control and Prevention. Ten great public health achievements—United States, 2001–2010. Maternal and infant health. *MMWR*. 2011;60(19):619–623.

8. Centers for Disease Control and Prevention. National Center on Birth Defects and Developmental Disabilities. Facts about critical congenital heart defects. Available at: http://www.cdc.gov/ncbddd/heartdefects/cchd-facts.html. Accessed July 11, 2016.

9. Centers for Disease Control and Prevention. Developmental monitoring and screening. Available at: http://www.cdc.gov/ncbddd/childdevelopment/screening.html. Accessed July 13, 2016.

10. Centers for Disease Control and Prevention. Colorectal cancer screening saves lives. CDC Publication #99-6948. Atlanta: CDC; revised July 2009.

11. American Diabetes Association. Screening for type 2 diabetes. *Diabetes Care*. 2004;27(Suppl 1):S11-S14.

12. Centers for Disease Control and Prevention. Diabetes report card 2014. Atlanta, GA: CDC; 2015.

13. Centers for Disease Control and Prevention. Prevalence of cholesterol screening and high blood cholesterol among adults—United States, 2005, 2007, and 2009. *MMWR*. 2012;61(35):697–702.

14. National Institutes of Health. U.S. National Library of Medicine. MedlinePlus. Cholesterol testing and results. Available at: https://medlineplus.gov/ency/patientinstructions/000386.htm. Accessed July 12, 2016.

15. National Heart, Lung, and Blood Institute. How is high cholesterol diagnosed? Available at: https://www.nhlbi.nih.gov/health/health-topics/topics/hbc/diagnosis. Accessed July 12, 2016.

16. Centers for Disease Control and Prevention. Cholesterol fact sheet. Available at: https://www.cdc.gov/dhdsp/data_statistics/fact_sheets/docs/fs_cholesterol.pdf. Accessed July 12, 2016.

17. Centers for Disease Control and Prevention. High blood pressure. Available at: https://www.cdc.gov/bloodpressure/. Accessed July 15, 2016.

18. Centers for Disease Control and Prevention. HIV testing. Available at: http://www.cdc.gov/hiv/testing/. Accessed July 15, 2016.

19. Kluger J, Park A. The Angelina effect. *Time*. May 27, 2013:28–33.

20. Spitzer RL, Williams JBW, Kroenke K. Public Health Questionnaire (PHQ) screeners. Screener overview. Available at: http://www.phqscreeners.com/select-screener/36. Accessed July 17, 2016.

21. American Psychological Association. Patient Health Questionnaire (PHQ-9 & PHQ-2). Available at: http://www.apa.org/pi/about/publications/caregivers/practice-settings/assessment/tools/patient-health.aspx. Accessed July 17, 2016.

22. Haynes RB. How to read clinical journals, II: to learn about a diagnostic test. *Can Med Assoc J*. 1981;124:703–710.

CHAPTER **10**

Infectious Diseases and Outbreak Investigation

INTRODUCTION

Infectious diseases remain important causes of morbidity and mortality in the United States and worldwide. During the past century, chronic health problems such as heart disease have replaced infectious diseases as the leading killers in developed countries and to a lesser extent in developing nations. Nevertheless, infectious diseases remain significant worldwide. For example, in the United States the category of influenza and pneumonia was the eighth leading cause of death in 2013 (56,979 deaths),[1] and infectious disease agents contributed to several of the other 14 leading causes of death. Additional examples of major infectious diseases are sexually transmitted diseases, such as those associated with human immunodeficiency virus (HIV); emerging infections, such as conditions linked to the Zika virus and the West Nile virus; and illnesses transmitted by food, including *Escherichia coli* infections. **Table 10-1** provides a summary of major terms that will be defined in this chapter.

According to World Health Organization (WHO) statistics, the category of infectious and parasitic diseases accounted for 11.5% of mortality worldwide in 2012. This level was a decline from 19.5% in 2002. See **Table 10-2** for data on the worldwide frequency of mortality from selected infectious diseases. **Figure 10-1** compares the global death rates for category A diseases (infectious and parasitic diseases) shown in Table 10-2.

TABLE 10-1 List of Important Terms Used in This Chapter

Agent	Immunity (passive vs. active)
Antigen	Incubation period
Attack rate	Index case
Bioterrorism attack	Infection
Carrier	Infectious disease
Case mapping	Infectivity
Contagious disease	Isolation
Communicable disease	Nosocomial infection
	Parasitic disease
Common-source epidemic	Point source epidemic
	Portal of entry
Direct vs. indirect transmission	Portal of exit
	Quarantine
Emerging infectious disease	Reservoir
	Resistance
Endemic	Sexually transmitted disease (sexually transmitted infection)
Enteric protozoal parasite	
Environment	Subclinical (inapparent) infection
Environmental determinant	
	Toxin
Epidemic curve	Vaccination (immunization)
Epidemiologic triangle	Vaccine preventable disease
Fomite	Vector
Generation time	Vehicle
Herd immunity	Virulence
Host	Zoonosis

TERMS USED TO DESCRIBE INFECTIOUS DISEASES

As we begin this chapter, here are several definitions of terms used for describing infectious diseases and related matters. These terms are *infectious disease, contagious disease, communicable disease, parasitic disease*, and *infection*.

- An **infectious disease** is defined as "[a] disease due to an infectious agent." Such agents include bacteria and viruses.[2]
- A **contagious disease** is "[a] disease transmitted by direct or indirect contact with a host that is the source of the pathogenic agent."[2]
- A **communicable disease** is "[a]n illness due to a *specific infectious* agent or its toxic products that arises through transmission of such agent or products from an infected person, animal, or reservoir to a susceptible host, either directly or indirectly through an intermediate plant or animal host, vector, or the inanimate environment."[2] Some writers use the terms infectious disease and communicable disease as synonyms. Technically speaking, these terms can have different meanings.
- A **parasitic disease** (for example, amebiasis) is an infection caused by a parasite, which "… is an animal or vegetable organism that lives on or in another and derives its nourishment therefrom."[3]
- An **infection** is defined as "[t]he entry and development or multiplication of an infectious agent in the body of persons or animals." [4(p698)]

TABLE 10-2 Number of Deaths from Selected Communicable Diseases, Worldwide[a], 2012 Estimates[b]

Cause	Number	Percentage of Total
Total deaths	55,843,142	100
A. Infectious and parasitic diseases (overall category A, i.e., all deaths from this cause)[†]	6,430,847	11.5
*HIV/AIDS	1,533,760	2.7
*Diarrheal diseases	1,497,647	2.7

TABLE 10-2 Number of Deaths from Selected Communicable Diseases, Worldwide[a], 2012 Estimates[b] (continued)

Cause	Number	Percentage of Total
*Tuberculosis	934,838	1.7
*Parasitic and vector diseases	786,166	1.4
**Malaria	618,248	1.1
B. Respiratory infections[†]	3,060,166	5.5

[†]A and B are names of cause categories used by the World Health Organization (WHO) for their global health estimates of deaths. Refer to WHO, *Methods and Data Sources for Country-Level Causes of Death: 2000–2012.* Global Health Estimates Technical Paper WHO/HIS/HIS/GHE/2014.7. Geneva, Switzerland: WHO; 2014.

*A subcategory of the overall cause category A (infectious and parasitic diseases).

**A subcategory of parasitic and vector diseases.

a. World population = 7,336,437,000 (U.S. Census Bureau estimate, July, 2016).

b. Data are for both sexes combined.

Data from World Health Organization. The World Health Report: 2003: shaping the future. Geneva, Switzerland: World Health Organization; 2003:154.

FIGURE 10-1 Global crude death rates from WHO cause category A (infectious and parasitic diseases), 2012.

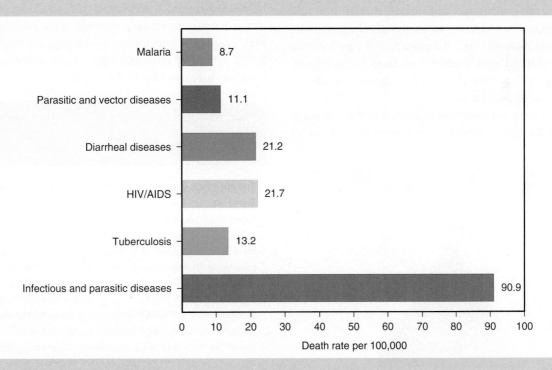

Data from World Health Organization. Available at: http://apps.who.int/gho/data/. Accessed August 2, 2016.

THE EPIDEMIOLOGIC TRIANGLE: AGENT, HOST, AND ENVIRONMENT

The **epidemiologic triangle**, which includes three major factors—agent, host, and environment—is one of the long-standing models used to describe the etiology of infectious diseases. Although this model has been applied to the field of infectious disease epidemiology, it also provides a framework for organizing the causality of some other types of health outcomes, such as those associated with the environment. Refer to **Figure 10-2** for an illustration of the epidemiologic triangle.

- An **agent** refers to "[a] factor (e.g., a microorganism, chemical substance, form of radiation, mechanical, behavioral, social agent or process) whose presence, excessive presence, or (in deficiency diseases) relative absence is essential for the occurrence of a disease. A disease may have a single agent, a number of independent alternative agents (at least one of which must be present), or a complex of two or more factors whose combined presence is essential for or contributes to the development of the disease or other outcome."[2]
- The **host** is "[a] person or other living animal, including birds and arthropods, that affords subsistence or lodgment to an *infectious agent* under natural conditions."[2] A human host is a person who is afflicted with a disease; or, from the epidemiologic perspective, the term *host* denotes an affected group or population.
- The term **environment** is defined as the domain in which disease-causing agents may exist, survive, or

originate; it consists of "[a]ll that which is external to the individual human host."[2]

Disease transmission involves the interaction of the three major components, as you will learn subsequently. Although the model provides a simplified account of the causality of infectious diseases, in reality the etiology of infectious diseases is often complex.

INFECTIOUS DISEASE AGENTS

With respect to infectious and communicable diseases, agents include specific microbes and vectors involved in the cycle of disease transmission. Examples of infectious agents are microbial agents such as bacteria, rickettsia, viruses, fungi, parasites, and prions. Infectious disease agents vary in their **infectivity**, which refers to the capacity of an agent to enter and multiply in a susceptible host and thus produce infection or disease. The term **virulence** refers to the severity of the disease produced, i.e., whether the disease has severe clinical manifestations or is fatal in a large number of cases.

Some infectious disease agents enter the body and cause illness when they multiply; they act directly. Other disease agents produce a toxin; it is the action of this toxin that causes illness. A **toxin** usually refers to a toxic substance (a material that is harmful to biologic systems) made by living organisms. Foodborne intoxications are examples of illness caused by the actions of microbial toxins. Refer to the example of botulism discussed later in this chapter.

The increasing antibiotic resistance of bacteria

The antibiotic penicillin was introduced into general use after World War II. Penicillin was so effective in controlling some types of bacterial infections that it became known as a "magic bullet." Since the introduction of penicillin, other antibiotics have been developed. Unfortunately, over time, bacteria have evolved resistance against many antibiotics, which are no longer effective against some bacterial agents. Outbreaks caused by drug-resistant organisms (e.g., methicillin-resistant *Staphylococcus aureus* [MRSA]) in hospitals are potential threats to patients and staff. Some common bacterial infections may no longer be treatable with antibiotics. Ultimately, antibiotics may not be able to protect us from bacterial diseases. Suspected causes for development of antibiotic resistance include overuse in humans and as growth promoters in farm animals destined for human consumption.

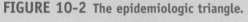

FIGURE 10-2 The epidemiologic triangle.

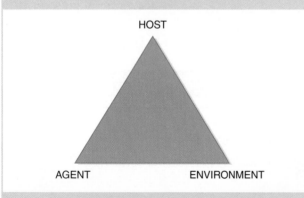

HOST

AGENT   ENVIRONMENT

The consequences of infectious diseases are manifested in diverse ways. A few examples are subclinical and clinically apparent infections, zoonotic illnesses, foodborne illnesses, infectious disease outbreaks that are associated with specific occupations, and infectious disease occurrences linked with water pollution. **Figure 10-3** illustrates four infectious disease agents: bacteria, viruses, fungi, and parasites (protozoa).

FIGURE 10-3 Four infectious disease agents. Upper left, *Bacillus anthracis* bacteria; lower left, Zika virus; upper right, dermatophytic fungus (causes ringworm infections of the skin and fungal infections of the nail bed); lower right, *Cryptosporidium parvum* oocysts.

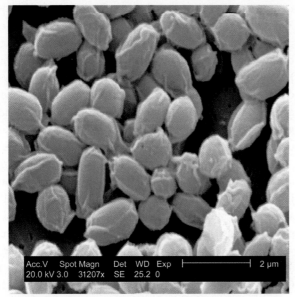

Courtesy of CDC/Laura Rose

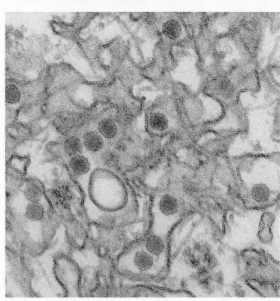

Courtesy of CDC/Dr. Libero Ajello

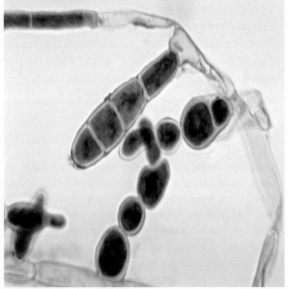

Courtesy of CDC/Cynthia Goldsmith

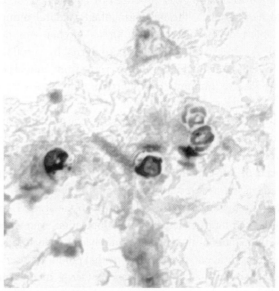

Courtesy of CDC/DPDx

Reprinted from Centers for Disease Control and Prevention. Public Health Image Library, ID# 10123 (upper left); ID# 20541 (lower left); ID# 4207(upper right); ID# 7829 (lower right). Available at: http://phil.cdc.gov/phil/details.asp. Accessed February 10, 2016.

HOST CHARACTERISTICS

A second component identified in the epidemiologic triangle is the host. Whether human or animal, hosts vary in their responses to disease agents. A host characteristic that can limit the ability of an infectious disease agent to produce infection is known as immunity, which refers to the host's ability to resist infection by the agent. **Immunity** is defined as "[a] status usually associated with the presence of antibodies or cells having a specific action on the microorganism concerned with a particular infectious disease or on its toxin."[4(p697)]

Susceptible hosts are those at risk (capable) of acquiring an infection. Generally speaking, immune hosts are at lowered risk of developing the infection, although they may be susceptible in some situations, for example, if they receive large doses of an infectious agent or they are under treatment with immunosuppressive drugs.

Immunity may be either active or passive, the former referring to immunity that the host has developed as a result of a natural infection with a microbial agent; active immunity also can be acquired from an injection of a vaccine (immunization) that contains an **antigen** (a substance that stimulates antibody formation). Examples of antigens are live or attenuated microbial agents. (Jenner's development of an immunization against smallpox was an early example of using a vaccination to protect against a disease.)

Active immunity is usually of long duration and is measured in years. **Passive immunity** refers to immunity that is acquired from antibodies produced by another person or animal. For instance, the newborn infant's natural immunity conferred transplacentally from its mother. Another example is artificial immunity that is conferred by injections of antibodies contained in immune serums from animals or humans. Passive immunity is of short duration, lasting from a few days to several months.

From the epidemiologic perspective, the immune statuses of both individual hosts and the entire population are noteworthy. The term **herd immunity** denotes the **resistance** (opposite of susceptibility) of an entire community to an infectious agent as a result of the immunity of a large proportion of individuals in that community to the agent. Herd immunity can limit epidemics in the population even when not every member of the population has been vaccinated.

A clinically apparent disease is one that produces observable clinical signs and symptoms. The term **incubation period** denotes the time interval between invasion by an infectious agent and the appearance of the first sign or symptom of the disease.

In some hosts, an infection may be **subclinical** (also called **inapparent**), meaning that the infection does not show obvious clinical signs or symptoms. For example, hepatitis A infections among children and the early phases of infection with HIV are largely asymptomatic. Nevertheless, individuals who have inapparent infections can transmit them to others; thus inapparent infections are epidemiologically significant and part of the spectrum of infection.

After an infectious organism has lodged and reproduced in the host, the agent can be transmitted to other hosts. The term **generation time** is defined as the time interval between lodgment of an infectious agent in a host and the maximal communicability of the host. The generation time for an infectious disease and the incubation time may or may not be equivalent. For some diseases, the period of maximal communicability precedes the development of active symptoms. Incubation period applies only to clinically apparent cases of disease, whereas generation time applies to both inapparent and apparent cases of disease.

A term related to inapparent infections is *carrier status*; a **carrier** is "[a] person or animal that harbors a specific infectious agent without discernible clinical disease and that serves as a potential source of infection."[4(p693)] When carrier status is longstanding, the host is called a chronic carrier.

A famous example of an infectious disease carrier was "Typhoid Mary" Mallon, who worked as a cook in New York City during the early 1900s and was alleged to be a typhoid carrier. Several cases of typhoid fever were traced to households where she was employed. Typhoid fever, caused by *Salmonella* bacteria (*S. typhi*), is a systemic infection associated with a 10 to 20% case fatality rate when untreated. After the first cases of typhoid were associated with her, Mallon was quarantined for 3 years on Brother Island in New York City and then released with the proviso that she no longer work as a cook.

What is quarantine?

Quarantine—Well persons who have been exposed to an infectious disease are prevented from interacting with those not exposed, for example, preventing medical personnel who have been exposed to Ebola virus from leaving their place of residence. This is different from isolation.

Isolation—Persons who have a communicable disease are kept away from other persons for a period of time that corresponds generally to the interval when the disease is communicable, for example, maintaining isolation of patients with Ebola in special isolation units.

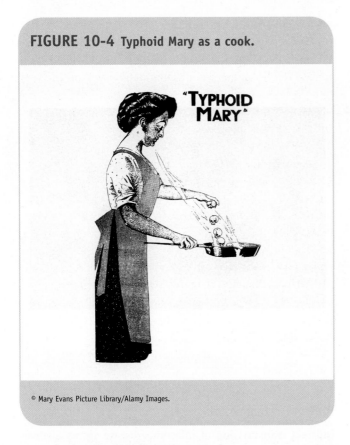

FIGURE 10-4 Typhoid Mary as a cook.

© Mary Evans Picture Library/Alamy Images.

Unfortunately, Mallon defied the quarantine order. Consequently, after she continued working as a cook and was linked to additional typhoid outbreaks, she again was confined to Brother Island until she died in 1938. Refer to **Figure 10-4** for an image of "Typhoid Mary."

The foregoing example illustrated an outbreak of typhoid fever. An outbreak of infectious disease may trigger an epidemiologic investigation. The term **index case** is used in an epidemiologic investigation of a disease outbreak to denote the first case of a disease to come to the attention of authorities.

ENVIRONMENT AND INFECTIOUS DISEASES

The third component of the epidemiologic triangle is the environment. The external environment is the sum of all influences that are not part of the host; it comprises physical, climatologic, biologic, social, and economic components. Here are some examples of how **environmental determinants** may act as potential influences associated with the occurrence of diseases and other health outcomes.

- Physical environment. The availability of clean and abundant water supplies is instrumental in maintaining optimal sanitary conditions; waterborne diseases

such as cholera are associated with pathogens that can contaminate water. Other pathogens such as fungi may be present naturally in the soil in some geographic areas. An example is the fungus *Coccidioides immitis*, found in California's San Joaquin Valley. This fungus is the agent for San Joaquin Valley fever.

- Climatologic environment. In warm, moist, tropical climates, disease agents and arthropod vectors such as the *Anopheles* mosquito, the vector for malaria, are able to survive and cause human and animal diseases. These same vectors and the diseases associated with them are not as common in drier, colder, temperate climates. However, with global warming observed in recent years, it may be possible for disease vectors to migrate to regions that formerly were much colder.
- Biologic environment. The biologic environment includes the presence of available plant and animal species that can act as reservoirs for disease agents. These species may be part of the cycle of reproduction of the disease agent. An example is the disease schistosomiasis, which depends on the presence of intermediate hosts (certain species of snails) in order to reproduce. Schistosomiasis, a major cause of illnesses including liver cirrhosis, is found in Africa, the Middle East, parts of South America and Asia, as well as some other geographic areas.
- Social and economic environments. While the world becomes increasingly urbanized as inhabitants search for improved opportunities, cities will become ever more crowded. The overcrowded urban environment can contribute to the spread of infections through person-to-person contact and creation of unsanitary conditions such as improper disposal of human wastes.

When an infectious disease agent is habitually present in an environment (either a geographic or population group), it is said to be **endemic**. In illustration, plague is endemic among certain species of rodents in the western United States. Another term to describe the presence of an infectious agent in the environment is a **reservoir**, which is a place where infectious agents normally live and multiply; the reservoir can be human beings, animals, insects, soils, or plants.

The term **zoonosis** refers to "[a]n infection … transmissible under natural conditions from vertebrate animals to humans."[4(p706)] An example of a zoonotic disease is rabies, a highly fatal viral disease that affects the brain (causing acute viral encephalomyelitis) and can be transmitted by the bite of an infected dog or other rabid animal. The concept called One Health "… recognizes that the health of humans is connected to the health of animals and the environment. There are many examples that show how the health of people is related to the health of animals and the environment. For instance, some diseases [zoonotic diseases] can be spread between animals and humans."[5]

HOW INFECTIOUS DISEASE AGENTS ARE TRANSMITTED

Now that the three elements of the epidemiologic triangle have been defined, the author will explain two methods for the spread of disease agents: directly from person to person and indirectly. Some modes of indirect transmission are by means of vehicles (defined later) and vectors. In order for infection to occur, the agent needs to move from the environment (an infected person or a reservoir) to a potential host. For an infected person, a **portal of exit** is the site from which the agent leaves that person's body; portals of exit include respiratory passages, the alimentary canal, the genitourinary system, and skin lesions.

Person to Person (Direct Transmission)

The term **direct transmission** refers to "[d]irect and essentially immediate transfer of infectious agents to a receptive portal of entry through which human or animal infection may take place. This may be by direct contact such as touching, kissing, biting, or sexual intercourse or by the direct projection (droplet spread) of droplet spray…"[2] See **Figure 10-5**, which illustrates that when one sneezes, potentially infectious droplets are dispersed over a wide area. When a person is infected with a microbial agent, such as a cold virus, and he or she sneezes, other individuals in the vicinity can inhale the virus-containing droplets. What happens next?

In order for an infectious agent to lodge in a host, it must gain access to a **portal of entry**, or site where the agent enters the body. Examples of portals of entry are the respiratory system (through inhalation), a skin wound (such as a break in skin), and the mucous membranes, which line some of the body's organs and cavities—e.g., nose, mouth, and lungs.

Depending on several factors—including the type of microbial agent, access to a portal of entry, the amount of the agent to which the potential host is exposed, and the immune status of the host—an active infection may result.

FIGURE 10-5 The model demonstrates that a sneeze releases a cloud of droplets into the nearby environment.

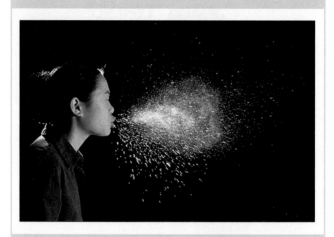

Photo courtesy of Andrew Davidhazy, Rochester Institute of Technology.

Indirect Transmission

Indirect transmission of infectious disease agents involves intermediary sources of infection, such as vehicles, droplet nuclei (particles), and vectors. The terms used to describe indirect transmission of disease agents by these sources are as follows:

- Vehicle-borne infections
- Airborne infections
- Vector-borne infections

Vehicle-Borne Infections

These infections result from contact with **vehicles**, which are contaminated, nonmoving objects. Vehicles can include fomites (defined later), unsanitary food, impure water, or infectious bodily fluids. For example, used injection needles may contain bloodborne pathogens. This was the case during a 2008 suspected hepatitis C virus (HCV) transmission by unsafe injection practices. In January 2008, the Nevada State Health Department reported three cases of acute hepatitis C to the Centers for Disease Control and Prevention (CDC). Investigations by state and local health departments in collaboration with CDC revealed that all three individuals had procedures performed at the same endoscopy clinic.

Endoscopy is a procedure for viewing the inside of a body cavity or organ (for example, the esophagus) by using an instrument such as a flexible tube. Laboratory and epidemiologic research findings suggested that syringes from single-use medication vials had been reused and that this unsafe practice could have been the cause of the outbreak. Health authorities notified approximately 40,000 patients who had been treated at the clinic of their possible exposure to HCV and other pathogens carried in blood. **Figure 10-6** portrays the unsafe injection practices that might have led to the outbrak.

A **fomite** is an inanimate object that carries infectious disease agents; fomites include the classroom doorknob, used towels found in a locker room, or carelessly discarded tissues. In hospitals, unsanitary linen contaminated with medical wastes can cause outbreaks of **hospital-acquired (nosocomial) infections**. For this reason, hospital epidemiologists seek to minimize exposure of patients and staff to these types of fomites by requiring hand-washing procedures, disposal of medical wastes in sealed bags (often red and marked "biohazard"), and frequent disinfection of floors and surfaces.

Foodborne diseases are those caused by ingestion of contaminated food. Such contamination can be from arsenic, heavy metals, toxins naturally present in foods, and toxic chemicals including pesticides. Other sources of contamination are microbial agents that have entered the food supply during growth and harvesting of crops, storage of ingredients, and preparation and storage of foods that are consumed. *Salmonella* bacteria are one of the most important causes of foodborne infections in the United States. This agent was identified as the cause of a foodborne disease outbreak during mid-2008. Initially, the source of the outbreak was thought to be *Salmonella*-contaminated tomatoes; later, however, authorities stated that the cause was *Salmonella* bacteria carried on jalapeño and serrano peppers imported from Mexico.

Waterborne infections are those caused by the presence of infectious disease agents that contaminate the water supply and in which water is the vehicle of infection. Examples of waterborne infections are bacterial infections (e.g., cholera, typhoid fever), parasitic infections (e.g., giardiasis, cryptosporidiosis) caused by enteric protozoal parasites, and viral infections (e.g., Norwalk agent disease, winter vomiting disease) caused by noroviruses. **Enteric protozoal parasites** are pathogenic single-celled microorganisms that can live in the intestinal tract; both giardiasis and cryptosporidiosis are diseases caused by these organisms. Waterborne infections take a great toll in morbidity and mortality in developing nations and present a hazard to tourists visiting these areas. In the United States, outbreaks of waterborne diseases occur sporadically, one case being the infamous 1993 cryptosporidiosis outbreak in Milwaukee, Wisconsin. The incident, which affected more

FIGURE 10-6 Unsafe injection practices and circumstances that likely resulted in transmission of hepatitis C virus (HCV) at clinic A—Nevada 2007.

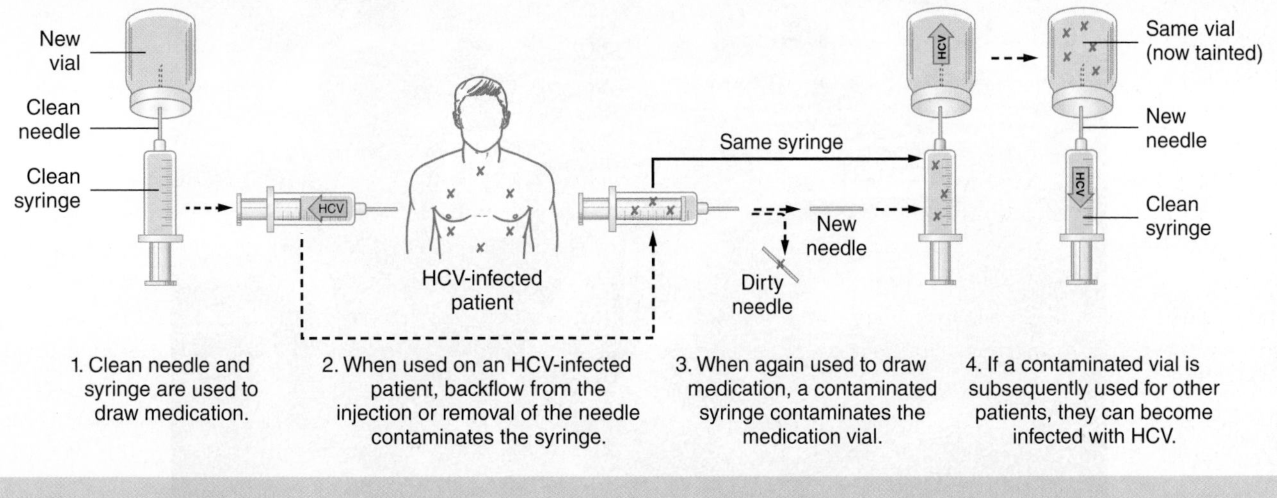

Reprinted from Centers for Disease Control and Prevention. Acute hepatitis C virus infections attributed to unsafe injection practices at an endoscopy clinic—Nevada, 2007. *MMWR.* 2008;57:516.

than 400,000 people, was attributed to inadequate treatment of the water supply during heavy precipitation.

Airborne Infections

Another type of indirect transmission involves the spread of droplet nuclei (particles) that are present in the air, for example, by stirring up dust that carries fungi or microbes. Some venues for the airborne transmission of disease agents are closed and poorly ventilated environments: movie theaters, doctors' examination rooms, classrooms, and motor vehicles. Passengers who are confined in closed environments, such as compartments of airplanes, are at theoretical risk of exposure to airborne infectious agents emitted by infected passengers.

On March 15, 2003, a 72-year-old man in Hong Kong, China boarded a Boeing 737-300 aircraft for a 3-hour flight that was bound for Beijing. This man (called the index case) had developed a fever on March 11; he was hospitalized when he arrived at his destination, was diagnosed with atypical pneumonia, and died on March 20. Between March 4 and March 9, the index case had visited his brother in a Hong Kong hospital. The brother, who died on March 9, was diagnosed with severe acute respiratory syndrome (SARS); several other patients on the same ward also were reported to have SARS. During the flight to Beijing, the index case shared the aircraft with 111 other passengers and 8 crew members. Investigations later revealed that 22 people (18% of the individuals on board the aircraft) were believed to have become infected with SARS and 5 subsequently died. A total of 65 of the 112 passengers were interviewed, and 18 of these (28%) met the WHO definition of a probable case of SARS.

The seat locations of the cases were mapped in relation to the index case. Passengers who sat closest to the index case had the highest risk of contracting SARS in comparison with passengers who sat farther away.[6] Nevertheless, the risk of airborne transmission of communicable disease agents in the closed environment of a jet plane is believed to be low because the cabin air is continuously recycled and highly filtered. Some conditions of potential concern are measles, tuberculosis, and meningitis, which can be transmitted by airborne respiratory droplets that are most likely to impinge upon passengers who are sitting next to or near an ill individual. **Figure 10**-7 shows the crowded seating arrangement of an aircraft.

FIGURE 10-7 A view of the interior of a jet aircraft.

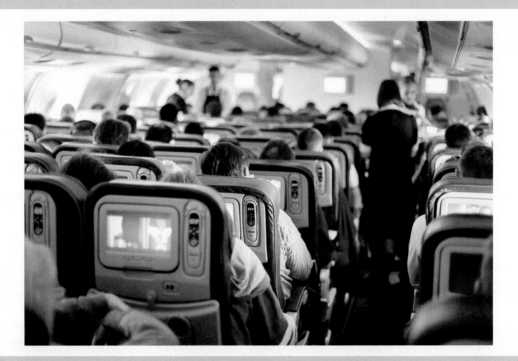

Vector-Borne infections

A **vector** is an animate, living insect or animal that is involved with the transmission of disease agents. Transmission of an infectious disease agent may happen when the vector feeds on a susceptible host. Examples of vectors are arthropods (insects such as lice, flies, mosquitoes, and ticks) that bite their victims and feed on the latter's blood. Rats are an example of a rodent species that can be a reservoir for fleas that transmit plague. **Figure 10-8** illustrates common vectors of infectious diseases.

EXAMPLES OF SIGNIFICANT INFECTIOUS DISEASES

Infectious diseases are often grouped into categories that are defined according to the method by which the disease is spread (e.g., foodborne) or by using other criteria, such as being vaccine-preventable or newly discovered. The categories are not mutually exclusive; several of the diseases could be included in more than one category. The following list presents categories of significant infectious diseases, some of which are discussed in the next section.

FIGURE 10-8 Four vectors of infectious diseases. Upper left, body lice; lower left, a deer tick; upper right, a female *Aedes aegypti* mosquito acquiring a blood meal; lower right, a flea.

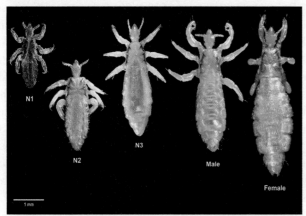

Courtesy of CDC/Joseph Strycharz, Ph.D.; Kyong Sup Yoon, Ph.D.; Frank Collins, Ph.D..

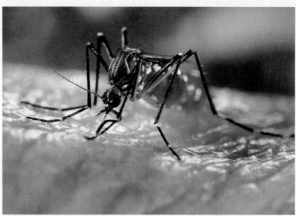

Courtesy of CDC/Prof. Frank Hadley Collins, Dir., Cntr. for Global Health and Infectious Diseases, Univ. of Notre Dame

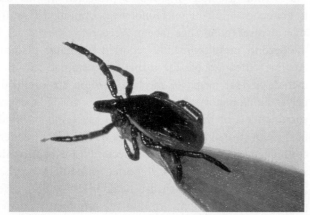

Courtesy of Centers for Disease Control and Prevention.

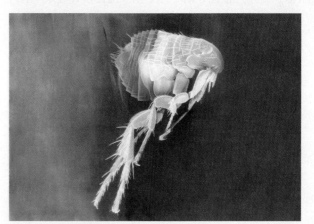

Courtesy of CDC/Janice Haney Carr

Reprinted from Centers for Disease Control and Prevention. Public Health Image Library, ID# 10854 (upper left); ID# 9255 (upper right); ID# 9959 (lower left); ID # 11436 (lower right). Available at: http://phil.cdc.gov/phil/details.asp. Accessed August 2, 2016.

- Sexually transmitted diseases
- Foodborne diseases
- Waterborne diseases (discussed earlier in the chapter)
  - Bacterial conditions (e.g., cholera and typhoid fever). Note that cholera and typhoid fever also can be transmitted in food.
  - Parasitic diseases (e.g., giardiasis and cryptosporidiosis; see previous example)
- Vector-borne (e.g., arthropod-borne) diseases
- Vaccine-preventable diseases
- Zoonotic diseases
- Emerging infections
- Bioterrorism-related diseases

Sexually Transmitted Diseases

Sexually transmitted diseases (STDs) are infectious diseases and related conditions (such as crab lice) that can be spread by sexual contact. They are also called **sexually transmitted infections (STIs)**. **Table 10-3** lists eight examples of STDs. In addition to those shown, many other infections may be transmitted through sexual contact; these diseases include salmonellosis, viral hepatitis B, and viral hepatitis C.

Human Immunodeficiency Virus (HIV) Infections

The first example of a sexually transmitted disease cited in this section is infection with HIV. Acquired immunodeficiency syndrome (AIDS) is a late clinical stage of infection with HIV. The term HIV/AIDS covers persons who are infected with HIV but who may not have been diagnosed with AIDS, as well as persons infected with HIV who have developed AIDS.

TABLE 10-3 Examples of Sexually Transmitted Diseases

Anogenital herpes infections (caused by herpes simplex virus type 2)

Chlamydial genital infections*

Crab lice

Gonococcal infections (gonorrhea)*

Human immunodeficiency virus (HIV) infections*

Lymphogranuloma venereum

Syphilis

Venereal warts

*Discussed in text.

The infectious agent of HIV is a type of virus called a retrovirus. Among the possible modes for transmission of the agent are unprotected sexual intercourse and contact with infected blood (e.g., through transfusions and accidental needle sticks). Transmission from infected mother to child (known as vertical transmission) is also possible. As noted, HIV can progress to AIDS, the term used to describe cases of a disease that began to emerge in 1981. Successful treatment programs have helped to limit the progression of HIV to AIDS. Because early infection with HIV is often asymptomatic, screening at-risk persons is essential for limiting the spread of this condition.

CDC conducts surveillance of HIV infection of all 50 states in the United States, the District of Columbia, and six dependent areas. Data stripped of identifying features are submitted to CDC, which later analyzes this information. CDC reported that from 2010 to 2014, the rate of diagnoses increased among persons age 25 to 29 years; this age group had the highest diagnosis rate in comparison with other age groups in 2014.[7] As shown in **Table 10-4**, annual rates of HIV diagnoses in the U.S. population tended to remain stable between 2010 and 2014; in 2014 the estimated numbers of cases among male adults or adolescents exceeded the number of female cases by a factor of more than four to one. Among males, the highest transmission category was male-to-male sexual contact; among females, transmission occurred most frequently among those who had heterosexual contact.

Gonococcal Infections

The second example of an STD presented in this text is gonococcal infections (gonorrhea). Among all notifiable diseases, gonorrhea (agent: *Neisseria gonorrhoeae*) is the second most frequently reported notifiable disease.[8] Possible outcomes of this sexually transmitted infection include several forms of morbidity; these are urethritis, pelvic inflammatory disease, pharyngitis, and gonococcal conjunctivitis of the newborn, which can result in blindness if not treated promptly. More severe and less frequent consequences of gonococcal infections are septicemia, arthritis, and endocarditis. Reported cases of gonorrhea in the United States reached a nadir in 2009 (98.1 cases per 100,000 population). In 2014 the rate then increased to 100.7 cases per 100,000 population. For 2013 and 2014, the incidence of gonorrhea was slightly higher among men than among women. **Figure 10-9** presents time trends in reported cases of gonorrhea since 1941.

TABLE 10-4 Estimated Diagnoses of Cases of HIV/AIDS, by Year of Diagnosis and Selected Characteristics—United States, 2011–2014

Transmission Category	Year of Diagnosis			
	2011	2012	2013	2014
Male adult or adolescent				
Male-to-male sexual contact	27,001	27,588	27,642	29,418
Injection drug use	1,819	1,642	1,575	1,590
Male-to-male sexual contact and injection drug use	1,393	1,342	1,216	1,217
Heterosexual contact[a]	3,883	3,617	3,545	3,285
Other[b]	50	69	57	60
Subtotal	34,146	34,259	34,034	35,571
Female adult or adolescent				
Injection drug use	1,284	1,178	1,073	1,045
Heterosexual contact[a]	7,833	7,439	7,213	7,242
Other[b]	49	39	55	41
Subtotal	9,166	8,656	8,340	8,328
Child (< 13 yrs at diagnosis)				
Perinatal	147	175	127	127
Other[c]	51	75	64	48
Subtotal	198	250	191	174
U.S. total	43,510	43,165	42,566	44,073

Note: These numbers do not represent reported case counts. Rather, these numbers are point estimates, which result from adjustments of reported case counts.
Data include persons with a diagnosis of HIV infection regardless of stage of disease at diagnosis.
[a]Heterosexual contact with a person known to have, or to be at high risk for, HIV infection.
[b]Includes hemophilia, blood transfusion, perinatal exposure, and risk factors not reported or not identified.
[c]Includes hemophilia, blood transfusion, and risk factors not reported or not identified.

Adapted and reprinted from Centers for Disease Control and Prevention. *HIV Surveillance Report*, 2014; vol. 26, pp 18–19. Available at: https://www.cdc.gov/hiv/pdf/library/reports/surveillance/cdc-hiv-surveillance-report-us.pdf. Published November 2015. Accessed December 6, 2016.

FIGURE 10-9 Gonorrhea: rates of reported cases, by year—United States, 1941–2014.

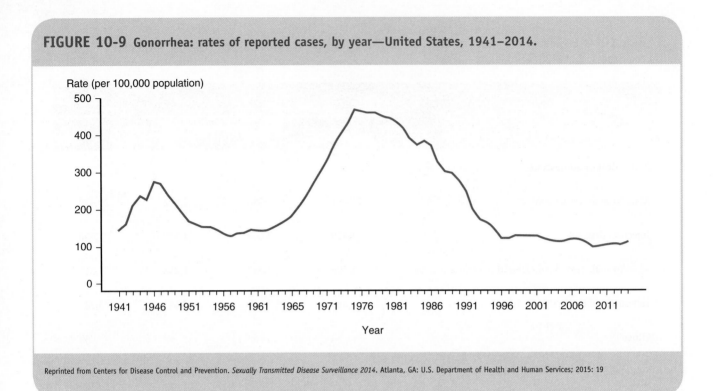

Reprinted from Centers for Disease Control and Prevention. *Sexually Transmitted Disease Surveillance 2014*. Atlanta, GA: U.S. Department of Health and Human Services; 2015: 19

Chlamydial Genital Infections

Chlamydial genital infections, which stem from the sexual transmission of the bacterial agent *Chlamydia trachomatis*, are the third example of an STD discussed here. The U.S. incidence rate of reported chlamydial infections was 456.1 cases per 100,000 population in 2014.[8]

Why is *C. trachomatis* a dangerous player? It is responsible for a large proportion of asymptomatic infections (up to 70% in women and 25% in men) with potentially devastating results. Among the sequelae of infections are male and female infertility. Among women, chlamydial infections are associated with chronic pelvic pain and preterm delivery; these infections can be transmitted to the fetus during pregnancy, possibly resulting in conjunctivitis and pneumonia among newborn infants. **Figure 10-10** portrays the geographic incidence of chlamydia among women in the United States; by region, the highest rate in 2014 was in the South (492.3 per 100,000 population).

Foodborne Illness

According to WHO, the global disease burden attributable to foodborne illness is vast in scope, affecting about 10% of the world's population and causing 420,000 deaths. (See **Figure 10-11**.) The most frequent illnesses associated with foodborne transmission are diarrheal conditions. Information on the frequent occurrence of foodborne illness in the United States is provided later in the chapter. Now, let's consider some of the biologic agents responsible for foodborne illness.

Biologic agents of foodborne illness include bacteria, parasites, viruses, and prions (linked to mad cow disease). A total of 31 pathogens have been identified. Some names of bacterial agents of foodborne illnesses can be found in **Table 10-5**.

From the worldwide perspective, foodborne illness is a major cause of morbidity. In the United States, "… each year roughly 1 in 6 Americans (or 48 million people) gets sick, 128,000 are hospitalized, and 3,000 die of foodborne diseases."[9]

The Foodborne Diseases Active Surveillance Network (FoodNet) monitors foodborne diseases in this country. FoodNet "… is a collaborative program of Centers for Disease Control and Prevention (CDC), 10 state health departments, the U.S. Department of Agriculture's Food Safety and Inspection Service (USDA-FSIS), and the Food and Drug Administration (FDA)."[10] The FoodNet surveillance program identified 19,507 laboratory-confirmed cases of foodborne infection in 2014.

FIGURE 10-10 Chlamydia: rates of reported cases, by state—United States and outlying areas, 2014.

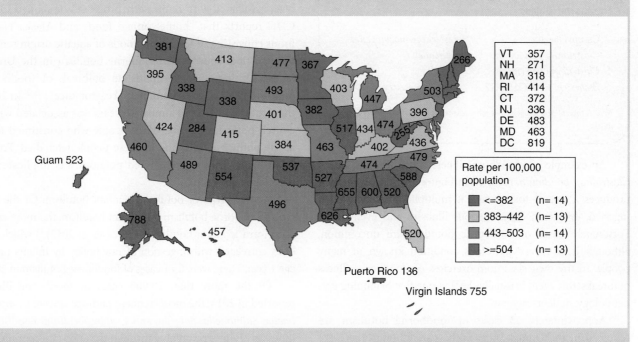

Reprinted from Centers for Disease Control and Prevention. *Sexually Transmitted Disease Surveillance 2014*. Atlanta, GA: U.S. Department of Health and Human Services; 2015; 9.

FIGURE 10-11 The global burden of foodborne diseases is substantial.

Every year foodborne diseases cause:

almost

in10
people to fall ill

33 million
healthy life years lost

Foodborne diseases can be deadly, **especially in children <5**

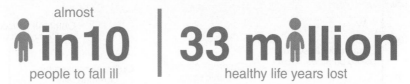

420 000
deaths

Children account for

almost **1/3**

of deaths from foodborne diseases

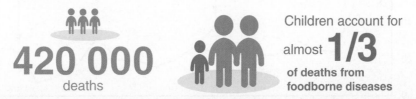

FOODBORNE DISEASES ARE PREVENTABLE.
EVERYONE HAS A ROLE TO PLAY.

Reproduced from World Health Organization. WHO estimates of the global burden of foodborne diseases. Infographic. Available at: http://www.who.int/foodsafety/areas_work/foodborne-diseases/ferg_infographics/en/. Accessed July 11, 2016.

TABLE 10-5 Examples of Bacterial Agents of Foodborne Illness

Campylobacter	Listeria monocytogenes
Clostridium botulinum	Salmonella
Clostridium perfringens	Shigella
Escherichia coli O157:H7	Staphylococcus aureus

Note: A total of 31 pathogens plus other agents are associated with foodborne illness.

An example of a foodborne illness is botulism caused by *Clostridium botulinum*, reported in **Figure 10-12**. *C. botulinum* produces a potent toxin when it multiplies in food. When ingested, this toxin causes serious illnesses and even death. Fortunately, cases of foodborne botulism are uncommon, although it is a very notorious condition known to many people. In my own classroom exercises on foodborne illness outbreaks, this agent is usually the first one that beginning epidemiology students suggest.

Approximately 25 cases of foodborne botulism are reported in the United States each year, although there are periodic increases in the number of cases as a result of outbreaks. (Refer to Figure 10-12.) Botulism outbreaks have been associated with improperly processed or canned foods. CDC reports that "home-canned foods and Alaska Native foods consisting of fermented foods of aquatic origin remain the principal sources of foodborne botulism in the United States. During 2006, a multistate outbreak of foodborne botulism was linked to commercial carrot juice."[11(p42)] In 2015, the largest outbreak in almost 40 years was associated with a church potluck.[12] A total of 29 people who consumed food at the potluck fell ill; one of these people later died. Potato salad made from home-canned potatoes was implicated as the suspected food.

Another type of botulism is infant botulism. Of the two types, foodborne botulism and infant botulism, the more common form is infant botulism (136 cases in 2013),[13] which has been correlated with ingestion of raw honey by infants under age 1 year. There were four cases of foodborne botulism in 2013.

Of the more than 19,000 cases of foodborne illness reported in 2014, the most frequent pathogens were *Campylobacter*, *Salmonella*, *Shigella*, and *Cryptosporidium*. Foodborne illness is highly preventable through the application of proper

FIGURE 10-12 Botulism, foodborne: number of reported cases, by year—United States, 1993–2013.

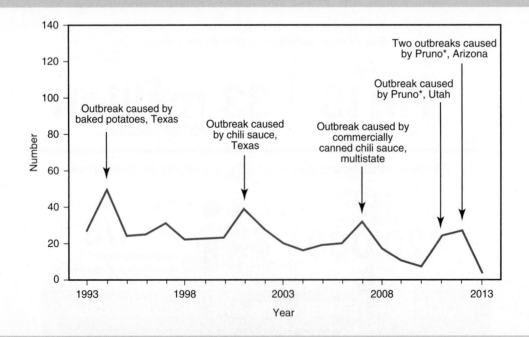

Reprinted from Centers for Disease Control and Prevention. Summary of notifiable infectious diseases and conditions—United States, 2013. *MMWR.* 2015;62(53):59.
* Pruno is an illicit alcoholic beverage brewed by prison inmates.

Preventing foodborne illness

Foodborne illness can be prevented through the following procedures:

- Thoroughly wash hands and surfaces where food is being prepared.
- Avoid cross-contamination—e.g., keep juices from raw chicken and meats away from other foods.
- Cook foods at correct temperatures that are sufficient to kill microorganisms (e.g., 180°F for poultry).
- Use proper storage methods (i.e., in a refrigerator below 40°F). Don't let your lunch stay in a hot car without refrigeration.

FIGURE 10-13 The Lyme disease bullseye.

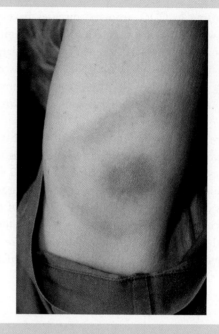

Reprinted from Centers for Disease Control and Prevention. Dengue hemorrhagic fever U.S.-Mexico border, 2005. *MMWR*. 2007;56:822.

food storage and handling techniques. Refer to the text box for tips about how to prevent foodborne illness.

Vector-Borne Diseases

Table 10-6 presents examples of vector-borne diseases, which include those caused by bacteria, viruses, and parasites. Four bacterially associated vector-borne conditions are Lyme disease, plague, tick-borne relapsing fever, and tularemia. The agent for Lyme disease is *Borrelia burgdorferi*, transmitted by a species of ticks. Lyme disease cases occur in most of the continental United States but have endemic foci on the Atlantic coast, Wisconsin, Minnesota, and sections of California and Oregon. **Figure 10-13** shows the distinctive "bullseye" skin lesions found in Lyme disease, which can cause arthritis and other serious conditions.

Arthropod-borne viral (arboviral) diseases are associated with significant morbidity (and mortality) in the United States.

The term arbovirus means "arthropod-borne virus." Responsible vectors for transmission of arboviruses include infected mosquitos and ticks.[14] Arboviruses can cause non-neuroinvasive diseases such as fevers and neuroinvasive diseases such as encephalitis and severe neurologic complications,[15] although the majority of cases are asymptomatic. Among the subtypes of arbovirus-associated diseases are the California serogroup virus diseases, Eastern equine encephalitis (EEE) virus disease,

TABLE 10-6 Examples of Vector-Borne Diseases (name of vector in parentheses)

Bacterial Diseases	Arthropod-Borne Viral (Arboviral) Diseases*	Parasitic Diseases
Lyme disease (tick)*	Eastern equine encephalitis (mosquito)	Malaria (mosquito)
Plague (flea)	West Nile encephalitis (mosquito)	Leishmaniasis (sandfly)
Tick-borne relapsing fever	Yellow fever (mosquito)	African trypanosomiasis (tsetse fly)
Tularemia (tick-borne in the United States)	Dengue fever (mosquito)	American trypanosomiasis (kissing bug)

*Discussed in text.

St. Louis encephalitis disease, and West Nile virus disease. The California serogroup viruses include the La Crosse virus and the Jamestown Canyon virus.[14]

According to CDC, arboviral diseases have seasonal patterns, with incidence increasing during summer and fall and peaking in the late summer.[16] In 2013, data for the United States revealed that West Nile virus was the most frequently reported cause of neuroinvasive arboviral disease, followed by La Crosse virus and Jamestown Canyon virus.[13]

Figure 10-14 shows time trends in the number of cases of three groups of neuroinvasive diseases from the following arboviruses: California serogroup viruses, the EEE virus, and the St. Louis encephalitis virus. (The number of cases of West Nile virus disease is not shown in the figure.) Of the three categories of virus-caused neuroinvasive diseases, those associated with the California serogroup viruses were reported most frequently between 2004 and 2013. EEE, which tended

to be an infrequently reported condition, is the most severe arboviral disease (50% case-fatality rate).

Referring back to Table 10-6, you will note that dengue fever is one of the types of arboviral diseases. Transmitted mainly by the *Aedes aegypti* mosquito, the dengue virus has caused epidemics in Asia and South and Central America. The virus also has appeared along the border of the United States and Texas.

A large proportion of dengue fever infections are asymptomatic. However, dengue fever is a potentially serious infection. The severe form, dengue hemorrhagic fever, causes bleeding at various sites of the body and can progress to life-threatening shock.

Figure 10-15 shows the epidemic curve for an outbreak of more than 1,600 cases of dengue fever that occurred along the U.S.-Mexico border in Matamoros, Mexico, and Cameron County in south Texas. Almost all of the cases took place in Matamoros, mainly between the months of July and November 2005, with the greatest number from August through October.

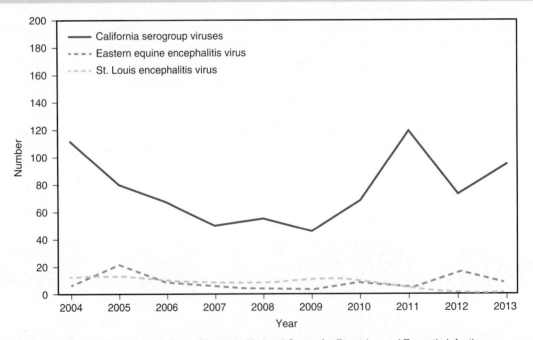

FIGURE 10-14 Arboviral diseases: number* of reported cases of neuroinvasive diseases, by year—United States, 2004–2013.

* Data from the Division of Vector-Borne Diseases, National Center for Emerging and Zoonotic Infectious Diseases (ArboNET Surveillance). Only reported cases of neuroinvasive disease are shown.

Reprinted from Centers for Disease Control and Prevention. Summary of notifiable infectious diseases and conditions—United States, 2013. *MMWR*. 2015;62(53):55.

FIGURE 10-15 Number of cases of dengue fever, by week of report—City of Matamoros, Mexico, and Cameron County, Texas, 2005.

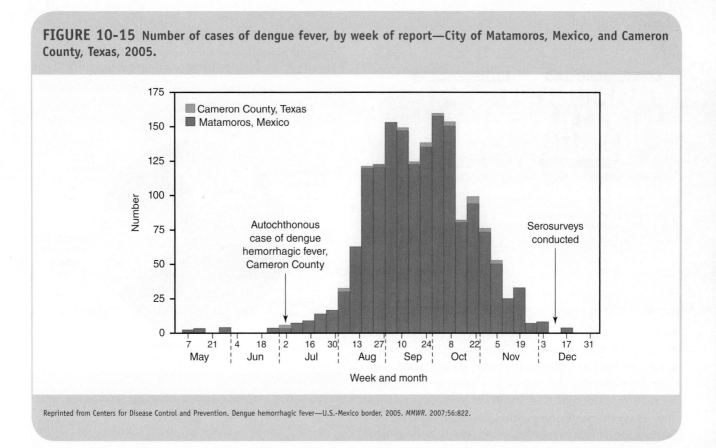

Reprinted from Centers for Disease Control and Prevention. Dengue hemorrhagic fever—U.S.-Mexico border, 2005. *MMWR*. 2007;56:822.

The presence of the *Aedes aegypti* mosquito as well as other favorable environmental conditions suggest that the spread of dengue fever is at least a theoretical possibility in south Texas.

Vaccine-Preventable Diseases

Vaccine-preventable diseases (VPDs) are conditions that can be prevented by **vaccination (immunization)**, a procedure in which a vaccine is injected into the body. Examples of diseases that can be prevented by vaccines include diphtheria, tetanus, whooping cough (pertussis), hepatitis A and hepatitis B, poliomyelitis, pneumococcal diseases, *Haemophilus influenzae* type B, rotavirus gastroenteritis, and measles.

Some vaccinations are given routinely to children beginning in early childhood (from birth to age 6 years). Others are administered to older children, teenagers, and young adults. In order to maintain immunity, booster shots of some vaccines, for example, the tetanus vaccine, are given periodically throughout life. Others, for conditions such as shingles and pneumonia, target older adults.

From the public health perspective, vaccination is a mainstay of the primary prevention of disease. Remarkable progress has been made in the elimination of once prevalent diseases such as smallpox and polio. When most people become vaccinated, the spread of a contagious disease is limited. This concept is also germane to herd immunity—when a large proportion of the population has immunity against a specific disease, the remaining nonimmune persons tend to be protected. **Figure 10-16** illustrates how vaccines help to protect the population.

With advances in medical science, the list of diseases that can be prevented through vaccination continues to grow. As a result of successful vaccination programs, some diseases, in illustration, poliomyelitis and measles, have shown marked drops in incidence over the span of recent years. Nevertheless, despite these advances, VPDs continue to impact the entire planet. From the global perspective, approximately 2.5 million children younger than age 5 years died by VPDs in 2002 (see **Figure 10-17**).

Measles is a noteworthy example of a VPD. Caused by the measles virus, the disease can produce a number of significant complications: middle ear infections, pneumonia, and encephalitis. Often a fatal disease in developing countries, the case fatality rate for measles infections can be as high as 30% in some regions.[4(p390)] In developed countries,

FIGURE 10-16 How vaccines protect.

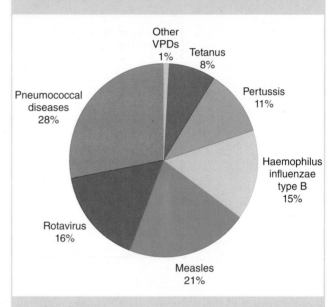

If only SOME get vaccinated...
...the virus spreads.

If MOST get vaccinated...
...spreading is contained.

👤 Healthy, non-vaccinated 👤 Healthy, vaccinated 👤 Not-vaccinated, sick, contagious

Reprinted from Centers for Disease Control and Prevention. What would happen if we stopped vaccinations? Available at: http://www.cdc.gov/vaccines/vac-gen/whatifstop.htm. Accessed Feb 10, 2016.

FIGURE 10-17 Percentage of deaths from vaccine-preventable diseases among children age less than 5 years, by disease—worldwide, 2002.

Other VPDs 1%
Tetanus 8%
Pertussis 11%
Haemophilus influenzae type B 15%
Measles 21%
Rotavirus 16%
Pneumococcal diseases 28%

Reprinted from Centers for Disease Control and Prevention. Vaccine preventable deaths and the global immunization vision and strategy, 2006–2015. *MMWR.* 2006;55(18):512.

measles occurs mainly among unimmunized persons. Large measles outbreaks occurred in 2014 among unvaccinated Amish residents in Ohio. In December of that same year, a measles outbreak befell at least 50 visitors to Disneyland in Anaheim, California. One reason for continuing measles outbreaks is that some Americans deliberately avoid protective immunizations because they mistakenly believe that vaccines cause autism.

The U.N. General Assembly adopted the Millennium Development Goals (MDG) in 2000.[17] One of the objectives of goal MDG4 was to increase global measles vaccination coverage of children. Between the introduction of the MDGs in 2000 and the year 2008, the number of deaths worldwide from measles dropped dramatically—by 78%.[18] Estimated global deaths declined from 733,000 to 164,000. According to CDC, reduced funding for measles control may have been responsible for stabilization of the downward mortality trend beginning in 2007.

By applying a statistical model developed by their staff members, WHO sources estimated a 79% decline in measles deaths between 2000 and 2014.[17] WHO proposed that during this time span the vaccination initiative prevented 17.1 million deaths, as shown in **Figure 10-18**.

Zoonotic Diseases

Zoonotic diseases were defined previously as diseases that can be transmitted from vertebrate animals to human beings. Examples of such diseases are the following:

- Rabies (discussed previously)
- Anthrax (discussed in the section on bioterrorism)

- Avian influenza (bird flu): A form of influenza caused by the H5N1 virus that began to appear in the late 1990s. It is a highly fatal condition that has been linked to transmission between poultry and human beings.
- Hantavirus pulmonary syndrome: An acute viral disease that produces a range of symptoms including fever, muscle pain, stomach ache, respiratory diseases, and low blood pressure. The case fatality rate is about 50%. Certain species of rodents (for example, deer mice) can serve as reservoirs for hantaviruses in the United States. The disease may be transmitted when aerosolized urine and droppings from infected rodents are inhaled.
- Toxoplasmosis: A protozoal infection transmitted from cats. Infection may occur when children ingest dirt that contains the protozoal oocysts from cat feces. Infection during pregnancy can cause death of the fetus.
- Tularemia (rabbit fever): The reservoir of tularemia is wild animals, particularly rabbits. This condition, which is caused by the bacterium *Francisella tularensis*, can in some cases cause fatalities when untreated. The disease can be transmitted by several

FIGURE 10-18 Global estimated measles mortality and measles deaths averted, 2000–2014.

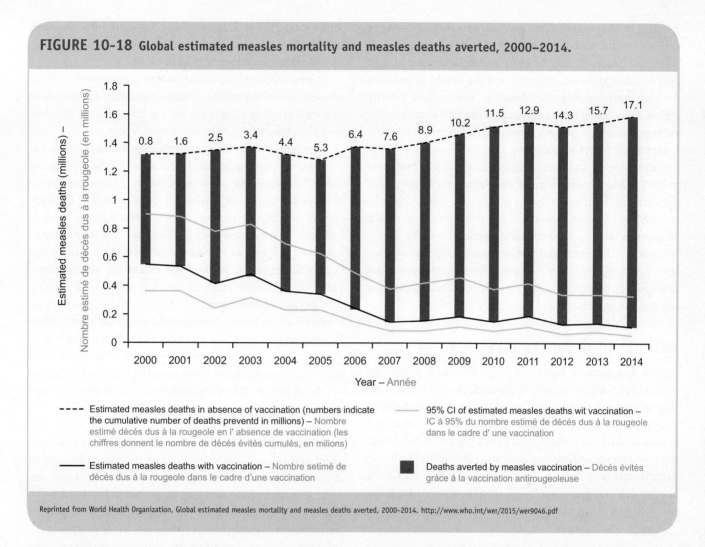

Reprinted from World Health Organization, Global estimated measles mortality and measles deaths averted, 2000–2014. http://www.who.int/wer/2015/wer9046.pdf

methods including tick bites; ingestion of inadequately cooked, contaminated food; and inhalation of microbe-laden dust.

As noted for tularemia, some zoonotic diseases are also foodborne illnesses. A second example is trichinosis (trichinellosis), which is associated with the agent *Trichinella spiralis*, the larva of a species of worm. Trichinosis can be acquired by eating raw or undercooked pork and pork products. A third example is variant Creutzfeldt-Jakob disease (vCJD), which has been linked to mad cow disease (bovine spongiform encephalopathy [BSE]). Consumption of meat from cattle that have developed BSE (caused by an agent known as a prion) is suspected of causing Creutzfeldt-Jakob disease in humans.

Emerging Infectious Diseases (Emerging Infections)

An **emerging infectious disease** is "[a]n infectious disease that has newly appeared in a population or that has been known for some time but is rapidly increasing in incidence or geographic range."[19] Examples of emerging infections are HIV infection, Ebola virus disease, hepatitis C, avian influenza, and *E. coli* O157:H7. In addition to being emerging infections, these diseases also fit into other categories (for example, foodborne, vector-borne, or sexually transmitted).

Bioterrorism-Related Diseases

In fall 2001, anthrax bacteria were distributed intentionally via the U.S. mail system causing 21 cases of illness. Since this attack, officials domestically and globally have developed a heightened awareness of and readiness for bioterrorism. CDC defines a **bioterrorism attack** as "… the deliberate release of viruses, bacteria, or other germs (agents) used to cause illness or death in people, animals, or plants. These agents are typically found in nature, but it is possible that they could be changed to increase their ability to cause disease, make them resistant to current medicines, or… increase their ability to be spread into the environment."[20]

CDC groups agents for bioterrorism according to how easily they may be disseminated and the degree of morbidity and mortality that they produce. The highest priority agents, called category A agents, cause the following diseases: anthrax, botulism, plague, smallpox, tularemia, and viral hemorrhagic fevers such as Ebola.

Consider the example of smallpox, which was eradicated in 1977. Although natural cases of smallpox no longer occur, the virus has been stockpiled in laboratories, which might be accessed by terrorists, who could use this agent in an attack. Smallpox is a contagious, untreatable disease preventable only by vaccination. The case fatality rate of severe smallpox is approximately 30%. **Figure 10-19** shows the characteristic appearance of a smallpox patient, who presents with raised bumps that later can produce permanent scarring and disfigurement.

METHODS OF OUTBREAK INVESTIGATION

Several examples of outbreaks were presented previously: typhoid fever, the salmonellosis outbreak in the United States that initially was suspected of being transmitted by tomatoes, and cryptosporidiosis from inadequately treated water in Wisconsin. In the United States, local health departments (often at the county level and sometimes at the city level), state health departments, and federal agencies (for example, CDC) are charged with the responsibility for tracking the cause of infectious disease outbreaks. Several procedures are common to

the investigation of such outbreaks. **Table 10-7** lists the steps involved in the investigation of an infectious disease outbreak.

Explanations of terms used in Table 10-7:

Clinical observations: The pattern of symptoms suggests possible infectious agents. Disease detectives are interested in a wide range of symptoms, such as fever, nausea, diarrhea, vomiting, headache, rashes, and stomach pain.

Epidemic curve: The term **epidemic curve** is defined as "[a] graphic plotting of the distribution of cases by time of onset."[2] An epidemic curve may reflect a **common-source epidemic**, which is defined as an "[o]utbreak due to exposure of a group of persons to a noxious influence that is common to the individuals in the group."[2] A **point source epidemic** is a type of common-source epidemic that occurs "when the exposure is brief and essentially simultaneous, [and] the resultant cases all develop within one incubation period of the disease…"[2] **Figure 10-20** illustrates an epidemic curve for a school gastroenteritis outbreak caused by norovirus, an agent for gastrointestinal illness. The beginning of the outbreak was on February 4, when three cases occurred; the number of cases declined to one on February 17, the apparent end of the outbreak. The number of cases peaked on February 7.

Incubation period: As noted previously, the incubation period is the time interval between invasion of an infectious agent and the appearance of the first signs or symptoms of disease. As part of the investigation of a disease outbreak, the incubation period for each affected person is estimated. From this information, the average and range of incubation periods for the affected group can be computed. In conjunction with information about symptoms, the incubation period provides clues regarding possible infectious disease agents that caused the outbreak. For example, in a foodborne illness outbreak caused by *Salmonella* bacteria, the incubation period would range from 6 to 72 hours, with most cases having an incubation period of 12 to 36 hours.

Attack rate: As a review, the formula for an **attack rate** is:

$$\text{Attack rate (\%)} = \frac{\text{Ill}}{\text{Ill} + \text{Well}} \times 100 \text{ during a time period}$$

Calculation example: Fifty-nine people ate roast beef suspected of causing a *Salmonella* outbreak. Thirty-four people fell ill; 25 remained well.

Number ill = 34

Number well = 25

Attack rate = 34/(34 + 25) × 100 = 57.6%

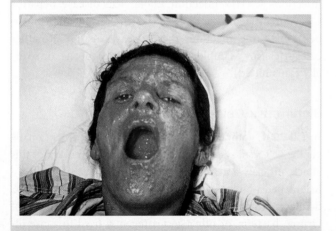

FIGURE 10-19 Smallpox victim.

Reprinted from Centers for Disease Control and Prevention. Public Health Image Library ID# 3333. Available at: http://phil.cdc.gov/phil/details.asp. Accessed February 8, 2016.

TABLE 10-7 Steps in the Investigation of an Infectious Disease Outbreak

Procedure	Relevant Questions and Activities
Define the problem.	Verify that an outbreak has occurred; is this a group of related cases that are part of an outbreak or a single sporadic case?
Appraise existing data.	Case identification: Track down all cases implicated in the outbreak. Clinical observations: Record the pattern of symptoms and collect specimens. Tabulations and spot maps: • Plot the epidemic curve. • Calculate the incubation period. • Calculate attack rates. • Map the cases (helpful for environmental studies).
Formulate a hypothesis.	Based on a data review, what caused the outbreak?
Confirm the hypothesis.	Identify additional cases; conduct laboratory assays to verify causal agent.
Draw conclusions and formulate practical applications.	What can be done to prevent similar outbreaks in the future?

Adapted from Friis RH, Sellers TA. *Epidemiology for Public Health Practice.* 5th ed. Burlington, MA: Jones & Bartlett Learning; 2014:511-512.

FIGURE 10-20 Number of identified cases (*n* = 103) in a school gastroenteritis outbreak, by date of symptom onset—District of Columbia, February 2–18, 2007.

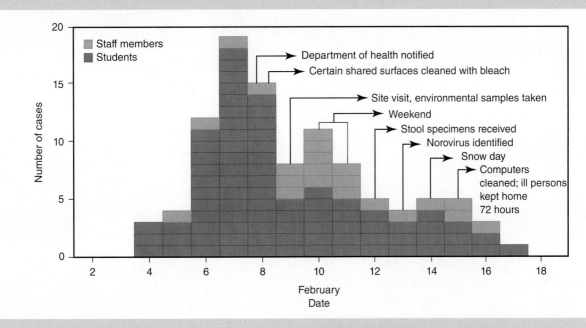

Case mapping: The process of **case mapping** involves plotting cases of disease on a map. Although mapping is a simple concept, it can yield powerful data. Early in the history of epidemiology (mid-1800s), John Snow used this method to show the location of cholera cases in London. Mapping procedures can be used to locate cases in relation to environmental exposures to pollution, identify contacts of cases of infectious diseases, and conduct many other innovative health research investigations. The process of case mapping is facilitated by computer hardware and software known as geographic information systems (GIS).

Hypothesis formulation and confirmation: With the foregoing types of information at hand, the epidemiologist is now in a position to suggest (hypothesize) the causative agent for the outbreak and attempt to confirm the hypothesis by trying to locate additional cases and conducting additional laboratory analyses.

Draw conclusions: Once the cause of an outbreak has been determined, the final stage in the investigation is to develop plans for the prevention of future outbreaks. For example, if the outbreak was a foodborne illness that occurred in a restaurant, the epidemiologist could recommend procedures to the management for improved methods of storing and preparing foods. Public health authorities in many localities are required to shut down restaurants that maintain unsanitary conditions until the deficiencies have been corrected.

CONCLUSION

At the beginning of the 1900s, infectious diseases were the leading causes of mortality in the United States. During the twentieth century, improvements in social conditions and advances in medical care led to a reduction in mortality caused by infectious diseases. At present (the first part of the twenty-first century), chronic diseases—heart disease, cancer, and stroke—are the leading causes of death in developed countries. Nevertheless, infectious diseases remain as significant causes of morbidity and mortality in both developed and developing countries. Infectious diseases take a particularly high toll in developing countries. Additionally, they remain a threat to all societies for several reasons. First, new types of diseases, known as emerging infections, are constantly evolving and imperiling public health; second, infectious disease outbreaks caused by acts of bioterrorism are a potential threat; and finally, some of the infectious disease agents, for example, bacteria, have mutated into forms that resist conventional antibiotic treatment, meaning that they could cause increased levels of morbidity and mortality. Foodborne illnesses, another infectious disease hazard, are capable of creating havoc until their sources have been identified and controlled. With the growing internationalization of the food supply, public health officials are experiencing formidable challenges in tracing the causes of foodborne disease outbreaks. Given these challenges, infectious disease epidemiology will remain an important application of epidemiology.

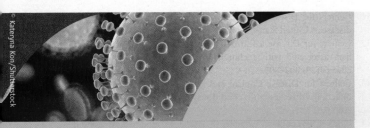

Study Questions and Exercises

1. Define the following terms:
   a. Infectious disease
   b. Parasitic disease
   c. Zoonotic disease

2. Explain what is meant by the epidemiologic triangle. Define the three elements of the triangle.

3. Describe the defense mechanisms that can protect a host from infection. Be sure to include the terms *immunity* (active or passive) and *herd immunity.*

4. Why are subclinical (also called inapparent) diseases significant for epidemiology and public health?

5. Describe the main differences between direct and indirect transmission of disease agents. Be sure to give examples.

6. What are vectors and how are they involved with the transmission of disease agents? Name three diseases transmitted by vectors.

7. Do the risk patterns for transmission of the HIV virus differ between men and women? Describe sex differences in transmission of the virus.

8. What is the mode of action of the foodborne illness botulism, that is, how does botulism cause its victims to become ill?

9. Describe the steps in investigating an infectious disease outbreak. Why do investigators collect information about clinical symptoms, attack rates, and the incubation period?

10. In your opinion, why are there so many worldwide deaths caused by vaccine-preventable diseases? What would you do in order to reduce this death toll?

Young Epidemiology Scholars (YES) Exercises

The Young Epidemiology Scholars: Competitions website provides links to teaching units and exercises that support instruction in epidemiology. The YES program, discontinued in 2011, was administered by the College Board and supported by the Robert Wood Johnson Foundation. The exercises continue to be available at the following website: http://yes-competition.org/yes /teaching-units/title.html. The following exercises relate to topics discussed in this chapter and can be found on the YES competitions website.

1. Fraser DW. An Outbreak of Legionnaires' Disease
2. Huang FI, Bayona M. Disease Outbreak Investigation
3. Klaucke D, Vogt R. Outbreak Investigation at a Vermont Community Hospital

REFERENCES

1. Xu JQ, Murphy SL, Kochanek KD, Bastian BA. Deaths: final data for 2013. *National Vital Statistics Reports.* 2016;64(2). Hyattsville, MD: National Center for Health Statistics.

2. Porta M, ed. *A Dictionary of Epidemiology.* 6th ed. New York, NY: Oxford University Press; 2014.

3. Centers for Disease Control and Prevention. About parasites. Available at: http://www.cdc.gov/parasites/about.html. Accessed August 9, 2016.

4. Heymann DL, ed. *Control of Communicable Diseases Manual.* 20th ed. Washington, DC: American Public Health Association; 2015.

5. Centers for Disease Control and Prevention. About One Health. Available at: https://www.cdc.gov/onehealth/about.html. Accessed July 28, 2016.

6. Olsen SJ, Chang H-L, Cheung TY-Y, et al. Transmission of the severe acute respiratory syndrome on aircraft. *N Engl J Med.* 2003;349:2416–2422.

7. Centers for Disease Control and Prevention. HIV surveillance report 2014. November 2015; vol 26. Available at: http://www.cdc.gov/hiv/library/reports/surveillance/. Accessed July 8, 2016.

8. Centers for Disease Control and Prevention. Sexually transmitted disease surveillance 2014. Atlanta, GA: U.S. Department of Health and Human Services; 2015.

9. Centers for Disease Control and Prevention. CDC estimates of foodborne illness in the United States. CDC 2011 estimates. Available at: http://www.cdc.gov/foodborneburden/pdfs/factsheet_a_findings_updated4-13.pdf. Accessed July 9, 2016.

10. Centers for Disease Control and Prevention. Foodborne Diseases Active Surveillance Network (FoodNet): FoodNet surveillance report for 2014 (final report). Atlanta, GA: U.S. Department of Health and Human Services, CDC. 2014.

11. Centers for Disease Control and Prevention. Summary of notifiable diseases—United States, 2006. *MMWR.* 2008;55(53):42.

12. Centers for Disease Control and Prevention. Large outbreak of botulism associated with a church potluck meal—Ohio, 2015. *MMWR.* 2015;64(29):802–803.

13. Centers for Disease Control and Prevention. Summary of notifiable infectious diseases and conditions—United States, 2013. *MMWR.* 2013;62(53):1–122.

14. Lindsey NP, Lehman JA, Staples JE, Fischer M. West Nile virus and other arboviral diseases—United States, 2013. *MMWR.* 2014;63(24):521–526.

15. Centers for Disease Control and Prevention. Arboviral diseases, neuroinvasive and non-neuroinvasive. 2015 case definition. Available at: https://wwwn.cdc.gov/nndss/conditions/arboviral-diseases-neuroinvasive-and-non-neuroinvasive/case-definition/2015/. Accessed July 11, 2016.

16. Centers for Disease Control and Prevention. Summary of notifiable diseases—United States, 2006. *MMWR.* 2008;55(53):48.

17. Perry RT, Murray JS, Gacic-Dobo M, et al. Progress towards regional measles elimination, worldwide, 2000–2014. *Wkly Epidemiol Rec.* 2015;46(13):623–631.

18. Centers for Disease Control and Prevention. Global measles mortality, 2000–2008. *MMWR.* 2009;58(47):1321–1326.

19. MedicineNet, Inc. Definition of emerging infectious disease. Available at: http://www.medicinenet.com/script/main/art.asp?articlekey=22801. Accessed August 9, 2105.

20. Centers for Disease Control and Prevention. Bioterrorism overview: what is bioterrorism? Available at: http://www.bt.cdc.gov/bioterrorism/pdf/bioterrorism_overview.pdf. Accessed August 9, 2015.

CHAPTER **11**

Social and Behavioral Epidemiology

LEARNING OBJECTIVES

By the end of this chapter you will be able to:

- Summarize the similarities and differences between social and behavioral epidemiology.
- Discuss the relationship between lifestyle and health status, giving two examples.
- Explain how the stress concept has been applied to population-based investigations.
- Describe the epidemiology of substance abuse and its linkage with adverse health outcomes.
- Contrast the descriptive epidemiology of two important mental disorders.

CHAPTER OUTLINE

INTRODUCTION

Epidemiologists have developed an increasing awareness of the association of social and behavioral factors with health and illness. Such factors that impact human health include social adversities (for example, poverty and discrimination), stress, and lifestyle practices such as tobacco use, binge drinking, and substance abuse. You will learn about the relationship between personal behavior and chronic diseases, including heart disease, cancer, and stroke. Preventing or limiting the effects of chronic diseases and other conditions related to unhealthy behavioral practices can be accomplished by encouraging people to change their lifestyles. Nevertheless, the impact of these factors on human health tends to be unrecognized and needs to be given more attention.

Correlated with the broad topic of social and behavioral factors related to health are mental disorders. Such disorders can be the consequence of social factors, including stress and social adversities. Mental disorders are also associated with choice of lifestyle, as in the case of depressive symptomatology that leads to inactivity and substance use disorders that are associated with abuse of legal and illegal drugs. Later in the chapter, the applications of epidemiology to the study of mental disorders will be covered in more detail. Refer to **Table 11-1** for a list of important terms used in this chapter.

TABLE 11-1 List of Important Terms Used in This Chapter

Autism	Passive smoking
Behavioral epidemiology	Posttraumatic stress disorder
Binge drinking	Psychiatric comorbidity
Body mass index (BMI)	Psychiatric epidemiology
Chronic strains	Social epidemiology
Coping skills	Social support
Lifestyle	Stress
Meth mouth	Stressful life events

DEFINING SOCIAL AND BEHAVIORAL EPIDEMIOLOGY

Social epidemiology is defined "… as the branch of epidemiology that studies the social distribution and social determinants of states of health."[1(p5)] Some of the topics that the discipline covers are the relationship between socioeconomic status and health, the effect of social relationships (e.g. social support) on health outcomes, the epidemiology of mental disorders (e.g., the association of stress with mental disorders), and how social factors affect the choice of health-related behaviors. Many social determinants are a function of how society is structured and are beyond the control of the individual; others are related to modifiable personal behavioral choices and lifestyle characteristics. The term **lifestyle** refers to how we live. Particularly relevant for social epidemiology is the growing phenomenon of inequities in people's health and society's role in regulating inequalities in health status.

Related to the discussion of social determinants of health is **behavioral epidemiology**, the study of the role of behavioral factors on health within a population. The contributions of unhealthful behaviors (e.g., consumption of high-fat foods, sedentary lifestyle, and cigarette smoking) to adverse health outcomes (e.g., obesity, diabetes, and asthma) have been documented. For examples, consult the Centers for Disease Control and Prevention's (CDC) program for surveillance of youth risk behaviors.[2] During the developmental stages of childhood and adolescence, both desirable and unhealthful behaviors that persist into adulthood are inculcated. For instance, teenage smoking and binge drinking represent individual behavioral decisions, which often continue later in life. Other lifestyle dimensions relate to dietary choices, substance abuse (e.g., methamphetamine and cocaine use),

and avoiding exercise. The role of peer pressure and advertising also are salient for the adoption of unhealthful behaviors.

STRESS AND HEALTH

The term **stress** has been defined in a number of ways, one being "… a physical, chemical, or emotional factor that causes bodily or mental tension and may be a factor in disease causation."[3] **Figure 11-1** symbolizes the effect of stress upon the human brain. The figure suggests that stress is a factor in depression and other mental disorders. As a general concept, stress has been studied in relation to a range of adverse health effects:

- Cardiovascular disease
- Substance abuse
- Mental disorders, including posttraumatic stress disorder
- Work-related anxiety and neurotic disorders
- Chronic diseases such as cancer and asthma
- Impaired immune function

FIGURE 11-1 Stress is hypothesized to impact the brain, causing adverse mental health effects such as symptoms of depression.

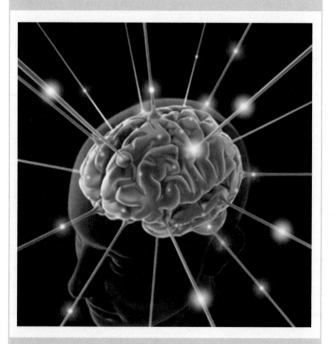

Reprinted from National Institute of Mental Health. Brain basics. Bethesda, MD: National Institutes of Health, NIMH; 6. Available at: http://www.nimh.nih.gov/health/educational-resources/brain-basics/nimh-brain-basics_132798.pdf. Accessed July 1, 2016.

Stressful life events are stressors (sources of stress) that arise from happenings such as job loss, financial problems, and death of a close family member. Events fall into homogeneous categories: health related, monetary, employment associated, and interpersonal. Stressful life events may be classified as either positive or negative. Those events that are associated with adverse life circumstances are called negative life events; examples of negative life events are being fired at work or being arrested and incarcerated. Examples of positive life events are graduation from school, marriage, and the birth of a child. According to the theory of stressful life events, the more salient the life event and the higher the frequency of these events, the greater the chance that an adverse health outcome will occur. Life events that are sustained over a long period of time are known as **chronic strains**.

Although several measures of stress exist, one common approach for its measurement is to tally the number of stressful life events that an individual has experienced during a defined time period. Some life event measures use a weighting scheme that assigns more importance to some events than others; other measures give equal weight to each item. Researchers Holmes and Rahe are credited with the development during the late 1960s of the life events approach to measurement of stress; their measure was a weighted checklist (the Schedule of Recent Experiences) that comprised 43 items.[4] Subsequently, longer checklists and other modifications have been developed. However, it has been noted that "…researchers still lack a coherent definition of stress or a classification of stressors, stress responses, and long-term effects of stress that can be applied across species and environments."[5]

Explorations of associations between stressful life events and physical and mental health outcomes encompass an extensive body of research literature. Representative examples are presented here. In one study of patients with schizophrenia, investigators detected an association between the experience of early life stresses (assessed by a life events scale) and substance abuse.[6] A prospective study tracked children with asthma, measuring the association between strongly negative life events and risk of a new asthma attack. Stressful life events were accompanied by new attacks immediately after the event; a delayed response after about 5 to 7 weeks also followed severe events.[7] In a Finnish cohort study, stressful life events were examined in relationship to breast cancer. The data came from 10,808 women in the Finnish Twin Cohort. Three negative life events (divorce or separation, death of a husband, and death of a close relative or friend) each predicted increased breast cancer risk.[8]

Posttraumatic Stress Disorder

The term **posttraumatic stress disorder** (PTSD) refers to "… an anxiety disorder that some people develop after seeing or living through an event that caused or threatened serious harm or death. Symptoms include flashbacks or bad dreams, emotional numbness, intense guilt or worry, angry outbursts, feeling 'on edge,' or avoiding thoughts and situations that remind them of the trauma. In PTSD, these symptoms last at least one month."[9] Many people believe that PTSD primarily affects soldiers who were involved in armed conflict. (See **Figure 11-2.**) However, also vulnerable are noncombatant civilians who are present in a theater of war. In illustration, PTSD was found to affect mothers responsible for child rearing who were exposed to traumatic events during armed conflict in Kabul Province, Afghanistan;[10] such events included shelling or rocket attacks, bomb explosions, and the murder of family members or relatives. As a result of armed conflict, these women experienced hardships in meeting their basic needs for food, water, and shelter. Their ability to take care of their children also was impaired.

Perhaps less widely recognized is that PTSD can impact people who have undergone traumatic events in the community where they live and not necessarily in a theater of war. Potentially violent events include gang conflict and school shootings. Another group that is vulnerable to the effects of PTSD includes first responders to a mass casualty event such as a terrorist attack, airplane crash, train collision, or serious motor vehicle crash.

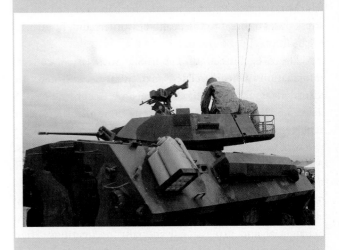

FIGURE 11-2 Military conflict: a setting for posttraumatic stress disorder.

The Veterans Health Study is a longitudinal investigation of the health of a representative sample of male veterans who are outpatients at hospitals operated by the Department of Veterans Affairs.[11] Data from this study indicated that 20% of the sample met the screening criteria of PTSD. In comparison with veterans who had not been so diagnosed, those who had PTSD reported higher levels of both health problems and healthcare utilization.[12] This generalization also applied to female veterans in other research.[13]

Is stress only a negative factor in one's health? Not all people who are under stress develop illnesses; in fact, for some people stress may be a positive experience that challenges them toward greater accomplishment. One of the factors associated with the ability to deal with stress is **social support**—the help that we receive from other people when we are under stress. Friends, relatives, and significant others often are able to provide material and emotional support during times of stress.

Coping skills are techniques for managing or removing sources of stress. Effective coping skills help to mitigate the effects of stress. Here is an example: Suppose that a person does not have enough money to pay for routine living expenses. Two effective coping skills would be to either lower one's expenses or find employment that provides a higher income. That individual might also request a loan from friends or family members.

Work-Related Stress

Stress, a common feature of most occupations, may result from work overload, time pressures, threat of job layoff and unemployment, interpersonal conflicts, and inadequate compensation. The National Institute for Occupational Safety and Health states that "The nature of work is changing at whirlwind speed. Perhaps now more than ever before, job stress poses a threat to the health of workers and, in turn, to the health [of] organizations."[14]

The U.S. Bureau of Labor Statistics (BLS) collects information on work-related anxiety, stress, and neurotic disorders associated with absenteeism.[15] According to BLS data, 5,659 absenteeism cases from these disorders were reported in 2001. Nearly 80% of the cases occurred among workers in their prime working years, age 25 to 54 years. About two-thirds happened among white, non-Hispanic women. The highest rates of anxiety, stress, and neurotic disorders were reported for the following two occupational categories: technical, sales, and administrative support; and managerial and professional specialty occupations. High rates were also reported for the finance, insurance, and real estate fields.

Between 1992 and 2001, absenteeism from anxiety, stress, and neurotic disorders declined by 25% (from 0.8 to 0.6 per 10,000 full-time workers). Nonetheless, despite these declines reported by the BLS for 2001, workplace stress is likely to remain a salient feature of many work settings. Numerous challenges to workers have transpired since the beginning of the present century. In fact, a survey conducted in 2012 by the American Psychological Association determined that about 41% of employed adults felt tense or stressed out during the workday—an increase of 5% over 2011.[16]

TOBACCO USE

Cigarette smoking and other forms of tobacco use (e.g., chew tobacco and inhalation of tobacco smoke from water pipes) increase the risk of many forms of adverse health outcomes. These conditions include lung diseases, coronary heart disease, stroke, and cancer. The second leading cause of death in the United States is cancer (malignant neoplasms); lung cancer is the leading cause of cancer death among both men and women. Lung cancer is causally associated with smoking, as are cancer of the cervix, kidney, oral cavity, pancreas, and stomach.

Between 1965 and 2005, the prevalence of adult current smokers in the United States declined sharply among men, from more than 50% to about 23%, and less steeply among women, from about 30% to about 19%.[17] For the period between 1999 and 2014, smoking prevalence among men declined from 25.2% to 19.0% and among women from 21.6% to 15.1%.[18] During the corresponding time period, a greater percentage of men than women tended to be current smokers within each of the following ethnic and racial groups: non-Hispanic blacks, non-Hispanic whites, Hispanics or Latinos, and Asians. In 2014 among these same racial and ethnic groups, the highest and lowest percentages of current male smokers were among non-Hispanic black men and Hispanic men, 22.0% versus 13.8%, respectively. [18] The highest and lowest percentages of female smokers were among non-Hispanic white women and non-Hispanic Asian women, 18.3% versus 5.1%, respectively. (Refer to **Figure 11**-3 for more information.)

Pregnant women who smoke risk damage (e.g., stillbirth, low birth weight, and sudden infant death syndrome) to their developing fetuses. From 1989 to 2004, the percentage of women who smoked during pregnancy showed a declining trend—from about 20% to about 10%.[17] These prevalence data were taken from mothers' self-reported smoking on certificates of live birth.

The National Survey on Drug Use and Health (NSDUH) is an annual survey that collects information on smoking.

FIGURE 11-3 Current cigarette smoking among adults age 18 years and over, by sex, race, and Hispanic origin—United States, 1999–2014.

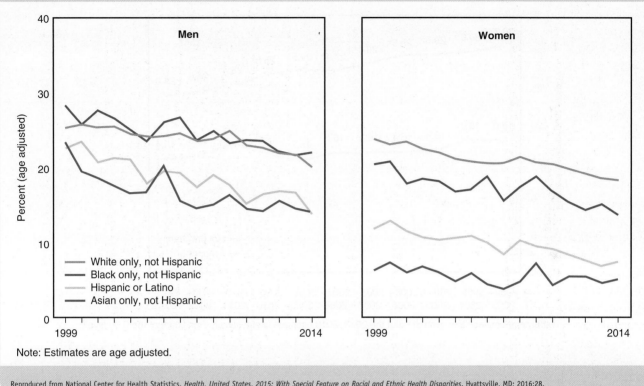

Note: Estimates are age adjusted.

Reproduced from National Center for Health Statistics. *Health, United States, 2015: With Special Feature on Racial and Ethnic Health Disparities.* Hyattsville, MD; 2016:28.

According to the NSDUH, the prevalence of smoking among pregnant women of childbearing age (15 to 44) did not decline significantly over an entire decade from 2002–2003 to 2012–2013. In 2002–2003, the prevalence of smoking among pregnant women was 18.0%; as of 2012–2013, the prevalence was 15.4% (not a significant difference). Among women of childbearing age (15 to 44) who were not pregnant, the prevalence of smoking declined from 30.7% to 24.0% between 2002–2003 and 2012–2013.[19] On a positive note, a smaller percentage of pregnant than nonpregnant women were current smokers. (Refer to **Figure 11-4** for time trends.)

Regarding the percentage of high school students who smoked, until the mid-1990s, smoking among high school students showed an increasing trend to a prevalence of almost 40%. Following this increase, prevalence has decreased. In 2002, the overall percentage of high school students (both sexes) who were current cigarette smokers was similar to the level among adult men in the United States. According to the National Youth Tobacco Survey (NYTS) conducted in 2002, the prevalence of current cigarette smokers was

22.5% (**Figure 11-5**), with 23.9% among male students and 21.0% among female students.[20] At the middle school level, the prevalence of current cigarette smoking was 9.8% and not significantly different between male and female students.

Almost a decade and a half later in 2015, the overall percentage of smoking (use of cigarettes during the past 30 days) among high school students had declined to 9.3% (10.7% versus 7.7% for males and females, respectively). In that same year, 2.3% of middle school students smoked (2.3% versus 2.2% for males and females, respectively).

Returning to 2002, we can examine the data for use of any tobacco product. Choices included cigars; cigarillos, or little cigars; chewing tobacco, snuff, or dip, such as Red Man, Levi Garrett, Beechnut, Skoal, Skoal Bandits, or Copenhagen; bidis; and kreteks. Among high school students, 28.2% were current users (32.6% for male students versus 23.7% for female students). The percentage of middle school students who were current users of any tobacco product was 13.3% (14.7% and 11.7% among males and females, respectively). Among both middle school and high school students, current

FIGURE 11-4 Past-month cigarette use among women age 15 to 44 years, by pregnancy status—combined years 2002–2003 to 2012–2013.

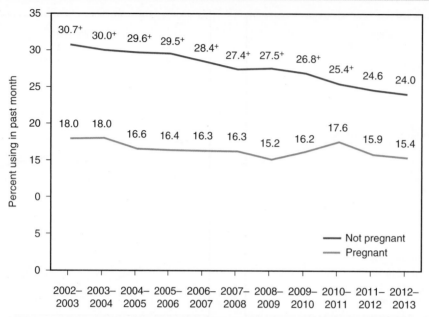

+ Difference between this estimate and the 2012–2013 estimate is statistically significant at the 0.05 level.

Reprinted from Substance Abuse and Mental Health Services Administration, Results from the 2013 National Survey on Drug Use and Health: summary of national findings, NSDUH Series H-48, HHS Publication No. (SMA) 14-4863. Rockville, MD: Substance Abuse and Mental Health Services Administration; 2014:51.

use of tobacco was most common for the following three products: cigarettes, followed by cigars and smokeless tobacco.

Regarding 2015 data, a total of 25.3% of high school students (30.0% for male students versus 20.3% for female students) reported use of any tobacco product.[21] The percentage of middle school students who used any tobacco product was 7.4% (8.3% versus 6.4% for male and female students, respectively. Refer to Figure 11-5, which shows data for the various kinds of tobacco products.

The NYTS collects information on tobacco use among high school and middle school students. It is unique in being the sole investigation devoted to tobacco use among this age group. **Figure 11-6** reflects data from the 2014 survey. According to the NYTS, about one-quarter of high school students were current users of any tobacco product. Consumption of e-cigarettes (electronic cigarettes) and use of hookahs has grown in popularity. In 2015, a total of 16.0% of high school students consumed electronic cigarettes and 7.2% used a hookah.

Controversies surround potential adverse health effects associated with both consumption of e-cigarettes and their contribution to smoking cessation. One point of view is that e-cigarettes serve as a gateway to cigarette smoking

and nicotine dependence. However, another point of view is that e-cigarettes might aid in smoking cessation. Further research needs to be conducted on the use of e-cigarettes in order to provide greater insight into this controversial topic. In many venues in the United States, smoking e-cigarettes is restricted in zones frequented by the public. Refer to Figure 11-5 and the infographic shown in **Figure 11-7** for more information. In late 2016, the first report from the U.S. Surgeon General on e-cigarette use concluded that they are a major public health concern. Among youth, e-cigarettes were the most commonly used tobacco product (as of 2016).

The NYTS (data from 2001–2002) queried middle school and high school students who currently smoke cigarettes regarding how they obtained cigarettes, for example, purchasing them in a store or from a vending machine, asking other people to purchase the cigarettes, borrowing them, or even stealing them. Middle school students acquired their cigarettes most typically by borrowing them from someone, having someone else buy them, or stealing them. High school students obtained their cigarettes by asking someone else to buy them, buying them in a store, or borrowing them from someone else.[20]

FIGURE 11-5 Estimated percentage of high school students who currently use any tobacco products,* two or more tobacco products,† and select tobacco products§—National Youth Tobacco Survey, 2011–2015.

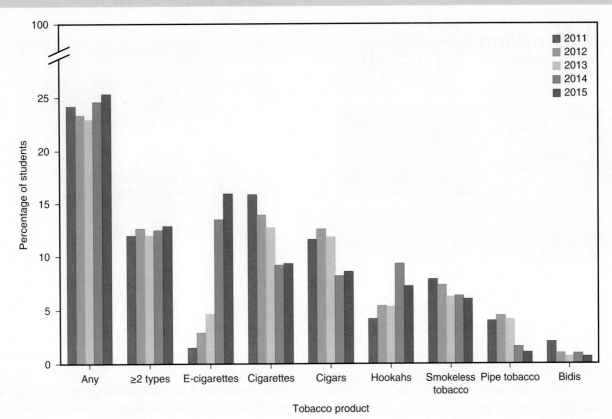

* Any tobacco product use is defined as past 30-day use of cigarettes, cigars, smokeless tobacco, e-cigarettes, hookahs, pipe tobacco, and/or bidis.
† ≥ Two tobacco product use is defined as past 30-day use of two or more of the following product types: cigarettes, cigars, smokeless tobacco, e-cigarettes, hookahs, pipe tobacco, and/or bidis.
§ E-cigarettes and hookahs demonstrated a nonlinear increase (p < 0.05). Cigarettes and smokeless tobacco demonstrated a linear decrease (p < 0.05). Cigars, pipe tobacco, and bidis demonstrated a nonlinear decrease (p < 0.05).

Reprinted from Singh T, Arrazola RA, Corey CG, et al. Tobacco use among middle and high school students—United States, 2011–2015. *MMWR*. 2016;65(14):365.

Exposure to Secondhand Smoke

The term **passive smoking**, also known as secondhand or side-stream exposure to cigarette smoke, refers to the involuntary breathing of cigarette smoke by nonsmokers in an environment where cigarette smokers are present. Exposure to secondhand smoke may occur in work settings, airports, restaurants, bars, and any other area where smokers gather. The U.S. Surgeon General's 2006 report titled *The Health Consequences of Involuntary Exposure to Tobacco Smoke* concluded, "Secondhand smoke exposure causes disease and premature death in children and in adults who do not smoke."[22(p9)] The adverse health effects of such exposure among adults include heart disease

and lung cancer. Among children, secondhand smoke increases the "risk for sudden infant death syndrome (SIDS), acute respiratory infections, ear problems, and more severe asthma. Smoking by parents causes respiratory symptoms and slows lung growth in their children"[22(p11)] (Refer to **Figure 11-8**.)

ALCOHOL CONSUMPTION

Data from the CDC's National Center for Health Statistics indicate that alcohol consumption is a significant cause of mortality in the United States. In 2014, the age-adjusted death rate for alcohol-induced causes was 8.5 per 100,000 persons, with a total of 30,722 U.S. deaths attributable to

FIGURE 11-6 Youth tobacco use.

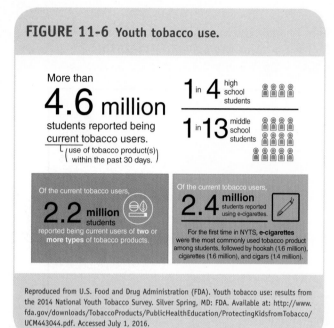

More than
4.6 million
students reported being
current tobacco users.
└ (use of tobacco product(s)
within the past 30 days.)

1 in 4 high school students
1 in 13 middle school students

Of the current tobacco users,
2.2 million students
reported being current users of **two** or **more types** of tobacco products.

Of the current tobacco users,
2.4 million students reported using e-cigarettes.
For the first time in NYTS, **e-cigarettes** were the most commonly used tobacco product among students, followed by hookah (1.6 million), cigarettes (1.6 million), and cigars (1.4 million).

Reproduced from U.S. Food and Drug Administration (FDA). Youth tobacco use: results from the 2014 National Youth Tobacco Survey. Silver Spring, MD: FDA. Available at: http://www. fda.gov/downloads/TobaccoProducts/PublicHealthEducation/ProtectingKidsfromTobacco/ UCM443044.pdf. Accessed July 1, 2016.

FIGURE 11-8 Secondhand smoke is dangerous to children. Smoking around children can cause sudden infant death.

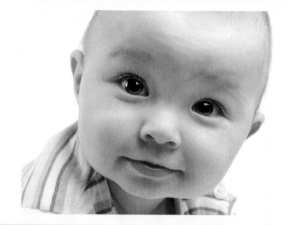

© Adam Borkowski/ShutterStock, Inc.

alcohol-induced causes. These causes included dependent use of alcohol, nondependent use, and unintentional alcohol poisoning. Deaths associated with the fetal alcohol syndrome and factors linked indirectly to alcohol use, for example, homicide, were excluded from the category of alcohol-induced deaths. The age-adjusted death rate for alcohol-induced causes among males was 2.8 times the rate among females. The rate for the Hispanic population was about 1.1 times the rate for the non-Hispanic population. Alcohol-induced death rates for Hispanic males were 1.3 times those of non-Hispanic males. [23]

See **Figure 11-9** for information on current, binge, and heavy alcohol use among people age 12 years and older in the United States. The definitions for binge drinking and heavy drinking vary according to sex. For men **binge drinking** is defined as drinking 5 or more drinks on one occasion; for women the number is 4 drinks. Heavy drinking among men is defined as 15 or more drinks per week; the figure is 8 or more drinks for women. [24] Alcohol use peaks at about age 21 to 25 years, when drinking becomes legal. As shown in the figure, almost 70% of people in this age group consumed alcohol. [19]

Binge Drinking

Alcohol consumption by people under age 21 is illegal in the United States. Nevertheless, a substantial amount of alcohol consumed in the United States is by people in this age group; much of this alcohol consumption takes place as binge drinking. Alcohol consumption by underage people is associated with numerous adverse consequences including problems at school, interpersonal difficulties, and legal problems stemming from involvement in automobile crashes. **Figure 11-10** shows the percentage of high school students who consumed five or more drinks of alcohol in a row (within a couple of hours) in 2015. Data are from the

FIGURE 11-7 The increasing use of e-cigarettes and hookahs from 2011 to 2014.

From 2011 to 2014, **e-cigarette** use

among high school students **increased** nearly **800%** and

 hookah use more than **doubled**.

Reproduced from U.S. Food and Drug Administration (FDA). Youth tobacco use: results from the 2014 National Youth Tobacco Survey. Silver Spring, MD: FDA. Available at: http://www. fda.gov/downloads/TobaccoProducts/PublicHealthEducation/ProtectingKidsfromTobacco/ UCM443044.pdf. Accessed July 1, 2016.

FIGURE 11-9 Current, binge, and heavy alcohol use among persons age 12 years or older, by age—2013.

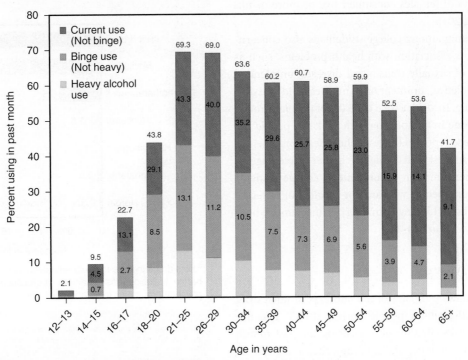

Note: The past-month binge alcohol use estimate for 12 or 13 year olds was 0.8 percent, and the past-month heavy alcohol use estimate was 0.1 percent.

Reprinted from Substance Abuse and Mental Health Services Administration, Results from the 2013 National Survey on Drug Use and Health: summary of national findings, NSDUH Series H-48, HHS Publication No. (SMA) 14-4863. Rockville, MD: Substance Abuse and Mental Health Services Administration; 2014:36.

FIGURE 11-10 Percentage of high school students who drank five or more drinks of alcohol in a row, by sex, grade, and race/ethnicity—2015.

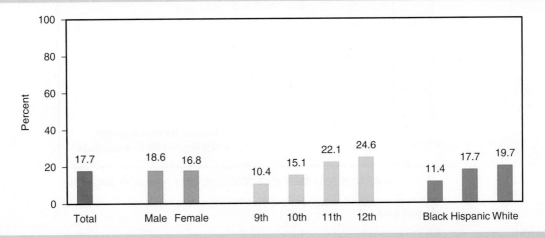

Adapted and reprinted from Centers for Disease Control and Prevention. 2015 Youth Risk Behavior Surveillance System Results. Atlanta, GA: CDC. Available at: http://www.cdc.gov/healthyyouth/data/yrbs/slides/2015/taodu_slides_yrbs.pptx. Accessed July 2, 2016.

2015 Youth Risk Behavior Surveillance System (YRBSS), which queried about consumption of alcohol between 1 and 30 days prior to the survey.[25] A total of 18.6% of male students and 16.8% of females consumed five or more drinks in a row during 2015.

Binge drinking among college students is also concerning because of its association with health problems, such as increased rates of sexually transmitted diseases, unintended pregnancies, violence, unintentional injuries, and possible alcohol poisoning. In 2013, a total of 39.0% of people enrolled in college full time in comparison with 33.4% of people not enrolled in college reported binge alcohol use. Consequently, these findings suggest that a slightly higher percentage of binge alcohol consumption occurs among college students than among young people who are not enrolled in college.[19] Between 2002 and 2013, binge drinking declined among both groups. (Refer to **Figure 11-11**.)

SUBSTANCE ABUSE

Figure 11-12 shows estimates of the numbers of illicit drug users—almost 25 million people during 2013.[19] The figure presents the distribution of use during the past month according to different types of illicit drugs, such as marijuana,

FIGURE 11-12 Past-month illicit drug use among persons age 12 years or older—2013.

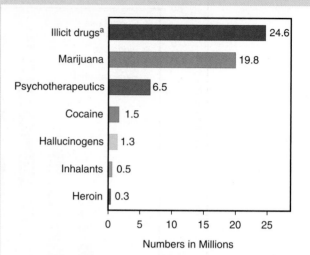

a Illicit drugs include marijuana/hashish, cocaine (including crack), heroin, hallucinogens, inhalants, or prescription-type psychotherapeutics used nonmedically.

Reproduced from Substance Abuse and Mental Health Services Administration, Results from the 2013 National Survey on Drug Use and Health: summary of national findings, NSDUH Series H-48, HHS Publication No. (SMA) 14-4863. Rockville, MD: Substance Abuse and Mental Health Services Administration; 2014:16.

FIGURE 11-11 Binge alcohol use among adults age 18 to 22 years, by college enrollment—2002–2013.

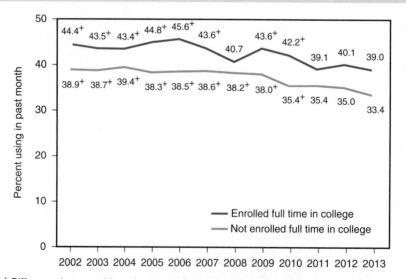

+ Difference between this estimate and the 2013 estimate is statistically significant at the 0.05 level.

Reprinted from Substance Abuse and Mental Health Services Administration, *Results from the 2013 National Survey on Drug Use and Health: Summary of National Findings*, NSDUH Series H-48, HHS Publication No. (SMA) 14-4863. Rockville, MD: Substance Abuse and Mental Health Services Administration; 2014:40.

psychotherapeutics, and heroin. Marijuana was the illicit drug used most commonly among all people age 12 years or older (19.8 million "past month" users during 2013). Of the 6.5 million people who abused psychotherapeutic drugs, a total of 5.2 million abused painkillers during the past month. Psychotherapeutic drugs include pain relievers, tranquilizers, stimulants, and sedatives.

Use of marijuana is also common among high school students. (Refer to **Figure 11-13**.) Among all groups shown in the figure, male students in 12th grade had the highest frequency of marijuana use. Approximately one-quarter of 12th grade male students reported using marijuana in 2014 in comparison with slightly less than one-fifth of female students at the same grade level. In general, the trends between 2000 and 2014 in marijuana use by sex and year in high school tended to show only slight fluctuations over time. Future epidemiologic research could assess whether loosening of laws prohibiting marijuana sales will change these trends.

Methamphetamine

Use of methamphetamine (also called methamphetamines) and other stimulants is fairly common in the United States. The Substance Abuse and Mental Health Services Administration reported that in 2013, a total of 595,000 persons age 12 years or older had used methamphetamine in the past month.[19] The figure for 2004 was 600,000 persons (0.2% of the population) who had reported past month use of methamphetamine.[26] At that time, the prevalence of methamphetamine use was higher among males than among females and highest among young adults age 18 to 25 years (1.6%). The number of people who reported past year use all forms of stimulant drugs decreased from 2002 and 2013.

Methamphetamine is a highly addictive substance that has powerful, stimulating effects on the body. In most cases the drug is produced and distributed illegally. Ingestion of large amounts of the drug can cause body temperature to rise

FIGURE 11-13 Use of marijuana in the past 30 days among 8th, 10th, 12th graders by sex and year—United States.

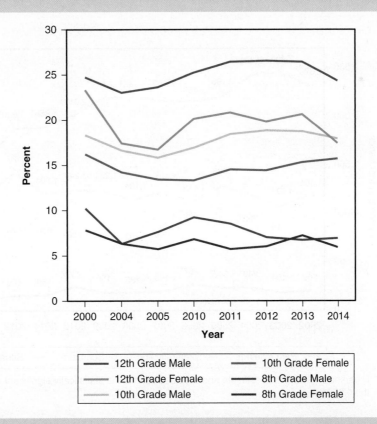

Data from National Center for Health Statistics. *Health, United States, 2015: With Special Feature on Racial and Ethnic Health Disparities.* Hyattsville, MD: NCHS; 2016.

to dangerous levels and can cause convulsions. Long-term use of methamphetamine can result in psychotic symptoms such as paranoia. Some users are affected with the "crank bug," a sensation of bugs crawling underneath or on top of the skin, causing victims to abrade their skin until it is raw and bleeding. Another consequence of methamphetamine use is known as **meth mouth**, a condition that contributes to decay and loss of teeth. The causes are reduced output of saliva, increased consumption of sugary, carbonated beverages, and neglect of personal hygiene (e.g., tooth brushing). Refer to **Figure 11-14** for a picture of meth mouth.

Nonmedical Use of Psychotherapeutic Drugs

Medical uses of psychotherapeutic drugs include the intake of prescribed drugs administered as pain relievers, tranquilizers, stimulants, and sedatives. Illicit use of these drugs means that they are being taken for nonmedical purposes. About 6.5 million persons used psychotherapeutic drugs illicitly in 2013 (Figure 11-12). Illicit users who are taking these drugs for the first time are classified as initiates. **Figure 11-15** reports data

FIGURE 11-14 Meth mouth.

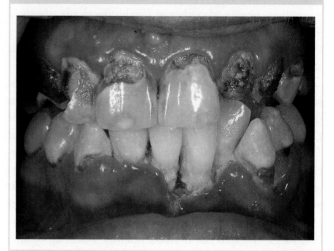

Courtesy of Stephan Wagner, DDS.

FIGURE 11-15 Past-year nonmedical psychotherapeutic initiates among persons age 12 years or older—2002–2013.

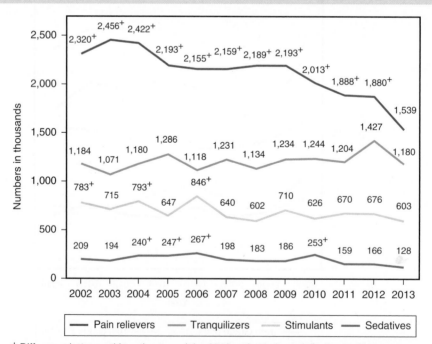

+ Difference between this estimate and the 2013 estimate is statistically significant at the 0.05 level.

on the numbers of initiates for four classes of drugs. Use of pain relievers declined between 2002 and 2013. During the same period, the use of tranquilizers tended to be stable; the trends for the remaining two classes of drugs showed small fluctuations over time.

The Youth Risk Behavior Survey investigated high school students' ever use of heroin or methamphetamines during 2015.[27] The percentage of ever use of heroin among U.S. high school students was 2.1%; the highest percentage of heroin use was among black males. For methamphetamines the percentage of ever use was 3.0% and highest among Hispanic males. (Refer to **Table 11-2**.)

An alarming phenomenon is the increasing abuse of a class of drugs called opioids. This phenomenon affects a cross-section of ages, social classes, races, and ethnicities in the United States. Opioid abuse has fueled an epidemic of drug dependency and early mortality. Refer to **Exhibit 11-1** for a description of this epidemic.

OVERWEIGHT AND OBESITY

Media reports inform us that both overweight and obesity are increasing in prevalence in the United States. Being overweight or obese can impact the quality of one's life and

TABLE 11-2 Percentage of High School Students Who Ever Used Heroin* and Who Ever Used Methamphetamines,[†] by Sex, Race/Ethnicity, and Grade—United States, Youth Risk Behavior Survey, 2015

| | Ever Used Heroin | | | | | | Ever Used Methamphetamines | | | | | |
| | Female | | Male | | Total | | Female | | Male | | Total | |
Category	%	CI[§]	%	CI	%	CI	%	CI	%	CI	%	CI
Race/Ethnicity												
White[¶]	0.8	(0.5–1.5)	1.7	(1.2–2.4)	1.3	(1.0–1.7)	1.7	(1.1–2.7)	2.5	(1.8–3.5)	2.1	(1.5–2.8)
Black[¶]	1.5	(0.6–3.6)	3.8	(1.9–7.5)	2.7	(1.3–5.6)	1.4	(0.9–2.3)	3.9	(2.1–7.4)	2.8	(1.5–5.1)
Hispanic	1.9	(1.2–3.0)	3.2	(2.1–5.0)	2.6	(1.8–3.8)	4.0	(2.9–5.5)	4.7	(3.3–6.6)	4.4	(3.3–5.9)
Grade												
9	1.4	(0.9–2.3)	2.0	(1.2–3.6)	1.8	(1.2–2.6)	2.2	(1.5–3.2)	1.9	(1.1–3.1)	2.0	(1.5–2.7)
10	1.5	(0.8–2.7)	3.3	(2.2–5.0)	2.4	(1.6–3.6)	2.5	(1.5–4.2)	4.2	(2.7–6.3)	3.3	(2.3–4.9)
11	0.9	(0.5–1.7)	2.3	(1.4–3.8)	1.9	(1.1–3.0)	2.3	(1.4–3.9)	2.8	(1.8–4.2)	2.8	(1.9–4.0)
12	1.0	(0.4–2.2)	2.8	(1.6–4.6)	1.9	(1.3–2.9)	1.8	(1.2–2.8)	5.6	(3.6–8.5)	3.8	(2.7–5.3)
Total	1.2	(0.9–1.8)	2.7	(1.9–3.8)	2.1	(1.5–2.8)	2.3	(1.7–3.0)	3.6	(2.6–4.9)	3.0	(2.4–3.8)

* Also called "smack," "junk," or "China White," used one or more times during their life.

[†] Also called "speed," "crystal," "crank," or "ice," used one or more times during their life.

[§] 95% confidence interval.

[¶] Non-Hispanic.

Reprinted from Centers for Disease Control and Prevention. Youth Risk Behavior Surveillance — United States, 2015. *MMWR Surveill Summ.* 2016; 65(6):111.

EXHIBIT 11-1 Prescription Opioid Overdose Epidemic

Patients taking prescription opioids are at risk for unintentional overdose or death and can become addicted. Up to one out of four people receiving long-term opioid therapy in a primary care setting struggles with addiction. Since 1999, overdose deaths involving prescription opioids have quadrupled and so have sales of these prescription drugs. From 1999 to 2014, more than 165,000 people have died in the U.S. from overdoses related to prescription opioids.

Opioid prescribing continues to fuel the epidemic. Today, at least half of all U.S. opioid overdose deaths involve a prescription opioid. In 2014, more than 14,000 people died from overdoses involving prescription opioids.

Most Commonly Overdosed Opioids

The most common drugs involved in prescription opioid overdose deaths include:

- Methadone
- Oxycodone (such as OxyContin)
- Hydrocodone (such as Vicodin)
- Oxymorphone (Opana)
- Fentanyl

Overdose Deaths

Among those who died from prescription opioid overdose between 1999 and 2014:

- Overdose rates were highest among people age 25 to 54 years.
- Overdose rates were higher among non-Hispanic whites and American Indian or Alaska Natives, compared to non-Hispanic blacks and Hispanics.
- Men were more likely to die from overdose, but the mortality gap between men and women is closing.

Additional Risks

Overdose is not the only risk related to prescription opioid use. Misuse, abuse, and opioid use disorder (addiction) are also potential dangers.

- In 2014, almost 2 million Americans abused or were dependent on prescription opioids.
- Every day, over 1,000 people are treated in emergency departments for misusing prescription opioids.

Adapted and reprinted from Centers for Disease Control and Prevention. Prescription overdose data. Atlanta, GA: CDC. Available at: http://www.cdc.gov/drugoverdose/data/overdose.html; and Guideline information for patients. Atlanta, GA: CDC. Available at: http://www.cdc.gov/drugoverdose/prescribing/patients.html. Accessed August 4, 2016.

increase the risk of chronic diseases such as coronary heart disease and diabetes. Obesity is related to higher healthcare costs and premature death.[28] Among the factors associated with overweight and obesity are inactivity (sedentary lifestyle) and consumption of high-calorie foods.

A measure of overweight and obesity, **body mass index (BMI)**, takes into account both a person's weight and height.

BMI is defined as body weight in kilograms divided by height in meters squared. A BMI of 25.0 to 29.9 classifies a person as being overweight; a BMI of 30 or higher classifies a person as being obese. (Refer to **Table 11-3**, which shows BMI levels for a person who is 5'9" tall.)

Figure 11-16 shows trends in child and adolescent obesity, which is defined as a "… body mass index greater

TABLE 11-3 Determining Overweight and Obesity

Height	Weight Range	BMI	Considered
5'9"	124 lbs or less	Below 18.5	Underweight
	125 lbs to 168 lbs	18.5 to 24.9	Healthy weight
	169 lbs to 202 lbs	25.0 to 29.9	Overweight
	203 lbs or more	30.0 or higher	Obese
	271 lbs or more	40.0 or higher	Extremely obese (Class 3 obese)

Adapted and reprinted from Centers for Disease Control and Prevention. Defining overweight and obesity. Atlanta, GA: CDC. Available at: http://www.cdc.gov/obesity/defining.html. Accessed June 20, 2016.

FIGURE 11-16 Trends in obesity among children and adolescents age 2–19 years, by sex—United States, selected years 1971–1974 through 2011–2012.

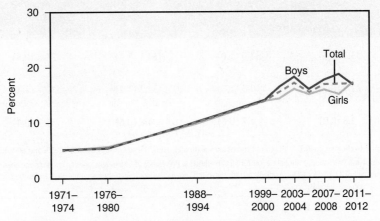

Note : Obesity is body mass index greater than or equal to the sex- and age-specific 95th percentile from the 2000 CDC growth charts.

than or equal to the sex- and age-specific 95th percentile from the 2000 CDC Growth Charts."[29] From the mid-1960s until 2003–2004, the percentages of children and adolescents who were obese has risen steadily. Almost 14% of children age 2 to 5 years were obese in 2003; nearly 19% of preadolescents and 18% adolescents were obese. This phenomenon has ominous implications for the future incidence of chronic diseases and reduced life expectancy in the United States.

Similar to the trends for children and teenagers, the levels of obesity among adults age 20 years and older have increased. The National Health and Nutrition Examination Survey III (NHANES III) in 1988 through 1994 found that 56% of U.S. adults were either overweight or obese (22.9% classified as obese); in 2003 through 2004, the NHANES survey indicated that 66.3% of adults were either overweight or obese with 32.2% counted as obese. By 2011 through 2012, a total of 68.5% of adults were overweight or obese. During this time period, the trend of increasing obesity held for both men and women, with a greater percentage of women tending to be obese than men. From 1988–1994 to 2011–2012, the prevalence of extremely obese adults increased from 2.8% to 6.4%. (Refer to **Table 11-4** and **Figure 11-17**.)

According to the 2011–2012 NHANES, the overall prevalence of obesity among adults in the United States was 35.1%. However, the prevalence of obesity showed substantial variations by region and state in the United States. (Refer to **Figure 11-18**.) Data for 2014 from Behavioral Risk Factor Surveillance System (BRFSS) demonstrated that in Arkansas, Mississippi, and West Virginia the prevalence of obesity was 35% or greater. The prevalence of obesity tended to be higher in the central regions of the country. Interestingly, in no state was the prevalence of obesity less than 20%.[30]

PSYCHIATRIC EPIDEMIOLOGY AND MENTAL HEALTH

Epidemiologic methods have been applied for many years to the study of mental health phenomena. The quest of this research has been to unravel the mysteries of mental disorders. The field of **psychiatric epidemiology** is concerned with the occurrence of mental disorders in the population. As with other health conditions, mental disorders have characteristic distributions according to the categories of person, place, and time. Psychiatric epidemiology studies the incidence and prevalence of mental disorders according to variables such as age, sex, and social class; the discipline measures

TABLE 11-4 Age-Adjusted* Prevalence of Overweight, Obesity, and Extreme Obesity among U.S. Adults, Age 20 Years and Over

	1988–1994 (*n* = 16,235)	1999–2000 (*n* = 4,117)	2003–2004 (*n* = 4,431)	2007–2008 (*n* = 5,550)	2011–2012 (*n* = 5,181)
Overweight	33.1 (0.6)	34.0 (1.0)	34.1 (1.1)	34.3 (0.8)	33.6 (1.3)
Obese	22.9 (0.7)	30.5 (1.5)	32.2 (1.2)	33.7 (1.1)	34.9 (1.4)
Extremely obese	2.8 (0.2)	4.7 (0.6)	4.8 (0.6)	5.7 (0.4)	6.4 (0.6)

*Age adjusted by the direct method to the year 2000 U.S. Bureau of the Census estimates using the age groups 20–39, 40–59, and 60 years and over.

Data from Centers for Disease Control and Prevention, National Center for Health Statistics. Prevalence of overweight, obesity, and extreme obesity among adults: United States, 1960-1962 through 2011-2012. Hyattsville, MD: NCHS, CDC. Available at: http://www.cdc.gov/nchs/data/hestat/obesity_adult_11_12/obesity_adult_11_12.pdf. Accessed July 3, 2016.

FIGURE 11-17 Trends in adult overweight, obesity, and extreme obesity among men and women age 20–24 years—United States, selected years 1960–1962 through 2011–2012.

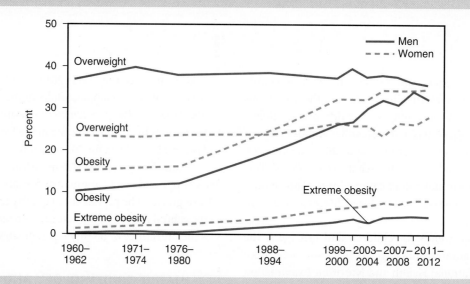

Reprinted from Centers for Disease Control and Prevention, National Center for Health Statistics. Prevalence of overweight, obesity, and extreme obesity among adults: United States, 1960-1962 through 2011-2012. Hyattsville, MD: NCHS, CDC: 3. Available at: http://www.cdc.gov/nchs/data/hestat/obesity_adult_11_12/obesity_adult_11_12.pdf. Accessed July 3, 2016.

the frequency of occurrence of mental disorders and factors related to their etiology.

The *Diagnostic and Statistical Manual of Mental Disorders, 5th edition,* referred to as the DSM-5, is used to classify psychiatric disorders. Anxiety disorders, mood disorders, impulse-control disorders, and substance use disorders are examples of groups of mental disorders defined by the manual. Epidemiologic research findings suggest that more than

one-quarter of the U.S. population is afflicted with a mental disorder during a given year.

Serious Mental Illness

In addition to the overall occurrence of mental disorders in the population, researchers have quantified the prevalence of a subset of disorders known as serious mental illness (SMI). In the National Survey on Drug Use and Health

FIGURE 11-18 Prevalence¶ of self-reported obesity among U.S. adults by state and territory, BRFSS, 2014.

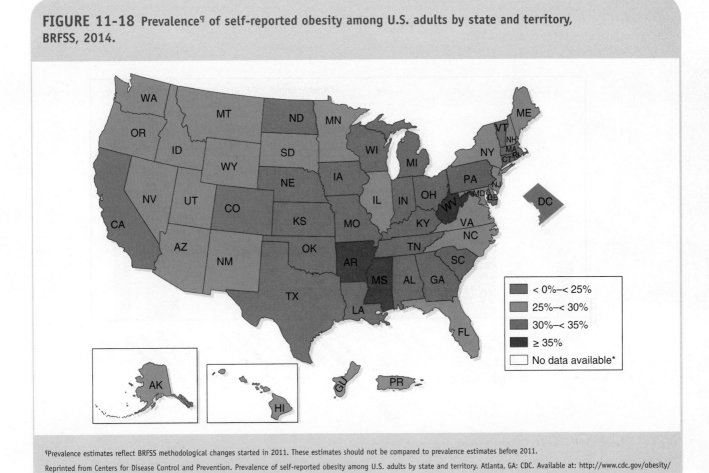

¶Prevalence estimates reflect BRFSS methodological changes started in 2011. These estimates should not be compared to prevalence estimates before 2011.

Reprinted from Centers for Disease Control and Prevention. Prevalence of self-reported obesity among U.S. adults by state and territory. Atlanta, GA: CDC. Available at: http://www.cdc.gov/obesity/downloads/data/overall-obesity-prevalence-map2014-508-compliant.pdf. Accessed April 18, 2016.

(NSDUH), "[s]erious mental illness (SMI) is defined as having a diagnosable mental, behavioral, or emotional disorder in the past year that results in serious functional impairment. These difficulties substantially interfere with a person's ability to carry out major life activities at home, at work, or in the community."[31(p10)] In the 2009 NSDUH, which surveyed adults age 18 years and older, investigators discovered that almost 5% of the American population had experienced an SMI during that year. SMIs were reported most frequently among respondents age 18 to 25 years, in comparison with other age groups; almost twice as many females as males were afflicted. Refer to **Figure 11-19** for more details.

Mood Disorders

As part of the NHANES III (conducted between 1988 and 1994), the Diagnostic Interview Schedule (DIS) was administered to almost 8,000 participants in order to obtain information on the lifetime prevalence of mood disorders. The DIS assesses the occurrence of major psychiatric disorders as defined in the DSM-IV (an earlier version of the DSM). One of the categories of disorders for which information was collected was mood disorders; these include the following:

1. Major depressive episode (MDE)
2. Major depressive episode with severity (MDE-s)
3. Dysthymia (a less severe form of depression)
4. Dysthymia with MDE-s
5. Any bipolar disorder
6. Any mood disorder

In the overall sample, for men and women combined, the most common diagnoses were MDE (8.6%), MDE-s (7.7%), and dysthymia (6.2%). The lifetime prevalence of MDE among women was higher than that among men (11.2% versus 6.0%).[32] The lifetime prevalence of mood disorders varied according to education level. A higher prevalence of mood disorders was found among less educated respondents

FIGURE 11-19 Percentage of persons age 18 years or older with past-year serious mental illness, by selected characteristics—United States, 2009.

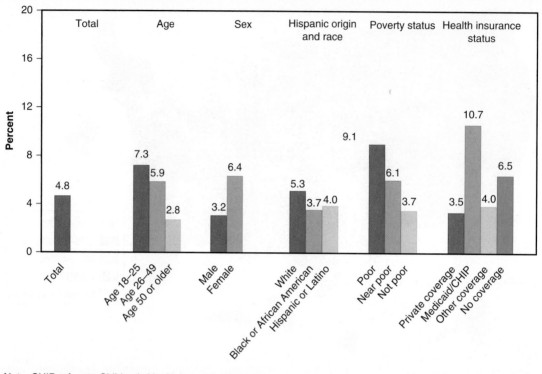

Note: CHIP refers to Children's Health Insurance Program

Reprinted from Substance Abuse and Mental Health Services Administration. *Mental Health, United States, 2010*. HHS Publication No. (SMA) 12-4681. Rockville, MD: Substance Abuse and Mental Health Services Administration; 2012:11.

than among more educated people. Additionally, the lifetime prevalence of mood disorders was higher among women than men. (Refer to **Figure 11-20**.)

Psychiatric Comorbidity

Comorbidity refers to the occurrence of two disorders or illnesses in the same individual. **Psychiatric comorbidity** is defined as the co-occurrence of two or more mental disorders. Another type of comorbidity is the association of substance use disorders (substance dependence or abuse) with serious mental illness. Data from the 2009 NSDUH indicate that substance dependence occurred among more than one-fourth of adults afflicted with SMI. (See **Figure 11-21**.) Also supporting of the notion of comorbidity, the 2006 NSDUH found that adults who had experienced a major depressive disorder episode within the past year were more likely to engage in illicit drug use, smoke cigarettes daily, and use alcohol heavily

in comparison with those who did not experience a major depressive episode.[33]

Children's Mental Health

Mental health issues are significant for children because such disorders are associated with impaired emotional, social, and behavioral development. During 2001 through 2003, approximately 12% (6.8 million) of children age 4 to 17 years were diagnosed with a disorder that affected behavior or learning. Frequently reported severe emotional or behavioral difficulties included a triad of disorders: attention deficit hyperactivity disorder (ADHD), learning disability, and developmental delay (found commonly among both boys and girls). "Among boys with severe/definite difficulties, 59% had ever been diagnosed with ADHD, 48% with learning disability, and 21% with developmental delay."[34(p193)] With the exception of ADHD (higher among boys), the

FIGURE 11-20 Lifetime prevalence (standard error) of mood disorders among 20- to 39-year-old respondents by sex and education.

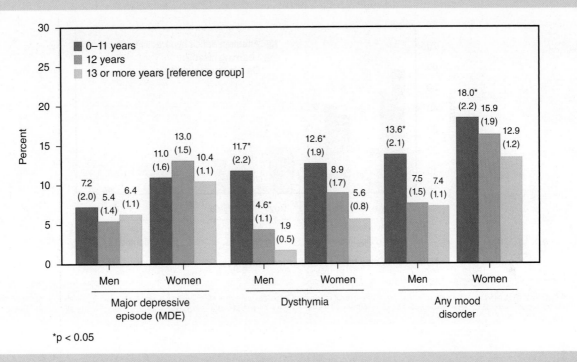

*p < 0.05

Reprinted from Jonas BS, Brody D, Roper M, Narrow W. Mood disorder prevalence among young men and women in the United States. In: Center for Mental Health Services. *Mental Health, United States, 2004*. Manderscheid RW and Berry JT, eds. DHHS Pub No. (SMA)-06-4195. Rockville, MD: Substance Abuse and Mental Health Services Administration; 2006:185.

FIGURE 11-21 Percentage of persons age 18 years or older with past-year serious mental illness or no mental illness, by past year substance dependence or abuse—United States, 2009.

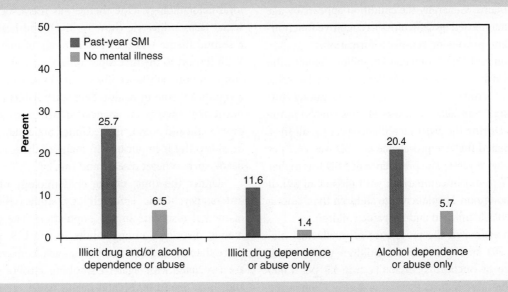

Reprinted from Substance Abuse and Mental Health Services Administration. *Mental Health, United States, 2010*. HHS Publication No. (SMA) 12-4681. Rockville, MD: Substance Abuse and Mental Health Services Administration; 2012:15.

FIGURE 11-22 Selected diagnosed disorders among children age 4 to 17 years, by level of emotional or behavioral difficulties and sex—United States, 2001–2003.

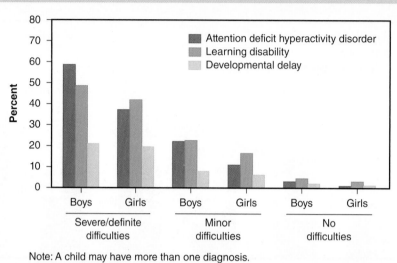

Note: A child may have more than one diagnosis.

Reprinted from Pastor PN, Reuben CA, Falkenstern A. Parental reports of emotional or behavioral difficulties and mental health service use among U.S. school-age children. In: Center for Mental Health Services. *Mental Health, United States, 2004*. Manderscheid RW and Berry JT, eds. DHHS Pub No. (SMA)-06-4195. Rockville, MD: Substance Abuse and Mental Health Services Administration; 2006:193.

corresponding percentages for girls were similar to those of boys. (Refer to **Figure 11-22**.)

Autism

Autism (autism spectrum disorder [ASD]) is a condition that impairs functioning in the social, communication, and behavioral domains. Generally the condition appears by age 3 years and is manifested by difficulties in cognitive functioning, learning, and processing sensory information.

The Autism and Developmental Disabilities Monitoring (ADDM) Network is an active surveillance system for ASD, which is used to estimate the prevalence of ASD among children age 8 years.[35] Surveillance covers 11 sites (states) in the United States. During the 2010 surveillance year for all sites, the CDC estimated that the prevalence of ASD was 14.7 per 1,000 children age 8 years. The prevalence of ASD was higher among boys (1 in 42) in comparison with girls (1 in 89). It was higher among non-Hispanic white children than among non-Hispanic black children and Hispanic children.

CDC also estimated the prevalence of intellectual disability (IQ ≤ 70) among 8-year-old children with autism. The prevalence of intellectual disability was 4.7 per 1,000 children—higher among boys than among girls. Comparing three racial/ethnic groups, CDC reported that the highest

prevalence of intellectual disability was among black children with ASD. (Refer to **Figure 11-23**.)

CONCLUSION

This chapter provided an overview of social and behavioral epidemiology. One theme was the association among social factors, lifestyle (how we live), and health outcomes; a second theme was the epidemiology of mental disorders. With respect to the first topic, tobacco use, excessive alcohol consumption, substance abuse, and experiencing stress play a significant role in health. Sedentary habits and unhealthy nutritional choices are associated with increasing levels of overweight and obesity in the United States. Lifestyle (directly or indirectly) is implicated in many of the leading causes of death, such as heart disease and cancer.

Under the topic of the epidemiology of mental disorders, psychiatric epidemiology studies the occurrence of mental disorders in the population. The prevalence of mental disorders among adults in the U.S. population is more than 25%. Some disorders, such as major depression, are associated with cigarette smoking, alcohol consumption, and illicit drug use. Mental health issues are common and significant for children in the United States. Autism, which

FIGURE 11-23 Estimated prevalence* of autism spectrum disorder among children age 8 years, by most recent intelligence quotient score and by sex and race/ethnicity—Autism and Developmental Disabilities Monitoring Network, seven sites,[†] United States, 2010.

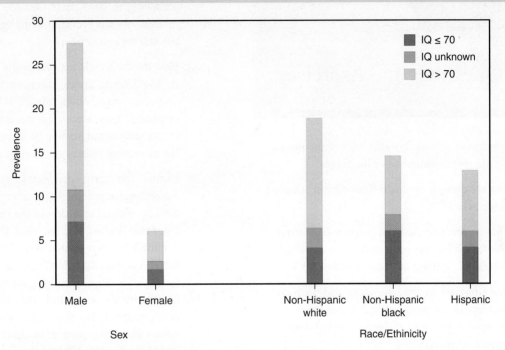

Abbreviation: IQ = intelligence quotient.
* Per 1,000 children aged 8 years.
[†] Includes sites that had intellectual ability data available for ≥ 70% of children who met the ASD case definition.

Reprinted from Centers for Disease Control and Prevention. Prevalence of autism spectrum disorder among children aged 8 years—Autism and Developmental Disabilities Monitoring Network, 11 sites, United States, 2010. *MMWR Surveill Summ.* 2014;63(No. SS-2):21.

appears early in life, is a serious disorder that affects many realms of functioning.

Our behavioral choices are modifiable factors that contribute to positive and negative health status. Although it is often difficult to change one's lifestyle, adoption of a desirable lifestyle would go a long way toward improving the health of both the individual and the population. Many successful interventions have been developed to encourage the adoption of healthful habits; examples are smoking cessation protocols and alcohol recovery programs, such as those operated by Alcoholics Anonymous. One of the greatest challenges for applied epidemiologists is to design programs that are successful for positive lifestyle modification.

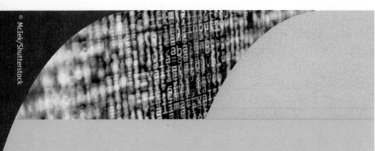

Study Questions and Exercises

1. Distinguish among stressful life events, negative life events, and positive life events.

2. How are chronic strains different from stressful life events?

3. What is meant by the term *posttraumatic stress disorder*? What are some situations in which posttraumatic stress disorder might occur?

4. How common are anxiety, stress, and neurotic disorders in the work setting? What has been the trend in the rates of these disorders during the past 10 years?

5. Describe three major health effects associated with tobacco use. In your opinion, why has the prevalence of current smokers declined sharply since 1965?

6. The following questions relate to cigarette smoking among middle school and high school students:
   a. How frequent is cigarette smoking among this group?
   b. What kinds of epidemiologic research studies would you conduct to further explore the issue of cigarette smoking?
   c. What types of data would you collect?
   d. How would you apply the results of your research?

7. Aside from the fact that alcohol consumption among people younger than 21 is illegal, what are some of the adverse consequences of binge drinking among this group?

8. What three kinds of illicit drugs are used most commonly by people age 12 years and older, according to 2013 data? Can you suggest any methods for the prevention of illegal substance use among young people?

9. How do the trends for overweight and obesity in the United States compare for children and adolescents versus adults? Why do levels of obesity vary across the country? To what extent should our society be concerned about the increasing rates of overweight and obesity?

10. Define the term *psychiatric epidemiology*. According to epidemiologic surveys, how common are mental disorders in the United States? Does this finding surprise you? How are gender and education related to the lifetime prevalence of mental disorders? Give an explanation for the associations you have stated.

11. Controversies surround the consumption of e-cigarettes: Do they have adverse health effects and consequences or do they promote smoking cessation? Propose one case-control study and one cohort study to explore this controversy.

12. In your opinion, what three public health policies could be formulated for the primary prevention of dependent alcohol use and unintentional alcohol poisonings? How might epidemiology contribute to the development of such policies?

13. What types of epidemiologic data would be helpful in exploring the prescription opioid overdose epidemic? Give five examples. Select one of these types of data and propose a cross-sectional study of hospital emergency room treatments for opioid overdoses. How could this study be linked with efforts to prevent overdoses?

14. How would one account for the more than doubling of the U.S. prevalence of extreme obesity over the past two decades? Formulate

three examples of quasi-experimental interventions for addressing the issue of extreme obesity.

15. Define the term *lifestyle* and describe how it can impact the health of populations, giving two examples. Using your own ideas, propose a theoretical model that maps the associations between lifestyle and health outcomes. In your opinion, how reasonable is it to expect that people can change their lifestyles? Consider both the individual and social environmental perspectives as they may pertain to lifestyle change.

16. Distinguish between social and behavioral epidemiology. Formulate a hypothetical cohort study of the relationship between stressful life events and adverse mental health outcomes. Be sure to include the impact of positive and negative life events.

Young Epidemiology Scholars (YES) Exercises

The Young Epidemiology Scholars: Competitions website provides links to teaching units and exercises that support instruction in epidemiology. The YES program, discontinued in 2011, was administered by the College Board and supported by the Robert Wood Johnson Foundation. The exercises continue to be available at the following website: http://yes-competition.org/yes/teaching-units/title.html. The following exercises relate to topics discussed in this chapter and can be found on the YES competitions website.

1. Huang FI, Baumgarten M. Adolescent Suicide: the Role of Epidemiology in Public Health

REFERENCES

1. Berkman LF, Kawachi I. A historical framework for social epidemiology. In: Berkman LF, Kawachi I, Glymour MM, eds. *Social Epidemiology*. 2nd ed. New York, NY: Oxford University Press; 2014.

2. Kann L, McManus T, Harris WA, et al. Youth risk behavior surveillance—United States, 2015. *MMWR Surveill Summ*. 2016;65(SS-6):1–178.

3. *Merriam-Webster Online Dictionary*. Stress. Available at: http://www.merriam-webster.com/dictionary/stress. Accessed June 30, 2016.

4. Holmes T, Rahe R. The social readjustment rating scale. *J Psychosom Res*. 1967;11(2):213–218.

5. National Institutes of Health, National Institute of Mental Health. Meeting summary: Cognition and stress: advances in basic and translational research. Available at: http://www.nimh.nih.gov/research-priorities/scientific-meetings/2007/cognition-and-stress-advances-in-basic-and-translational-research/index.shtml. Accessed August 3, 2016.

6. Scheller-Gilkey G, Thomas SM, Woolwine BJ, Miller AH. Increased early life stress and depressive symptoms in patients with comorbid substance abuse and schizophrenia. *Schizophr Bull*. 2002;28(2):223–231.

7. Sandberg S, Järvenpää S, Penttinen A, et al. Asthma exacerbations in children immediately following stressful life events: a Cox's hierarchical regression. *Thorax*. 2004;59:1046–1051.

8. Lillberg K, Verkasalo PK, Kaprio J, et al. Stressful life events and risk of breast cancer in 10,808 women: a cohort study. *Am J Epidemiol*. 2003;157(5):415–423.

9. National Institutes of Health, National Institute of Mental Health. NIMH Fact Sheet. Post-traumatic stress disorder research. Available at: https://infocenter.nimh.nih.gov/pubstatic/OM%2009-4299/OM%2009-4299.pdf. Accessed August 3, 2016.

10. Seino K, Takano T, Mashal T, et al. Prevalence of and factors influencing posttraumatic stress disorder among mothers of children under five in Kabul, Afghanistan, after decades of armed conflicts. *Health Qual Life Outcomes*. April 23, 2008;6:29.

11. Hankin CS, Spiro A 3rd, Miller DR, Kazis L. Mental disorders and mental health treatment among U.S. Department of Veterans Affairs outpatients: the Veterans Health Study. *Am J Psychiatry*. 1999;156(12):1924–1930.

12. Calhoun PS, Bosworth HB, Grambow SC, Dudley TK, Beckham JC. Medical service utilization by veterans seeking help for posttraumatic stress disorder. *Am J Psychiatry*. 2002;159(12):2081–2086.

13. Dobie DJ, Maynard C, Kiviahan DR, Dudley TK, Beckham JC. Post-traumatic stress disorder screening status is associated with increased VA medical and surgical utilization in women. *J Gen Intern Med*. 2006;21(Suppl 3):S58–S64.

14. Centers for Disease Control and Prevention. National Institute for Occupational Safety and Health (NIOSH). Stress… at work. NIOSH Publication No. 99-101. Available at: http://www.cdc.gov/Niosh/stresswk.html. Accessed August 23, 2015.

15. National Institute for Occupational Safety and Health (NIOSH). Worker health chartbook, 2004. Cincinnati, OH: DHHS (NIOSH) Publication No. 2004-146; 2004.

16. American Psychological Association. Workplace survey. Available at: https://www.apa.org/news/press/releases/phwa/workplace-survey.pdf. Accessed July 1, 2016.

17. National Center for Health Statistics. *Health, United States, 2006, With Chartbook on Trends in the Health of Americans*. Hyattsville, MD: National Center for Health Statistics; 2006.

18. National Center for Health Statistics. *Health, United States, 2015: With Special Feature on Racial and Ethnic Health Disparities*. Hyattsville, MD: National Center for Health Statistics; 2016:28.

19. Substance Abuse and Mental Health Services Administration. *Results from the 2013 National Survey on Drug Use and Health: summary of national findings*. NSDUH Series H-48, HHS Publication No. (SMA) 14-4863. Rockville, MD: Substance Abuse and Mental Health Services Administration; 2014.

20. Marshall L, Schooley M, Ryan H, et al. Youth tobacco surveillance—United States, 2001–2002. *MMWR Surveill Summ*. 2006;55(SS-3):1–56.

21. Singh T, Arrazola RA, Corey CG, et al. CDC tobacco use among middle and high school students—United States, 2011–2015. *MMWR*. 2016;65(14):361–367.

22. U.S. Department of Health and Human Services. *The Health Consequences of Involuntary Exposure to Tobacco Smoke: A Report of the Surgeon General*. Washington, DC: U.S. Department of Health and Human Services, Centers for Disease Control and Prevention, Coordinating Center for Health Promotion, National Center for Chronic Disease Prevention and Health Promotion, Office on Smoking and Health; 2006.

23. Kochanek KD, Murphy SL, Xu J, et al. Deaths: final data for 2014. *National Vital Statistics Reports*. 2016;65(4). Hyattsville, MD: National Center for Health Statistics.

24. Centers for Disease Control and Prevention. Alcohol and public health fact sheets—alcohol use and your health. Available at: http://www.cdc.gov/alcohol/fact-sheets/alcohol-use.htm. Accessed July 2, 2016.

25. Centers for Disease Control and Prevention. 2015 Youth Risk Behavior Surveillance System Results. Available at: http://www.cdc.gov/healthy youth/data/yrbs/slides/2015/taodu_slides_yrbs.pptx. Accessed July 2, 2016.

26. U.S. Department of Health and Human Services, Substance Abuse and Mental Health Services Administration, Office of Applied Studies. The NSDUH Report: methamphetamine use, abuse, and dependence: 2002, 2003, and 2004. September 16, 2005.

27. Centers for Disease Control and Prevention. Youth Risk Behavior Surveillance—United States, 2015. *MMWR Surveill Summ*. 2016;65(6): 1–174.

28. Centers for Disease Control and Prevention. State-specific prevalence of obesity among adults—United States, 2007. *MMWR*. 2008;57:766–768.

29. Centers for Disease Control and Prevention, National Center for Health Statistics. Prevalence of overweight and obesity among children and adolescents: United States, 1960–1962 through 2011–2012. Available at: http://www.cdc.gov/nchs/data/hestat/obesity_child_11_12/obesity_child_11_12.pdf. Accessed August 3, 2016.

30. Centers for Disease Control and Prevention. Prevalence of self-reported obesity among U.S. adults by state and territory. Available at: http://www.cdc.gov/obesity/downloads/data/overall-obesity-prevalence-map2014-508-compliant.pdf. Accessed April 18, 2016.

31. Substance Abuse and Mental Health Services Administration. *Mental Health, United States, 2010*. HHS Publication No. (SMA) 12-4681. Rockville, MD: Substance Abuse and Mental Health Services Administration; 2012.

32. Jonas BS, Brody D, Roper M, Narrow W. Mood disorder prevalence among young men and women in the United States. In: Manderscheid RW, Berry JT, eds. Center for Mental Health Services. *Mental Health, United States, 2004*. DHHS Pub No. (SMA)-06-4195. Rockville, MD: Substance Abuse and Mental Health Services Administration; 2006.

33. Substance Abuse and Mental Health Services Administration. *Results from the 2006 National Survey on Drug Use and Health: national findings*. (Office of Applied Studies, NSDUH Series H-32, DHHS Publication No. SMA 07-4293). Rockville, MD: Substance Abuse and Mental Health Services Administration; 2007.

34. Pastor PN, Reuben CA, Falkenstern A. Parental reports of emotional or behavioral difficulties and mental health service use among U.S. school-age children. In: Manderscheid RW, Berry JT, eds. Center for Mental Health Services. *Mental Health, United States, 2004*. DHHS Pub No. (SMA)-06-4195. Rockville, MD: Substance Abuse and Mental Health Services Administration; 2006.

35. Centers for Disease Control and Prevention. Prevalence of autism spectrum disorder among children aged 8 years—Autism and Developmental Disabilities Monitoring Network, 11 sites, United States, 2010. *MMWR*. 2014;63(SS-2):1–22.

CHAPTER **12**

Special Epidemiologic Applications

INTRODUCTION

Scientists utilize epidemiologic methods and concepts with respect to a wide range of health-related phenomena. Earlier, we discussed the most familiar applications of epidemiology, for example, descriptive epidemiologic investigations of infectious disease outbreaks and studies of the role of social and behavioral factors in health. This chapter presents health-related applications not discussed previously, including cutting-edge molecular and genetic techniques. Other uses are in the fields of environmental epidemiology and injury epidemiology, which fit epidemiologic methods to the study of various types of injuries, such as intentional and unintentional injuries; the latter are a leading cause of death in the United States. In addition, several uses are indirectly related to health; examples cited in this chapter include screen-based media use (e.g., television and computer games) and "sewage epidemiology." See **Table 12-1** for a list of important terms used in this chapter.

MOLECULAR AND GENETIC EPIDEMIOLOGY

The application of molecular and genetic methods to the study of diseases in the population is an exciting development that has expanded in recent years. Traditionally, epidemiologic research has uncovered associations between exposures and health outcomes, often without fully developing an explanation for the observed linkages. This type of epidemiologic research is called "black box" epidemiology: the associations are "black boxes" in which the mechanisms for the relationships are hidden and unknown. Molecular and genetic methods have increased the ability of scientists to peer inside these black boxes in order to expand the knowledge base of disease causality.

Jointly coordinated by the U.S. Department of Energy and the National Institutes of Health, the **Human Genome Project (HGP)** was completed in 2003. **Figure 12-1** portrays the logo of the HGP. One of the goals of the HGP was to

TABLE 12-1 List of Important Terms Used in This Chapter

Autosomal dominant	Human Genome Project
Autosomal recessive	Injury epidemiology
Congenital malformation	Ionizing radiation
Dioxin	Nanotechnology
Dichloro-diphenyl-trichloroethane (DDT)	Molecular epidemiology
Disaster	Occupational epidemiology
Disaster epidemiology	Pharmacoepidemiology
Environmental epidemiology	Physical dating violence
Forensic epidemiology	Polychlorinated biphenyls (PCBs)
Genetic epidemiology	Sewage epidemiology
Genetic marker (of susceptibility)	Sex-linked disorder
Global warming	Traumatic brain injury
Heavy metal	Unintentional injury

FIGURE 12-1 Human Genome Project.

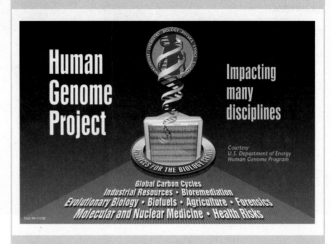

Reprinted from Office of Biological and Environmental Research of the U.S. Department of Energy Office of Science. Available at: https://public.ornl.gov/site/gallery/detail.cfm?id=411&restsection=HGPArchive. Accessed January 6, 2016.

identify all of the genes (20,000 to 25,000) in human DNA. This project will continue to provide valuable information for epidemiologic research for many years. As an example, the HGP will aid in studying genetic and environmental interactions. The fields of both molecular and genetic epidemiology make use of genetic methods.

Molecular epidemiology is a subfield of epidemiology that uses molecular biology to improve measurements of exposures and disease. A variety of biologic measures of exposure and disease can be employed. For example, molecular epidemiology uses molecular markers (identified as genetic markers) in addition to genes to establish exposure-disease relationships. "A **genetic marker** of susceptibility is a host factor that enhances some step in the progression between exposure and disease such that the downstream step is more likely to occur. The term genetic marker is used here in reference to susceptibility genes."[1] Certain genes are markers for exposure and do not confer risk on their own; health effects occur in conjunction with specific exposures. When these genes are present, the person may have increased susceptibility to specific exposures. While more detailed

information is beyond the scope of this text, an example is the linkage between the gene *CYP2D6* and susceptibility to the effects of exposure to benzo[a]pyrene, a hazardous chemical released by incomplete combustion of petroleum-based chemicals.

The field of **genetic epidemiology**, which has a narrower focus than molecular epidemiology, is concerned with "... the identification of inherited factors that influence disease, and how variation in the genetic material interacts with environmental factors to increase (or decrease) risk of disease."[2(p536)] Examples of research questions addressed by genetic epidemiology are whether diseases cluster in families and whether the patterns of diseases within families are consistent with the laws of inheritance.

Genetic factors have been implicated in a wide range of conditions. According to the World Health Organization, insufficient data are available regarding epidemiology of genetic disorders, despite growing knowledge about their importance in chronic and infectious diseases.[3] Examples of conditions that are known or believed to have a genetic basis are:

- Hemophilia: The inherited form of hemophilia is a **sex-linked disorder**. It is caused by an abnormal gene carried on an X chromosome. (Note that hemophilia also occurs in an acquired form, which is not discussed here.) Hemophilia is a bleeding disorder in which the blood does not clot normally. This rare condition has a prevalence of approximately 18,000 persons (almost always males) in the United States.[4] How is the condition inherited? Females have two X chromosomes. In most cases, females who are carriers of the abnormal gene for hemophilia are not themselves affected. Males have an X and a Y chromosome. The affected male inherits the abnormal gene on the X chromosome from his mother, if she has the carrier trait. A father who has hemophilia can transmit the affected gene on his X chromosome to his daughter, who usually will not be affected but will be a carrier. The father's son also will not be affected; he cannot inherit the trait from his father because he receives only a Y chromosome from his father.

- Tay-Sachs disease: This condition is an uncommon inherited disease. Infants born with Tay-Sachs disease at first appear normal and later in the first year of life develop severe neurologic symptoms such as blindness, deafness, and inability to swallow.[5] This highly fatal condition causes the death of most patients by age 4 years. People of Eastern European and Ashkenazi [Eastern European] Jewish descent have a higher incidence of the disease than other groups. The affliction is caused by a genetic mutation that is inherited in an autosomal recessive pattern. (**Autosomal recessive** denotes those diseases for which two copies of an altered gene are required to increase risk of the disease; **autosomal dominant** refers to a situation in which only a single copy of an altered gene located on a nonsex chromosome is sufficient to cause an increased risk of disease.) In order for a child to be affected, he or she must receive the gene from both parents.

- Sickle cell disease: This condition encompasses a group of inherited disorders that affect red blood cells.[6] The most common and severe variation of sickle cell disease is called sickle cell anemia. This genetic disorder is caused by a mutation that causes a person's red blood cells to have abnormal hemoglobin called hemoglobin S: the red blood cells appear to be sickle shaped.

Sickle cell anemia is caused by an autosomal recessive gene. People who inherit one copy of the gene are carriers of the trait but usually will not be affected. If a child inherits the trait from both parents

(two copies of the sickle gene), the individual will have sickle cell anemia.

The mutation is thought to have evolved as a protection against malaria. The trait is found among people whose ancestors came from sub-Saharan Africa, Saudi Arabia, India, and some Mediterranean countries, as well as several other countries.

- **Inherited cancers** associated with *BRCA1* and *BRCA2* genes: Breast cancer gene one (*BRCA1*) and breast cancer gene two (*BRCA2*) are human genes that create proteins instrumental in suppression of tumors.[7] Inherited harmful mutations in *BRCA1* and *BRCA2* have been linked to increased risk of breast and ovarian cancer among women. Estimates suggest that about 5 to 10% of all breast cancers are associated with mutations in these genes. Furthermore, such mutations are found in up to 25% of inherited breast cancers. Although mutations in *BRCA1* and *BRCA2* genes are uncommon in the general population, researchers have identified several factors that increase their risk: ethnicity (for example, Ashkenazi Jewish background); personal history (for example, diagnosis of breast cancer among women younger than age 50 years; development of cancer in both breasts; having both breast and ovarian cancer); and family history (for example, occurrence in a family of multiple cases of breast cancers or of cases of both breast and ovarian cancer).

Healthcare providers use genetic tests for detection of mutations in *BRCA1* and *BRCA2* genes. See Chapter 9 for more information. A positive test result shows the presence of a harmful mutation, which is related to an increased risk of cancer. Because these mutations are rare in the general population, testing is usually applied only to individuals who do not have cancer, but are at possible risk because of their family or individual history. The test is unable to verify that a woman who tests positively will go on to develop breast or ovarian cancer in the future, and some of these women never acquire these diagnoses. Further population-based research would help to compare risks of breast, ovarian, and other cancer diagnoses among women with and without harmful mutations in these genes. Note also that men with *BRCA2* mutations (and to a lesser degree *BRCA1* mutations) have increased risks of some forms of cancer including prostate cancer and male breast cancer.

- Down syndrome: The most common chromosomal disorder, Down syndrome is caused by a chromosomal abnormality associated with the presence of an extra chromosome 21 (either all or part). The prevalence of Down syndrome is 14.2 cases per 10,000 live births.[8] One of the noteworthy epidemiologic characteristics of Down syndrome is its association with age of mother; its prevalence among newborns rises with increasing maternal age, as demonstrated in **Figure 12-2**. The prevalence of Down syndrome births begins to increase among mothers who are in their early thirties; the rate exceeds 120 cases per 10,000 live births among mothers who are age 40 years and older. In addition, the prevalence of the condition is higher among Hispanics than among whites or blacks. People with Down syndrome are quite varied in their abilities. They also tend to share distinctive facial and bodily characteristics, as shown in **Figure 12-3**.

- Congenital malformations (birth defects): **Congenital malformations** are defects present at birth. Birth defects include both structural birth defects and those that are produced by chromosomal abnormalities (e.g., Down syndrome). "Major structural birth

FIGURE 12-3 Girl with Down syndrome.

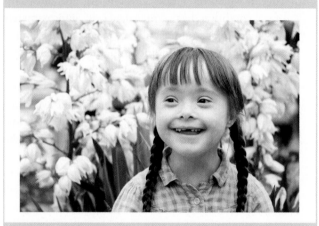

Denis Kuvaev/Shutterstock, Inc.

defects are defined as conditions that (1) result from a malformation, deformation, or disruption in one or more parts of the body; (2) are present at birth; and

FIGURE 12-2 Maternal age and prevalence of Down syndrome—United States, January 1, 2006 through December 31, 2010.

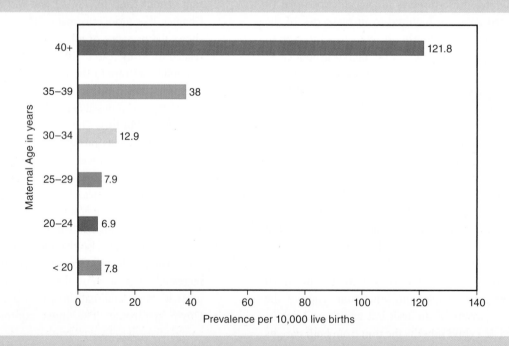

Data from Mai CT, Kucik JE, Isenburg J, et al. Selected birth defects data from population-based birth defects surveillance programs in the United States, 2006 to 2010: featuring trisomy conditions. *Birth Defects Res A Clin Mol Teratol.* 2013;97(11):709-725.

FIGURE 12-4 A photograph of a child with cleft feet, or "lobster claw" feet.

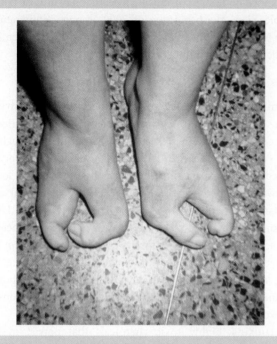

Reprinted from Centers for Disease Control and Prevention. Public Health Image Library, ID# 2631. CDC/Allan J. Ebbin, MD, MPH. Available at: http://phil.cdc.gov/phil/home.asp. Accessed July 5, 2016.

(3) have a serious, adverse effect on health, development, or functional ability."[9(p1302)] An example of a congenital malformation is a cleft foot, a rare inherited anomaly called partial adactyly. (See **Figure 12-4.**)

ENVIRONMENTAL EPIDEMIOLOGY

The term **environmental epidemiology** refers to the study of diseases and conditions (occurring in the population) that are linked to environmental factors. Examples of topics included under the purview of this field are health effects of exposure to air pollution, global warming, pesticides and toxic chemicals, **heavy metals** (e.g., lead, mercury, and arsenic [technically a crystalline metalloid]), contaminated drinking water, and radiation.

Air Pollution

Epidemiologic research has examined a number of adverse health outcomes as possible consequences of exposure to air pollution—mortality, coronary heart disease, chronic obstructive pulmonary disease, asthma, and lung cancer. Air

pollution represents potential health risks to the residents of cities (e.g., Beijing and Mexico City) in developing countries of the world as well as in the United States (e.g., the Los Angeles Basin and Houston, Texas). With the growing use of fossil fuels such as coal and oil to power increasing numbers of industries and automobiles, the threat of air pollution will escalate as an environmental health issue. Epidemiologic approaches to the study of air pollution include the following:

- Observations of the health effects of extreme air pollution episodes: Several noteworthy severe air pollution episodes are historically important; two examples are the event in Donora, Pennsylvania, in 1948, and the incident in London, England, during 1952; both were linked to increases in morbidity and mortality.
  - Donora is a small town located on the Monongahela River about 30 miles south of Pittsburgh. An atmospheric condition known as an inversion layer caused a thick layer of fog combined with particles from industrial and other facilities to descend on Donora. The industrial sources of the contaminants were iron and steel mills, factories that burned coal, coke ovens, and metal works. Other emitters of smoke included coal-fired home stoves. This episode caused widespread illnesses, hospitalizations, and deaths in the small town.
  - Between December 5 and December 9, 1952, a severe air pollution event confronted London, England. London's normally foggy climate, in combination with the heavy combustion of coal and other fossil fuels, meant that "pea-souper" fogs were common. The particularly heavy air pollution episode in December of 1952 resulted in a "killer fog" that was reported to have caused in excess of 3,000 deaths.
- Studies of associations between mortality and increased air pollution levels at much lower levels than those recorded in extreme air pollution events: Several research studies conducted in the 1970s and 1980s showed that increased pollution levels (from particles in the air) were correlated with increased daily mortality.
- Examinations of total communities: Noteworthy is the Tucson Epidemiological Study of Airway Obstructive Disease, which tracked the etiology and natural history of chronic obstructive pulmonary disease and other conditions.

- Studies of the possible associations between air pollution and specific diseases and adverse health outcomes.
  - Coronary heart disease exacerbates the risk of adverse health effects of air pollution.
  - Asthma, one of the most common chronic diseases in the United States, has increased in prevalence, despite improving air quality.
- Examinations of traffic patterns and **air pollution health effects**: Residents who live near heavily traveled motorways, highways, and city streets may have increased risk of mortality and other adverse health effects.

Global Warming

The term **global warming** refers to the gradual increase in the Earth's temperature over time. Global warming is a controversial topic because some have argued that it is merely a transitory phenomenon and is not supported by scientific evidence. Nevertheless, historical data indicate that the Earth's temperature has warmed approximately 0.6°C since the end of the nineteenth century and about 0.4°C within the past 25 years. Some estimates suggest that the Earth's temperature may increase by about 1.5° to 4°C by the mid-twenty-first century. Factors that are believed to contribute to global warming include the use of fossil fuels such as coal and petroleum-based fuels that release greenhouse gases—carbon dioxide, methane, chlorofluorocarbons, and nitrous oxide. Additionally, widespread deforestation in many parts of the world, particularly the Brazilian Amazon jungle, has reduced the capacity of trees in the forest ecosystem to absorb carbon dioxide from the atmosphere.

The potential impacts of global warming include receding glaciers, alterations in the geographic distribution of insect vectors, and extreme changes in Earth's climate. Over the past half century, glaciers in many parts of the world have receded; you can observe this phenomenon if you visit or view photographs of glaciers in North America, Europe, and elsewhere on the globe. It may be possible for disease-carrying arthropods such as the *Aedes aegypti* mosquito, which is endemic to warmer climate regions, to migrate northward and disseminate diseases such as malaria and Zika virus disease. (However, the potential relationship between global warming and the spread of diseases such as malaria has not been established definitively and remains a controversial matter.[10] An alternative explanation for the spread of malaria during recent years could be the failure of mosquito control programs.) Finally, evidence suggests that global warming is associated with extreme climatic conditions including heat waves and severe rainstorms. During mid-1995, Chicago, Illinois, experienced episodes of heat-related mortality caused by abnormal heat waves. In August 2003, a blistering heat wave descended on France, producing a death toll of almost 15,000 people. Since the beginning of 2000, average temperatures have increased globally. By the end of this century, scientists predict increasing numbers of extreme heat events.

Toxic Chemicals

Chemicals and pesticides are used extensively in industry, at home, and in agriculture; two examples are **DDT** (**dichloro-diphenyl-trichloroethane**, a pesticide from the organochlorine family) and dioxins. DDT, a highly effective agent for the control of malaria-bearing mosquitoes, became a focus of awareness because of its possible adverse animal and human health effects. For example, in North America DDT endangered bird species such as the brown pelican. Concerns about the safety of DDT led to its prohibition in 1972 in the United States. With the discontinuance of DDT spraying, the *Anopheles* mosquito has reestablished itself, with corresponding increases in malaria cases in formerly endemic regions of the world.

Dioxins, highly toxic chemicals that persist in the environment, have been associated with disruption of the immune, endocrine, reproductive, and nervous systems. They have been reported to cause cancer in laboratory animals. **Polychlorinated biphenyls (PCBs)** are classified as dioxin-like chemicals. They are shown to cause cancer in laboratory animals, and they have been designated as probable human carcinogens. Agent Orange, the defoliant used in the Vietnam War, was found to contain minute levels of dioxins. Returning veterans from the battle theater reported unusual adverse health outcomes including cancer and skin rashes among themselves and birth defects among their children.

Heavy Metals

Industrial sites, metal smelters, some mining operations, and coal-fired power plants can release heavy metals into the environment, endangering the health of people who live near such facilities. Also at risk are employees who come into contact with heavy metals in their work environment. Heavy metals from these sources also can permanently contaminate the soil. Other sources of release of heavy metals into the environment are waste disposal sites. Used electronic equipment and old automobile tires that have been deposited in these sites contain toxic heavy metals, for example, lead, mercury, cadmium, and arsenic. Improperly designed disposal sites can allow toxic metals to leach into the groundwater, which often is used for human consumption.

Lead

This potent neurotoxin is associated with serious central nervous system effects and other adverse health consequences, even when uptake occurs at low levels. Lead exposure can occur through ingestion and inhalation. Children, who are particularly vulnerable to the effects of lead, may come into contact with the toxic metal from lead-based paints applied to playground equipment and by ingesting paint chips that are peeling off the interior surfaces of older buildings. Among children, lead exposure is associated with intellectual impairment and behavioral deficits.

In previous eras, lead was dispersed widely into the environment. Formerly lead was an additive in paints and motor vehicle fuels, before its use was prohibited for these purposes. Lead is also a component of automobile batteries and solder used in electronics. Fortunately, most of the lead in automobile batteries is now recycled. In 2016, Flint, Michigan, gained national and global attention because the public water supply was found to have high levels of lead contamination.

Mercury

A highly toxic metal that is a particular hazard to the unborn children of pregnant women, mercury is released into the environment as a by-product of industrial processes. Certain types of fish (e.g., shark, swordfish, tilefish, king mackerel, and canned albacore) are believed to contain unhealthful mercury levels; frequent consumption of such fish may expose one to unacceptably high levels of mercury.

Nuclear Facilities

Nuclear facilities include weapons production plants, test sites, and nuclear power plants. Past releases of radioactive materials from these installations have exposed populations to varying amounts of ionizing radiation, often at low levels. **Ionizing radiation** is an intense form of radiation that has enough energy to remove tightly bound electrons from atoms, thus creating ions (electrically charged atoms). A role for environmental health epidemiologists includes studying the long-term effects of exposures to ionizing radiation. One of the potential outcomes of such exposures is development of various forms of cancer, such as thyroid cancer. Several past releases from nuclear facilities in the United States, Ukraine, and Japan are covered in this section.

A well-publicized incident in the United States was the unintentional release of radiation into the community from the Three-Mile Island nuclear power plant in Pennsylvania on March 28, 1979. This release occurred as a result of a partial meltdown of the reactor core. Apparently, ionizing radiation exposure levels from this accident were very low and adverse health effects were difficult to document.

A much more serious accident (involving explosions and fires) occurred at the nuclear power plant in Chernobyl, Ukraine, on April 26, 1986. This accident caused substantial radiation exposure of the population nearby as well as in many neighboring European countries. In fact, the Chernobyl accident resulted in the second largest major exposure of a large population to radiation. (The largest radiation exposure occurred in 1945 among the Japanese population. This happened when atomic bombs were detonated over Hiroshima and Nagasaki.)

The most common adverse health effect associated with Chernobyl was an increase in thyroid cancer among people who were exposed as children.[11] According to an editorial that marked the twenty-fifth anniversary of the catastrophe at Chernobyl, more than 6,000 cases have been attributed to childhood exposure to radioactive iodine (iodine-131) from the release, with additional cases expected in the future.[12] Another serious adverse outcome has been an epidemic of stress (the psychosocial effect) among the numerous Europeans who resided in a wide swath of the impacted continent and who were obliged to endure this event.

On March 11, 2011, the Great East Japan Earthquake caused major damage to the Fukushima Daiichi nuclear power plant located in northern Japan.[13] A meltdown in the reactor cores in Units 1 through 3 led to breaching of containment vessels and explosions in some of the facility's buildings. The environmental consequences of these explosions included atmospheric release of radioactive materials that settled on the land and nearby ocean. Authorities ordered immediate evacuation of people within a 20-km radius of the plant.

An ongoing concern of the Fukushima disaster has been environmental and human health effects. In response, research has evaluated the health effects of radiation exposure among workers and the exposed population.[13] Investigators were unable to observe any early adverse radiation-linked health effects among either workers or residents. However, data suggest that anxiety and stress-related disorders have proliferated in response to community members' fears of risks from radiation exposures and concerns about stigmatization.

The aforementioned cases demonstrate some of the challenges inherent in studying the health effects of radiation exposures of the population to radiation. Among these challenges for epidemiology are that exposures may occur at low levels and that the latency period (time period between initial exposure and a measurable response) for cancers to develop can range from 10 to 60 years. Given these long latencies at these exposure levels, epidemiologists encounter difficulties in differentiating cancers induced by unintentional releases of ionizing radiation from those caused by other exposures. Optimally, epidemiologic studies should include very large numbers of exposed subjects and take place over long time periods. The high costs of such research may not be economically feasible. Certainly, a nuclear "accident" incites panic among the general public, many of whom may not be familiar with the health effects of ionizing radiation. Such public responses have been a topic of social epidemiologic investigations and are a valuable topic for future research.

EPIDEMIOLOGY AND OCCUPATIONAL HEALTH

Occupational epidemiology focuses on adverse health outcomes associated with the work environment. In many instances, the work environment can present health hazards to workers employed in a variety of positions. Sometimes these hazards are similar to those that are found in the general environment. However, in the work environment, the levels of exposures that occur among employees are often much higher than exposure levels that the general population encounters in the ambient environment.

Applications of epidemiology to occupational health include the study of adverse health effects related to environmental exposures that occur at work. The field of occupational health and safety is closely related to environmental epidemiology and focuses on identifying, preventing, and remediating adverse health effects related to the occupational environment. Potential work-related hazards include high noise levels, fumes and dusts, toxic chemicals, and dangerous biological agents. Another topic of occupational epidemiology is occurrence and prevention of occupational injuries. Occupational injuries and illnesses are major causes of morbidity and mortality and have significant economic impacts on society because of lost work time and the cost of treating occupational illnesses, some of which may last a lifetime.

The U.S. Department of Labor, Bureau of Labor Statistics (BLS) tallies cases of occupational injuries and illnesses in private industry. According to the BLS (2014 data), most cases reported were nonfatal occupational injuries, with the remainder (about 5%) attributable to illnesses.[14] The leading occupational illnesses were skin diseases, hearing loss, and respiratory conditions (refer to **Figure 12-5**). The skin, auditory system, and respiratory system are the sites that come into the most direct contact with occupationally associated disease-causing agents. The other category of

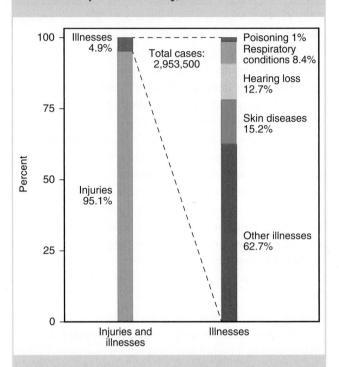

FIGURE 12-5 Distribution of nonfatal occupational injury and illness cases, by category of illness—private industry, 2014.

Reprinted from U.S. Bureau of Labor Statistics. 2014 survey of occupational injuries and illnesses. Summary Estimates Charts Package. Washington, DC: U.S. Department of Labor, BLS; October 29, 2015:5. Available at: http://www.bls.gov/iif/oshwc/osh/os/osch0054.pdf. Accessed March 23, 2016.

illnesses comprised afflictions such as repetitive motion disorders and systemic diseases.

Workers in many industries are exposed to hazardous agents. One example is the high-tech industry that manufactures semiconductors and electronic equipment. Semiconductor chip manufacturing requires the use of dangerous solvents, acids, and gases. Many of these agents are potentially carcinogenic; some of the solvents used in high-tech manufacturing processes may contaminate nearby groundwater, posing a hazard to residents of the area. Fortunately, exposures of employees and the community to hazardous agents are largely preventable. Methods for limiting exposures include requiring workers to use personal protective devices, designing safer manufacturing processes, and controlling emissions from factories.

A topic of increasing concern is the use of nanomaterials (substances on a near-atomic scale) in products such as medicines and electronic devices. Although a small body of suggestive evidence has been developed regarding adverse effects of nanomaterials among exposed workers, the health effects of nanomaterials are not understood fully. Contributions of epidemiology regarding nanomaterials might include conducting systematic reviews of past epidemiologic research; determining needed areas of research; and implementing screening programs for employees who work with these materials. Refer to **Exhibit 12-1** for information on nanomaterials.

Figure 12-6 shows geographic variation in the incidence rates for occupational injuries and illnesses by state in the United States. The BLS defined this incidence rate as "the total recordable case (TRC) incidence rate per 100 full-time workers."[15] Data for private industry and public sector estimates were available for 41 participating states and the District of Columbia in 2014. The U.S. national average for injuries and illness in 2014 was 3.2 cases per 100 workers. The incidence rate of 8 states was not statistically different from the average. A total of 19 states had rates that were significantly higher; the District of Columbia and 14 states had lower rates.

UNINTENTIONAL INJURIES

Injury epidemiology studies the distribution and determinants of injuries (both intentional and unintentional) in the population. Use of the term **unintentional injury** is preferred to accident; when most people use the term *accident* they are implying that a random, unpreventable event has occurred. "Epidemiological studies have demonstrated that the risk of accidents is often predictable and that many accidents and *disasters* are preventable."[16] Consequently, scientific works should not use the term accident.

As of 2013, unintentional injuries were the fourth most frequent cause of mortality in the United States. During that year, more than 130,000 deaths from unintentional injuries (5% of total deaths) were recorded.[17] The crude and age-adjusted death rates for this cause were 41.3 and 39.4 per 100,000 population, respectively. The category of unintentional injuries includes transport injuries (motor vehicle injuries, other land transport injuries, and injuries that occur on water and in the air and space) and nontransport injuries (unintentional poisoning, falls, and accidental discharges of firearms).

EXHIBIT 12-1   New Technologies: Nanotechnology and Use of Nanoparticles

Nanotechnologies hold much potential for groundbreaking progress in diverse fields, for example medicine, energy production, and products for the consumer. In fact, nanotechnologies "... may revolutionize life in the future."[a(pvii)] The word **nanotechnology** denotes "... the manipulation of matter on a near-atomic scale [1 to 100 nanometers in length] to produce new structures, materials and devices."[b] These near-atomic scale materials are called nanomaterials. Because of their tiny size, nanomaterials have unique effects on physical, chemical, and biological behaviors.

Those likely to be first exposed to nanomaterials are research workers. It is possible that nanomaterials may affect human health adversely, as some preliminary evidence has suggested. Engeman and colleagues state "... the potential adverse human health effects of manufactured nanomaterial exposure are not yet fully understood, and exposures in humans are mostly uncharacterized."[c(p487)] The National Institute of Occupational Safety and Health (NIOSH) has developed a list of 10 critical topic areas for research on nanotechnology. Among the critical research topics are toxicity of nanomaterials, risk assessments with respect to their use, and epidemiologic studies and surveillance of workplace exposures to nanomaterials.[d] Several ethical issues need to be resolved with respect to workers involved with nanoparticles. These ethical issues "... are linked to identification and communication of hazards and risks by scientists, authorities, and employers; acceptance of risk by workers; implementation of controls; choice of participation in medical screening; and adequate investment in toxicologic and exposure control research...."[e(p5)]

---

[a]Centers for Disease Control and Prevention, National Institute for Occupational Safety and Health (NIOSH). General safe practices for working with engineered nanomaterials in research laboratories. DHHS (NIOSH) Pub. No. 2012-147; 2012.

[b]Centers for Disease Control and Prevention. Workplace safety and health topics. Nanotechnology: overview. Available at: http://www.cdc.gov/niosh/topics/nanotech/. Accessed August 7, 2016.

[c]Engeman CD, Baumgartner L, Carr BM, et al. The hierarchy of environmental health and safety practices in the U.S. nanotechnology workplace. *J Occup Environ Hyg.* 2013;10:487–495.

[d]Centers for Disease Control and Prevention, National Institute for Occupational Safety and Health (NIOSH). Nanotechnology: 10 critical topic areas. Available at: http://www.cdc.gov/niosh/topics/nanotech/critical.html. Accessed August 7, 2016.

[e]Schulte PA, Salamanca-Buentello F. Ethical and scientific issues of nanotechnology in the workplace. *Environ Health Perspect.* 2007;115(1):5–12.

FIGURE 12-6 State nonfatal occupational injury and illness incidence rates compared to the national rate—private industry, 2014.

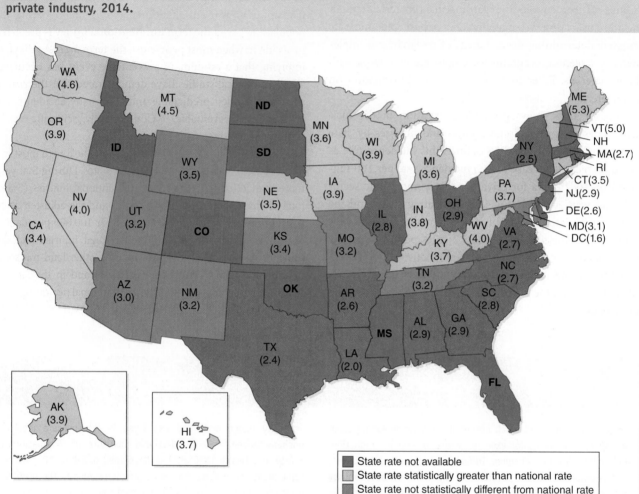

Reprinted from U.S. Bureau of Labor Statistics. 2014 survey of occupational injuries and illnesses. Summary Estimates Charts Package. Washington, DC: U.S. Department of Labor, BLS; October 29, 2015:15. Available at: http://www.bls.gov/iif/oshwc/osh/os/osch0054.pdf. Accessed March 23, 2016.

Figure 12-7 illustrates time trends in age-adjusted death rates for four causes of injury death—poisoning, motor-vehicle traffic, firearms, and falls—from 1999 to 2014. According to Centers for Disease Control and Prevention (CDC), these four mechanisms of injury death in 2013 were associated with 76.3% of total deaths from injuries.[17]

Poisoning

CDC noted that "In 2004, for the first time since 1968, when such data first became available, the number of reported poisoning deaths (30,308) and the age-adjusted poisoning death rate (10.3 per 100,000 population) exceeded the number of firearm deaths (29,569) and the firearm death rate (10.0), respectively. During 1999–2004, the poisoning death rate increased 45%, whereas the firearm death rate declined 3%; during the same period, no change occurred in the rate (14.7%) for motor-vehicle traffic deaths."[18(p1363)] Since 1999 (Figure 12-7), age-adjusted death rates from poisoning have continued to increase to 16.2 per 100,000 in 2014.[19] A total of 51,966 poisoning deaths occurred in 2014.

Motor Vehicle Traffic Deaths

Motor vehicle fatalities have exhibited a declining trend since the mid-1960s, when the death rate was close to 30.0 per

FIGURE 12-7 Age-adjusted death rates* for leading causes of injury death, by year—United States, 1999–2014.

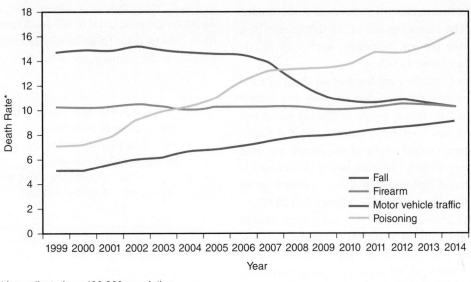

*Age-adjusted per 100,000 population

Data from Centers for Disease Control and Prevention. National Center for Health Statistics. Underlying cause of death 1999-2014. CDC WONDER Online Database; 2015. Data are from the multiple causes of death files, 1999-2014, as compiled from data provided by the 57 vital statistics jurisdictions through the Vital Statistics Cooperative Program. Available at: http://wonder.cdc .gov/ucd-icd10.html. Accessed March 25, 2016.

100,000 persons. In 2013, the death rate was 10.5 per 100,000 persons, with 33,804 total fatalities.[17] In comparison with all other age groups, people who were age 15 to 24 years had the largest number of deaths from this cause followed by people who were age 25 to 34 years. **Figure 12-8** illustrates the destruction that can be caused by a severe automobile crash.

Firearms

The death rate from firearms has tended to reflect slight variations over time, with a rate of 10.3 per 100,000 in 2014. Comparisons of 1999 mortality rates with 2014 rates show no differences between these two years. A total of 33,563 people were killed by firearms in 2013; this figure amounts to 10.3 deaths per 100,000 people. Because firearms continue to be a major determinant of injury mortality, their contribution to the death toll is a riveting public health issue. Well-formulated epidemiologic research might suggest policy initiatives to address firearm violence, which has received a continuous flow of media attention, especially following a series of mass shootings in recent years in the United States.

FIGURE 12-8 An overturned car with first responders.

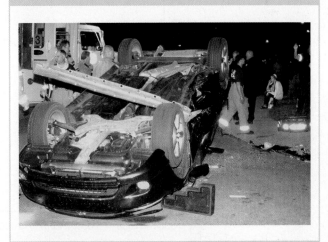

© Jack Dagley/ShutterStock, Inc.

Falls

Deaths from falling reflect a consistently increasing trend over time. In 2014 the total number of deaths from falls was 33,018; the death rate from falls was 9.1 per 100,000. Given this mounting death toll, effective interventions are needed to prevent falls. The increasing rate of fall deaths may be a consequence of the nation's increasing number of elderly individuals, who are prone to falling.

According to CDC, falls are the leading cause of fatal and nonfatal injuries for persons age 65 years and older.[20] The prevalence of falls among people in this age group was estimated by using data from the 2006 Behavioral Risk Factor Surveillance System. Overall, 15.9% of the sample reported falling during the preceding 3 months; among those who fell, 31.3% were injured at least one time. Among persons age 80 years and older, the prevalence of falls increased to 20.8%.

In the CDC study, race and ethnicity were related to falling, with the greatest prevalence occurring among American Indian/Alaska Natives; the highest prevalence of injuries among those who fell occurred among Hispanics.

The prevalence of falling was similar for men and women, although women had a greater percentage of fall-related injuries than men.

Over time, the number of deaths from falls has continued to increase, especially among older adults. **Figure 12-9** shows the growing trend in fall death rates among the elderly from 2004 to 2013. The following facts highlight some of the possible serious consequences of falls:

- One out of five falls causes serious injuries such as broken bones or acute injury.
- More than 95% of hip fractures are caused by falling, usually by falling sideways.
- Adjusted for inflation, the direct medical costs for fall injuries are $34 billion annually.

Reproduced from Centers for Disease Control and Prevention. Important facts about falls. Available at: http://www.cdc.gov/homeandrecreationalsafety/falls/adultfalls.html. Accessed January 7, 2016.

FIGURE 12-9 Unintentional fall death rates, adults age 65 years and over.

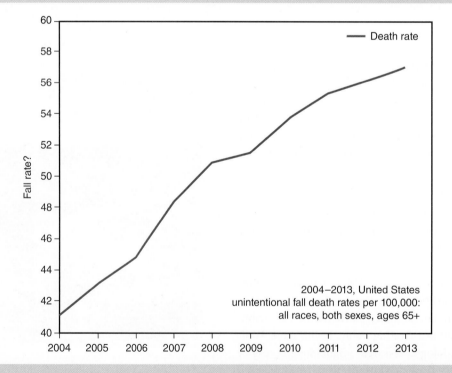

2004–2013, United States
unintentional fall death rates per 100,000:
all races, both sexes, ages 65+

Reproduced from Centers for Disease Control and Prevention. Important facts about falls. Available at: http://www.cdc.gov/homeandrecreationalsafety/falls/adultfalls.html. Accessed January 7, 2016.

Children—Injury Mortality

Several other categories of unintentional injuries are significant causes of mortality for subgroups of the population; these include all types of injuries among children and young adults, and sports-related injuries among children.

The crude death rate for unintentional injuries among children age 0 to 10 years in the United States (2013) is shown in **Figure 12-10**. The highest death rates from injuries among children and young adults occur during the first 5 years of life and then decline to their minimum level at age 10, after which death rates increase with increasing age. These data suggest the need for improved interventions for reducing the toll of unintentional injuries during early childhood.

Traumatic Brain Injuries among Children and Adults

Traumatic brain injuries can be one of the unfortunate results of children's participation in sports. Almost 40 million children and adolescents take part in organized sports in the United States. Participation in these activities incurs the risk of **traumatic brain injuries (TBIs)**, which can cause long-lasting adverse health effects such as behavioral changes and memory loss.

Here are some facts about sports- and recreation-related traumatic brain injuries:[21] Between 2001 and 2005, almost 208,000 people received emergency room treatment for concussions and other TBIs annually.

- Children between age 5 and 18 years comprised 65% of these visits.
- Boys and young men age 10 to 19 years had the highest rates of TBIs.

Figure 12-11 rank orders sports and recreation activities associated with the greatest number of TBI-related emergency department visits by children and teenagers between 2001 and 2009. These pursuits included bicycling, playground activities, baseball, basketball, football, soccer, and

---

FIGURE 12-10 Rate of injury death among children age 0 to 10 years—United States, 2013.

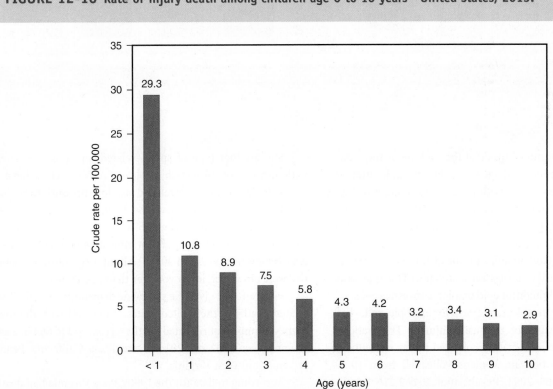

Reproduced from Centers for Disease Control and Prevention, National Center for Health Statistics. Underlying cause of death. 1999-2014. CDC WONDER Online Database; 2015. Data are from the Multiple cause of death files, 1999-2014, as compiled from data provided by the 57 vital statistics jurisdictions through the Vital Statistics Cooperative Program. Available at: https://wonder.cdc.gov/ucd-icd10.html. Accessed July 6, 2016.

FIGURE 12-11 Three most common activities associated with emergency department visits for nonfatal traumatic brain injuries related to sports or recreational activities, by age group and sex.

Age →	≤ 4		5–9		10–14		15–19	
Rank	Boys	Girls	Boys	Girls	Boys	Girls	Boys	Girls
1	Playground N = 3,187 (35.3%)	Playground N = 2,297 (47.8%)	Bicycling N = 5,997 (23.6%)	Playground N = 3,445 (12.2%)	Football N = 8,988 (20.7%)	Bicycling N = 2,051 (12.2%)	Football N = 24,431 (19.9%)	Soccer N = 2,578 (16.0%)
2	Bicycling N = 1,608 (17.8%)	Bicycling N = 775 (14.4%)	Playground N = 4,790 (18.9%)	Bicycling N = 2,351 (20.7%)	Bicycling N = 8,302 (19.1%)	Basketball N = 1,863 (11.1%)	Bicycling N = 20,285 (16.5%)	Basketball N = 2,446 (14.6%)
3	Baseball N = 656 (7.3%)	Baseball N = 321 (6.0%)	Baseball N = 2,227 (8.8%)	Baseball N = 541 (4.7%)	Basketball N = 4,000 (9.2%)	Soccer N = 1,843 (11.0%)	Basketball N = 9,568 (7.8%)	Gymnastics N = 1,513 (9.1%)

Data from Centers for Disease Control and Prevention. Nonfatal traumatic brain injuries related to sports and recreation activities among persons aged ≤ 19 years—United States, 2001-2009. *MMWR.* 2011;60(39):1337-1342.

gymnastics. The figure shows that the ranking of these pastimes varies by gender and age group. For example, after age 10, football was associated with the greatest number of injuries for boys; bicycling and soccer caused the greatest number of injuries among girls. Much debate has been reported in the media regarding concussions from football and other collision sports. (Concussions and head trauma are also an occupational hazard of professional athletes.) This is an issue that will require thoughtful epidemiologic investigations.

Participation in collegiate sports, for example, volleyball, is sometimes a cause of traumatic injuries. The National Collegiate Athletic Association collected injury surveillance data for participation in women's volleyball from 1988–1989 through 2003–2004. Results indicated 2,216 injuries reported from 50,000 games and 4,725 injuries from 90,000 practices. The majority of reported injuries affected the lower extremities; ankle injuries were the most frequently reported type of injury.[22]

Still another type of sports-related injury is associated with the use of all-terrain vehicles (ATVs). ATVs have a motor for high-speed travel and use low-pressure tires that enable travel off road. They have been a source of injuries to children and adults. The U.S. Consumer Product Safety Commission collected reports of almost 14,000 ATV-related deaths between 1982 and 2014.[23] About 3,100 of these fatalities were among children younger than age 16 years.

Figure 12-12 gives the statewide distribution of all ATV-related deaths in the United States. The states with the four highest numbers of reported deaths—from 554 to 664 in each state between 1982 and 2014—were Texas, California, Pennsylvania, and West Virginia.

According to data for the 1990s, West Virginia had death rates from ATV crashes that were about eight times higher than the national average.[24] The state enacted several laws to reduce ATV fatalities; these laws reduced the distance that is permitted for ATVs to travel on paved roads, reduced the

FIGURE 12-12 Number of reported ATV-related fatalities, by state—1982–2011.

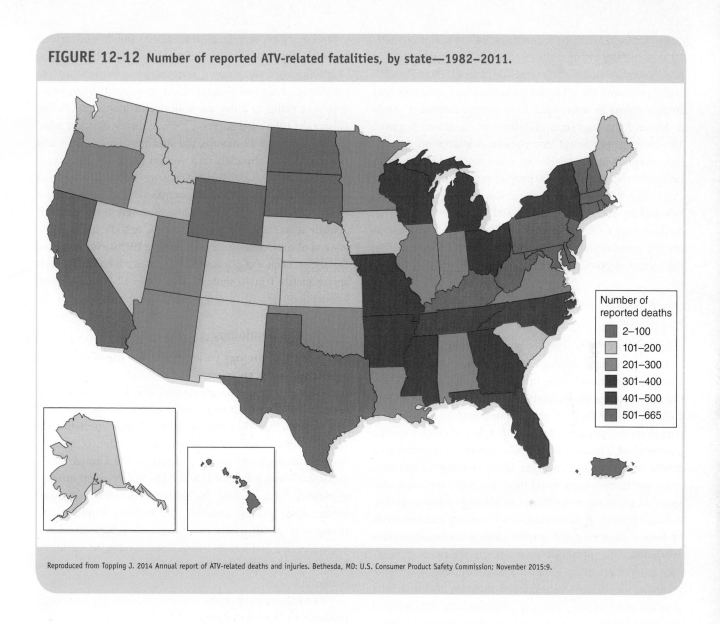

Number of
reported deaths

- 2–100
- 101–200
- 201–300
- 301–400
- 401–500
- 501–665

Reproduced from Topping J. 2014 Annual report of ATV-related deaths and injuries. Bethesda, MD: U.S. Consumer Product Safety Commission; November 2015:9.

speed of the vehicle, and required helmet use. Nevertheless, between 1999 and 2006, fatal ATV crashes increased by about 14% per year. During this period, 250 people died from ATV crashes in West Virginia. Between 1982 and 2011, a total of 594 people died. Factors related to ATV fatalities were lower socioeconomic status, being single or divorced, and having lower levels of education.

Postscript

In recent years, the strides that have been made in prevention of some types of unintentional injuries confirm that they are highly preventable. For example, laws that require seat belts and air bags in cars have contributed to a decline in motor vehicle driver and passenger deaths. Other examples include the improved design of helmets for bicyclists and sports participants. Descriptive epidemiologic studies can aid in the development of policies and procedures to prevent unintentional injuries. This is an area that will require much additional research and the leadership of government and public health officials.

OTHER APPLICATIONS OF EPIDEMIOLOGY

Sewage Epidemiology

Sewage epidemiology refers to monitoring levels of excreted drugs in the sewer system in order to assess the level of illicit drug use in the community. Sewage wastewater systems contain measurable levels of human metabolic end-products of drugs that have been consumed, from both prescription medications and illicit drugs. The substances that are measured in wastewater are called drug target residues (DTRs). Zuccato et al.[25] measured the DTRs for cocaine, opiates, cannabis, and amphetamines in wastewater from sewage treatment plants in Milan, Italy; Lugano, Switzerland; and London, England. The investigators found that cocaine consumption rose on the weekends in Milan. Heroin consumption (measured in milligrams per day per 1,000 people) varied among the three cities. The highest consumption was 210 mg in London, followed by 100 mg in Lugano, and 70 mg in Milan. This methodology could be used to test for levels of drug use in specific communities and even at the household level, raising the specter of privacy issues.

Descriptive Epidemiology of Screen-Based Media Use

It is well known that levels of obesity in the population are increasing in many developed areas of the world; obesity is also a growing health issue in the developing world. Of particular concern is the increasing prevalence of obesity among children and youth. This phenomenon may be attributed in part to contemporary sedentary lifestyles; research into this development is known as the **epidemiology of screen-based media use**. Instead of engaging in active free-time pursuits, more and more youths spend their free hours watching television (TV), using smartphones, or playing computer games. A Swedish study determined that TV viewing and low levels of leisure time physical activity during adolescence were associated with metabolic syndrome in adulthood.[26] However, in older research, Marshall et al. conducted a systematic review of journal articles published between 1949 and 2004 in order to assess the frequency of adolescents' media-based inactivity. Media-based activities included viewing TV, playing video games, and using computers. The investigators concluded that TV viewing had not increased during the 50-year span of their review and that watching TV and other using other media are "… being unfairly implicated in the 'epidemic' of youth sedentariness."[27(p345)]

Physical Dating Violence

"Dating violence is defined as physical, sexual, or psychological violence within a dating relationship."[28(p532)] The CDC examined the occurrence of physical dating violence by using information from the Youth Risk Behavior Surveillance System (YRBSS). Developed by the CDC, the YRBSS is a biennial school-based survey of health risk behaviors of students in the ninth through twelfth grades. The survey produces a representative sample of students in public and private schools. **Physical dating violence** was defined as being "… physically hurt on purpose (counting being hit, slammed into something, or injured with an object or weapon) by someone they were dating or going out with one or more times during 12 months before the survey…"[29(p11)] A survey question asked "[d]uring the past 12 months, did your boyfriend or girlfriend ever hit, slap, or physically hurt you on purpose?" The overall prevalence of physical dating violence was 9.6% and was higher among females (11.7%) than among males (7.4%). Factors related to physical dating violence victimization were being currently sexually active, having attempted suicide, episodic heavy drinking, and physical fighting. Results from the 2015 survey suggested that the prevalence of physical dating violence is high and affects approximately 1 in 10 students. (See **Table 12-2** for additional information.)

Forensic Epidemiology

Forensic epidemiology pertains to "[t]he use of epidemiological reasoning, knowledge, and methods in the investigation of public health problems that may have been caused by or associated with intentional and/or criminal acts."[16] An impetus for the development of this specialization was the 2001 bioterrorism attack (distribution of anthrax bacteria through the postal system) in the United States. Since this event, public health and law enforcement officials worldwide have become increasingly alert for additional bioterrorism attacks; advance preparedness would enable responsible jurisdictions to respond to future attacks in a coordinated fashion and thus limit the impact of intentional dissemination of harmful biologic and other agents on society.

Forensic epidemiology applies standard epidemiologic methods to detect and respond to bioterrorism and other criminal acts that can affect the population. These methods include detection of unusual occurrence of disease (e.g., smallpox), use of ongoing surveillance systems, case identification and confirmation, and development of a descriptive epidemiologic profile of a group of cases. During a bioterrorism attack, surveillance systems might detect an increase in the number of patients who present with infectious diseases in hospital emergency rooms, increases in ambulance services, and increases in the sales of antibiotics.

A specific type of surveillance, known as a *syndromic surveillance system*, records information on syndromes of diseases (e.g., influenza-like conditions) reported in ambulatory care settings; information from syndromic surveillance systems can aid in the detection of disease clusters from natural disease outbreaks and bioterrorism attacks.

TABLE 12-2 Percentage of High School Students Who Experienced Physical Dating Violence, by Sex, Race/Ethnicity, and Grade—United States, Youth Risk Behavior Survey, 2015

Characteristic	Total %	Total (95% CI)	Male %	Male (95% CI)	Female %	Female (95% CI)
Overall	9.6	(8.8–10.6)	7.4	(6.5–8.5)	11.7	(9.9–13.8)
Grade level						
9	8.1	(6.8–9.5)	5.3	(3.5–7.9)	11.1	(8.3–14.7)
10	9.6	(8.0–11.5)	8.2	(6.3–10.7)	10.9	(8.7–13.6)
11	10.1	(8.6–11.8)	7.9	(6.6–9.5)	11.6	(9.0–14.7)
12	10.5	(8.6–12.7)	8.2	(6.4–10.6)	12.9	(9.9–16.5)
Race/Ethnicity						
White, non-Hispanic	9.0	(7.5–10.7)	5.9	(4.8–7.2)	11.9	(9.2–15.2)
Black, non-Hispanic	10.5	(8.4–13.0)	9.0	(6.0–13.4)	12.2	(9.1–16.2)
Hispanic	9.7	(8.0–11.7)	8.0	(6.2–10.2)	11.4	(9.2–14.1)

Reproduced from Kann L, McManus T, Harris WA, et al. Youth Risk Behavior Surveillance—United States, 2015. *MMWR Surveill Summ*. 2016;65(No. SS-6):71.

By applying the information gathered during a forensic epidemiologic investigation, officials can formulate and implement plans for response to bioterrorism-associated events. **Figure 12-13** shows an investigative team at the scene of a crime.

Pharmacoepidemiology

Pharmaceuticals may be thought of as being a two-edged sword. On the one hand, they have contributed dramatically to reducing the scourges that plague humanity and, consequently, are one of the keystones of public health progress. However, on the other hand, they have been linked in some notorious situations to unanticipated side effects. **Pharmacoepidemiology** is "[t]he study of the distribution and determinants of drug-related events in populations and the application of this study to efficacious treatment."[16] An example of an untoward result of the use of a drug was treatment of morning sickness with thalidomide during the 1950s. Some of the mothers who were treated with thalidomide gave

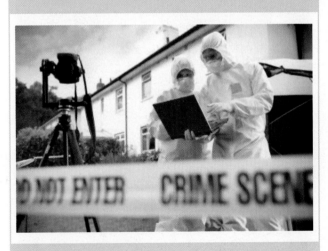

FIGURE 12-13 Forensic epidemiology team investigates public health aspects of criminal acts.

Monty Rakusen/Cultura/Getty Images.

birth to children with defects that included severe limb deformities, as demonstrated in **Figure 12-14**.

Disaster Epidemiology

CDC defines the term **disaster epidemiology** as "... the use of epidemiology to assess the short- and long-term adverse health effects of disasters and to predict consequences of future disasters."[30] A **disaster** refers to "... a serious disruption of the functioning of society, causing widespread human, material or environmental losses, that exceeds the local capacity to respond, and calls for external assistance."[30] Disasters can result from either a natural process, e.g., a severe earthquake or hurricane; or a human-caused tragedy, e.g., a jumbo jet crash with mass casualties or a terrorist attack. Specific examples of disasters are the aftermaths of the Northridge earthquake in California in 1994, Hurricane Katrina in 2005, and the Haitian earthquake in 2010. Note that for an event to be considered a disaster, it must outstrip the resources available in a particular geographic area to cope with the event. Thus, in a tiny community a small-scale event might be declared a disaster because of the community's limited resources.

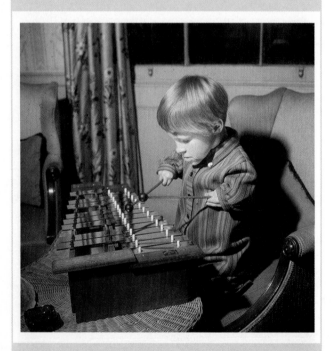

FIGURE 12-14 Child afflicted with thalidomide-induced deformities.

A further issue for consideration is how epidemiology might help in responding to a disaster. CDC stresses how epidemiology can apply a scientific approach to a disaster. "Epidemiology should be an important component during a disaster response because its methods can provide scientific situational awareness. Epidemiologic activities can be used to identify health problems, establish priorities for decision-makers, and evaluate the effectiveness of response activities."[31] Mortality and morbidity can skyrocket following a disaster. Epidemiology can play a central role in limiting infectious disease outbreaks that may occur following a disaster and minimizing mortality. For more information about disaster epidemiology, refer to **Exhibit 12-2**.

Extreme Epidemiology

Extreme epidemiology pertains to the study of population health outcomes in climatically extreme regions such as the Earth's polar zones and tropical regions.[32] Sports fans use "extreme" to refer to activities such as skydiving, mountain climbing without safety gear, and rafting over waterfalls. Extreme epidemiology has nothing to do with extreme sports.

Representative topics covered by this newly coined field include the surveillance of infectious diseases in the Arctic, studies of unintentional injuries among indigenous populations in the Canadian Arctic, protection of the population from extreme temperatures (either frigid or hot), and the impact of climate change on these regions. The journal *Public Health* (August 2016, Volume 137) published a special issue devoted to extreme epidemiology in Arctic and other cold climates. Refer to this issue of the journal for more information.

CONCLUSION

This chapter presented information on additional uses of epidemiology not covered previously. Examples of these uses were taken from the fields of molecular and genetic epidemiology, environmental health, occupational health, and injury epidemiology. Miscellaneous uses of epidemiology were also described. The examples presented demonstrate that epidemiology is a growing field with many applications—both inside and outside the worlds of medicine and public health. Additionally, with society's increasing awareness of epidemiology, the number of applications of this discipline is likely to increase. Many opportunities exist for additional study as well as for employment in positions that use epidemiologic skills. The author hopes that what you have learned will motivate you to consider the many research and employment possibilities that exist in the discipline of epidemiology; these opportunities can be found in both the public sector and within private industry.

EXHIBIT 12-2 Disaster Epidemiology

Disaster epidemiology brings together various topic areas of epidemiology, including acute and communicable disease, environmental health, occupational health, chronic disease, injury, mental health, and behavioral health. Disaster epidemiology provides situational awareness; that is, it provides information that helps us to understand what the needs are, plan the response, and gather the appropriate resources. The main objectives of disaster epidemiology are to prevent or reduce the number of deaths, illnesses, and injuries caused by disasters, provide timely and accurate health information for decision-makers, and improve prevention and mitigation strategies for future disasters by collecting information for future response preparation.

During a disaster, public health workers aid in responding by conducting surveillance. This term denotes the systematic collection, analysis, and interpretation of data regarding deaths, injuries, and illnesses caused by the disaster. Such data enable public health officials to track and identify any adverse health effects (for example, their extent and scope) in the community. Surveillance allows officials to assess the human health impacts of a disaster and evaluate potential problems related to planning and prevention. Public health surveillance during a disaster allows for the detection of potential disease outbreaks and the tracking of disease and injury trends. A common myth is that epidemics are inevitable during a disaster. However, epidemics do not spontaneously occur; public health surveillance can mitigate the likelihood of outbreaks through early detection and response. Additionally, conducting health surveillance allows for the ability to make informed decisions about action items, such as allocating resources, targeting interventions to meet specific needs, and planning future disaster response. While each disaster is different, there are many similarities, and we can apply knowledge learned from each response to the next disaster.

Adapted and reprinted from Centers for Disease Control and Prevention. Disaster epidemiology. Available at: http://www.cdc.gov/nceh/hsb/disaster/epidemiology.htm. Accessed March 9, 2016.

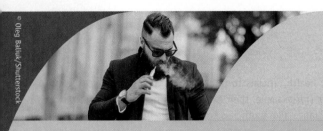

Study Questions and Exercises

1. Define the following types of epidemiology and give at least one example of the application of each type:
   a. Molecular and genetic epidemiology
   b. Environmental epidemiology
   c. Occupational epidemiology
   d. Injury epidemiology

2. Compare and contrast the genetic basis for hemophilia and sickle cell anemia.

3. Give an example of a disease that has a genetic mutation in one of the *BRCA1* or *BRCA2* genes.

4. Why should you be concerned about the health effects of air pollution? What types of adverse health outcomes and conditions have been associated with air pollution? Are there examples of significant air pollution in your own community? Using your own ideas, suggest epidemiologic research studies that might be helpful for discerning the health effects of air pollution in your community.

5. What caused the extreme air pollution episodes in Donora, Pennsylvania, and London, England? Could episodes such as these occur today in the developed world? On the Internet, research air pollution in Beijing, China. List the similarities between the air pollution in the Chinese capital and the episodes in Donora and London.

6. Why are dioxins regarded as potentially dangerous chemicals? What hazards do they present for the environment? In your opinion, what risk management techniques could be applied to dioxin exposure and, more generally, to chemicals that persist in the environment?

7. If you are presently employed, what type of occupational exposures do you have in your work? Name three types of occupational injuries and illnesses that occur in the work environment. In your opinion, what could be done to prevent them?

8. Define the term *global warming* and describe some of its potential consequences.

9. Name some adverse health effects associated with mercury and lead exposures. How might you be exposed to these toxic metals?

10. How can nuclear facilities place you at risk of exposure to ionizing radiation? State one possible health effect associated with ionizing radiation.

11. Using your own ideas, suggest reasons for the trends in the following types of unintentional injury deaths:
    a. Increases in poisoning deaths
    b. Decreases in motor vehicle traffic deaths
    c. Only slight changes in firearm deaths
    d. Increasing numbers of deaths from falls

12. What are the leading causes of traumatic brain injuries among children and teenagers? Using you own ideas, suggest preventive measures.

13. Define each of the following types of epidemiology and give one example of each.
    a. Sewage epidemiology
    b. Forensic epidemiology
    c. Pharmacoepidemiology
    d. Disaster epidemiology

14. What unusual applications of epidemiology have you heard about that were not mentioned in this chapter?

Exercises

1. Invite a trauma specialist to your classroom and ask him or her to discuss the types of injuries treated in the hospital trauma center.

2. Arrange a debate in your classroom to discuss the causes and consequences of unintentional injuries. Assume that little can be done to prevent such events because they are random occurrences. Ask one group of students to present the pro side of this assumption and another group to present the con side of the assumption.

Young Epidemiology Scholars (YES) Exercises

The Young Epidemiology Scholars: Competitions website provides links to teaching units and exercises that support instruction in epidemiology. The YES program, discontinued in 2011, was administered by the College Board and supported by the Robert Wood Johnson Foundation. The exercises continue to be available at the following website: http://yes-competition.org/yes/teaching-units/title.html. The following exercises relate to topics discussed in this chapter and can be found on the YES competitions website.

1. McCrary F, Baumgarten M. Casualties of War: the Short- and Long-Term Effects of the 1945 Atomic Bomb Attacks on Japan

REFERENCES

1. Schulte PA, Lomax GP, Ward EM, Colligan ML. Ethical issues in the use of genetic markers in occupational epidemiologic research. *J Occup Environ Med*. 1999;41(8):630–646.

2. Friis RH, Sellers TA. *Epidemiology for Public Health Practice*. 5th ed. Burlington, MA: Jones & Bartlett Learning; 2014.

3. World Health Organization. Control of genetic diseases: Report by the Secretariat. Geneva, Switzerland: WHO. Available at: http://apps.who.int/gb/archive/pdf_files/EB116/B116_3-en.pdf. Accessed September 1, 2015.

4. National Institutes of Health, National Heart, Lung, and Blood Institute. What is hemophilia? Bethesda, MD: NIH, NHLBI. Available at: http://www.nhlbi.nih.gov/health/health-topics/topics/hemophilia. Accessed July 19, 2016.

5. National Institutes of Health, National Institute of Neurological Disorders and Stroke. NINDS Tay-Sachs disease information page. Bethesda, MD: NIH, NINDS. Available at: http://www.ninds.nih.gov/disorders/taysachs/taysachs.htm. Accessed August 5, 2016.

6. National Institutes of Health, National Heart, Lung, and Blood Institute. What is sickle cell disease? Bethesda, MD: NIH, NHLBI. Available at: http://www.nhlbi.nih.gov/health/health-topics/topics/sca. Accessed August 5, 2016.

7. National Institutes of Health, National Cancer Institute. *BRCA1* and *BRCA2:* cancer risk and genetic testing. Rockville, MD: NIH, NCI. Available at: http://www.cancer.gov/about-cancer/causes-prevention/genetics/brca-fact-sheet. Accessed July 5, 2016.

8. Mai CT, Kucik JE, Isenburg J, et al. Selected birth defects data from population-based birth defects surveillance programs in the United States, 2006 to 2010: featuring trisomy conditions. *Birth Defects Res A Clin Mol Teratol*. 2013;97(11):709–725.

9. Centers for Disease Control and Prevention. Improved national prevalence estimates for 18 selected major birth defects—United States, 1999–2001. *MMWR*. 2006;54:1301–1305.

10. Nabi S, Qader S. Is global warming likely to cause an increased incidence of malaria? *Libyan J Med*. 2009;4(1):18–22. doi: 10.4176/090105.

11. Baverstock K, Williams D. The Chernobyl accident 20 years on: an assessment of the health consequences and the international response. *Environ Health Perspect*. 2006;114:1312–1317.

12. Baverstock K. Chernobyl 25 years on. *BMJ*. 2011;342:d2443.

13. International Atomic Energy Agency. The Fusushima Daiichi Accident. Vienna, Austria: IAEA; 2015.

14. U.S. Bureau of Labor Statistics. 2014 survey of occupational injuries and Illnesses. Summary Estimates Charts Package. Washington, DC: U.S. Department of Labor, BLS; October 29, 2015:5. Available at: http://www.bls.gov/iif/oshwc/osh/os/osch0054.pdf. Accessed March 23, 2016.

15. U.S. Bureau of Labor Statistics. 2014 survey of occupational injuries and illnesses. Summary Estimates Charts Package. Washington, DC: U.S. Department of Labor, BLS; October 29, 2015:15. Available at: http://www.bls.gov/iif/oshwc/osh/os/osch0054.pdf. Accessed March 23, 2016.

16. Porta M, ed. *A Dictionary of Epidemiology*. 6th ed. New York, NY: Oxford University Press; 2014.

17. Xu JQ, Murphy SL, Kochanek KD, Bastian BA. Deaths: final data for 2013. *National Vital Statistics Reports*. 2016;64(2). Hyattsville, MD: National Center for Health Statistics.

18. Centers for Disease Control and Prevention. QuickStats: age-adjusted death rates for leading causes of injury death, by year—United States, 1979–2004. *MMWR*. December 22, 2006;55(50):1363.

19. Centers for Disease Control and Prevention, National Center for Health Statistics. Underlying cause of death 1999–2014. CDC WONDER Online Database; 2015. Data are from the multiple causes of death files, 1999–2014, as compiled from data provided by the 57 vital statistics jurisdictions through the Vital Statistics Cooperative Program. Available at: http://wonder.cdc.gov/ucd-icd10.html. Accessed March 25, 2016.

20. Centers for Disease Control and Prevention. Self-reported falls and fall-related injuries among persons aged ≥ 65 years—United States, 2006. *MMWR*. March 7, 2008;57(09):225–229.

21. Centers for Disease Control and Prevention. Nonfatal traumatic brain injuries related to sports and recreation activities among persons aged ≤ 19 Years—United States, 2001–2009. *MMWR*. October 7, 2011;60(39):1337–1342.

22. Agel J, Palmieri-Smith RM, Dick R, Wojtys EM, Marshall SW. Descriptive epidemiology of collegiate women's volleyball injuries: National Collegiate Athletic Association Injury Surveillance System, 1988–1989 through 2003–2004. *J Ath. Train*. 2007;42(2):295–302.

23. Topping J. 2014 annual report of ATV-related deaths and injuries. Bethesda, MD: U.S. Consumer Product Safety Commission; November 2015.

24. Centers for Disease Control and Prevention. All-terrain vehicle fatalities—West Virginia, 1999–2006. *MMWR*. March 28, 2008;57(12):312–315.

25. Zuccato E, Chiabrando C, Castiglioni S, et al. Estimating community drug abuse by wastewater analysis. National Institutes of Health, National Institute of Environmental Health Sciences. *Environ Health Perspect*. August 2008;116(8):1027–1032.

26. Wennberg P, Gustafsson PE, Dunstan DW, et al. Television viewing and low leisure-time physical activity in adolescence independently predict the metabolic syndrome in mid-adulthood. *Diabetes Care*. July 2013;36(7):2090–2097.

27. Marshall SJ, Gorely T, Biddle SJH. A descriptive epidemiology of screen-based media use in youth: a review and critique. *J Adolesc*. June 2006;29(3):333–349.

28. Centers for Disease Control and Prevention. Physical dating violence among high school students—United States, 2003. *MMWR*. May 19, 2006;55(19):532–535.

29. Kann L, McManus T, Harris WA, et al. Youth Risk Behavior Surveillance—United States, 2015. *MMWR*. 2016;65(SS-6):1–178.

30. Centers for Disease Control and Prevention. Disaster epidemiology. Atlanta, GA: CDC. Available at: http://www.cdc.gov/nceh/hsb/disaster/epidemiology.htm. Accessed March 9, 2016.

31. Centers for Disease Control and Prevention (CDC). *Community Assessment for Public Health Emergency Response (CASPER) Toolkit*. 2nd ed. Atlanta, GA: CDC; 2012.

32. Johnson RM. Extreme epidemiology. *Public Health*. August 2016;137:3-4.

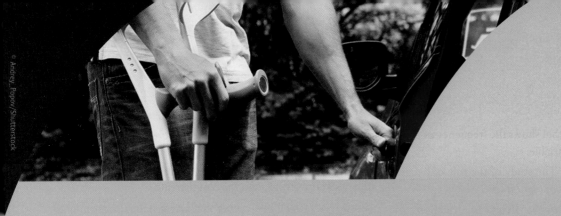

Glossary

A

Adjusted rate Rate of morbidity or mortality in a population in which statistical procedures have been applied to permit fair comparisons across populations by removing the effect of differences in the composition of various populations; an example is age adjustment.

Agent In the epidemiologic triangle, the causative factor for a disease; in infectious diseases, a microorganism such as a virus or bacterium; other agents include chemicals, radiation, and societal influences.

Age-specific rate Frequency of a disease in a particular age stratum divided by the total number of persons within that age stratum during a time period.

American Community Survey A survey conducted by the U.S. Census Bureau to collect detailed population information; previously this information was collected by the Census Bureau's long questionnaire, which has been eliminated in the decennial census.

Analyses of bivariate association Analyses that examine relationships between two variables.

Analytic epidemiology A type of epidemiology that examines causal (etiologic) hypotheses regarding the association between exposures and health conditions. The field of analytic epidemiology proposes and evaluates causal models for etiologic associations and studies them empirically.

Analytic epidemiologic study Concerned with the etiology (causes) of diseases and other health outcomes. Examines causal (etiologic) hypotheses regarding the association between exposures and health conditions; proposes and evaluates causal models for etiologic associations and studies them empirically. Identifies mechanisms of causation of disease; tests specific etiologic hypotheses. Includes case-control studies, cohort studies, and some types of ecologic studies.

Antigen A substance that stimulates antibody formation.

Association A linkage between or among variables.

Attack rate An alternative form of the incidence rate that is used when the nature of a disease or condition is such that a population is observed for a short time period. The attack rate is calculated by the formula ill/(ill + well) × 100 (during a time period). The attack rate is not a true rate because the time dimension is often uncertain.

Attributable risk A measure of risk difference. In a cohort study, refers to the difference between the incidence rate of a disease in the exposed group and the incidence rate in the nonexposed group. It is the rate of disease associated with an exposure.

Autosomal dominant A situation in which a single copy of an altered gene located on a nonsex chromosome is sufficient to cause an increased risk of disease.

Autosomal recessive Denotes those diseases for which two copies of an altered gene are required to increase risk of disease.

Availability of the data Refers to the investigator's access to data (e.g., patient records and databases in which personally identifying information has been removed).

B

Bar chart   A type of graph that shows the frequency of cases for categories of a discrete variable.

Behavioral epidemiology   The study of the role of behavioral factors in health at the population level.

Bias (also, systematic errors)   Refers to deviations of results, or inferences, from the truth.

Big data   Vast electronic storehouses of information that include Internet search transactions, social media activities, data from health insurance programs, and electronic medical records from receipt of healthcare services.

Bioterroristm attack   The deliberate release of viruses, bacteria, or other germs (agents) used to cause illness or death in people, animals, or plants.

Bisphenol A (BPA)   A chemical ingredient used in the manufacture of plastics and resins that is used extensively in food containers, on ATM receipts, and in many other applications. It is no longer used in baby bottles and sippy cups.

Blinding (also, masking)   An aspect of study design wherein the subject is not aware of his or her group assignment of placebo or treatment; seeks to alleviate bias in study results.

Body mass index (BMI)   Measures overweight and obesity. Defined as body weight in kilograms divided by height in meters squared.

C

Carrier   An asymptomatic person or animal that harbors a specific infectious agent and serves as a potential source of infection.

Case-control study   A study that compares individuals who have a disease with individuals who do not have the disease in order to examine differences in exposures or risk factors for the disease.

Case fatality rate   Number of deaths caused by a disease among those who have the disease during a time period.

Case mapping   Portraying the geographic distribution of cases of a disease or health condition by showing their location on a map; a technique used by John Snow to map cholera cases.

Case reports   Accounts of a single occurrence of a noteworthy health-related incident or small collection of such events.

Case series   A larger collection of cases of disease, often grouped consecutively and listing common features such as the characteristics of affected patients.

Causal association   An association between an exposure and a health outcome that has been substantiated by the criteria of causality, e.g., using Sir Austin Bradford Hill's causal criteria.

Cause   In epidemiology, a specific exposure related to a disease; also, independent variable. Includes necessary and sufficient causes.

Cause-specific rate   Measure that refers to mortality (or frequency of a given disease) divided by the population size at the midpoint of a time period times a multiplier.

Cholesterol   A waxy material that can be found throughout the body; travels through the bloodstream.

Chronic strains   Life events that are sustained over a long period of time.

Clinical trial   A research activity that involves the administration of a test regimen to humans to evaluate its efficacy or its effectiveness and safety.

Clustering (case clustering)   An unusual aggregation of health events grouped together in space or time.

Cohort   A population group, or subset thereof (distinguished by a common characteristic), that is followed over a period of time; examples are birth cohorts and age cohorts.

Cohort study (also, prospective or longitudinal study): population-based; exposure   Tracks the incidence of a specific disease or other outcome over time. *Exposure cohort study*: Collects data and follows a group of subjects who have received a specific exposure. The incidence in the exposed group is compared with the incidence in groups that are not exposed, that have different levels of exposure, or that have different types of exposures. *Population-based cohort study*: Tracks a total population or a representative sample of a population for various outcomes, e.g., chronic diseases. An example is the Framingham Heart Study in Massachusetts.

Common-source epidemic   An outbreak due to exposure of a group of persons to a noxious influence that is common to the individuals in the group.

Communicable disease   An illness due to a specific infectious agent or its toxic products that arises through transmission of that agent or products from an infected person, animal, or reservoir to a susceptible host, either directly or indirectly through an intermediate plant or animal host, vector, or the inanimate environment.

Concomitant variation   A type of association in which the frequency of an outcome increases with the frequency of exposure to a factor.

Confidence interval (CI) estimate   A range of values that with a certain degree of probability contain the population parameter, e.g., the 95% CI. An example is the confidence interval about a sample mean.

Confounding   Distortion of an association between an exposure and an outcome because of the influence of a third variable not considered in the study design or analysis.

Congenital malformation   A type of defect present at birth; for example, cleft foot.

Contagion   A theory that proposes that infections are caused by transferable seed-like beings, seminaria or germs, which could cause infection.

Contagious disease   A disease transmitted by direct or indirect contact with a host that is the source of the pathogenic agent.

Contingency table   A type of table that tabulates data according to two dimensions.

Continuous data   Data that have an infinite number of possible values along a continuum.

Continuous variable   A type of variable that is composed of continuous data. Examples of continuous variables are blood cholesterol, height, and weight.

Convenience sampling   Sampling that uses available groups selected by an arbitrary and easily performed method.

Coping skills   Techniques for managing or removing sources of stress.

Correlation coefficient (Pearson correlation coefficient [r])   A measure of the strength of association used with continuous variables. Pearson correlation coefficients (r) range from –1 to 0 to +1.

Cost-effectiveness (cost-benefit) analysis (CEA)   An economic analysis that computes a ratio (called the cost-effectiveness [CE] ratio) by dividing the costs of an intervention by its outcomes expressed as units, for example, deaths averted. These CE ratios, when compared with alternative programs and interventions, help to identify the least costly alternatives.

Count   Total number of cases of a disease or other health phenomenon being studied.

Crossover design   Any change of treatment for a patient in a clinical trial that involves a switch of study treatments.

Cross-sectional study (also, prevalence study)   A type of descriptive study (e.g., a population survey) designed to estimate the prevalence of a disease or exposure.

Crude birth rate   Number of live births during a specified period of time per the resident population during the midpoint of the time period (expressed as rate per 1,000).

Crude death rate   Number of deaths in a given year divided by the reference population (during midpoint of the year) times 100,000. Synonyms: death rate, mortality rate, crude mortality rate.

Crude rate   A type of rate that has not been modified to take into account any of the factors, such as the demographic makeup of the population, that may affect the observed rate. A summary rate based on the actual number of events in a population over a given time period. An example is the crude death rate, which approximates the proportion of the population that dies during a time period of interest.

Cumulative incidence (incidence proportion)   Number of new cases over a time period divided by the total population at risk during the same time period. Used when all individuals in the population (as in a fixed or closed population) are at risk throughout the time period during which they were observed.

Cyclic trends (cyclic fluctuations)   An increase or decrease in the frequency of a disease or health condition in a population over a period of years or within each year. The increases and decreases in the frequency of a disease or other phenomenon over a period of several years or within a year.

D

Data mining   The gathering and exploring of large troves of data in order to discern heretofore unrecognized patterns and associations in the data.

Decision analysis   Developing a set of possible choices and stating the likely outcomes linked with those choices, each of which may have associated risks and benefits.

Demographic transition   Historical shift from high birth and death rates found in agrarian societies to much lower birth and death rates found in developed countries.

Descriptive epidemiologic study   A type of study designed to portray the health characteristics of a population with respect to person, place, and time. Such studies are utilized to estimate disease frequency and time trends and include case reports, case series, and cross-sectional surveys.

Descriptive epidemiology   Epidemiologic studies that are concerned with characterizing the amount and distribution of health and disease within a population.

Determinant   A collective or individual risk factor (or set of factors) that is causally related to a health condition, outcome, or other defined characteristic.

Deterministic model   A model of causality that claims a cause is invariably followed by an effect.

Dichotomous data   Binary data. Example sex: male/female.

Direct transmission   Spread of infection through person-to-person contact.

Disaster   A serious disruption of the functioning of society, causing widespread human, material, or environmental losses, that exceeds the local capacity to respond, and calls for external assistance.

Disaster epidemiology   The use of epidemiology to assess the short- and long-term adverse health effects of disasters and to predict consequences of future disasters.

Discrete data   Data that have a finite or countable number of values.

Discrete variable   A variable made up of discrete data; e.g., variables that use data such as household size (number of persons who reside in a household) or number of doctor visits.

Disease management   A method of reducing healthcare costs by providing integrated care for chronic conditions (e.g., heart disease, hypertension, and diabetes).

Distribution   Variations in the occurrence of diseases and other health outcomes in populations, with some subgroups of the populations more frequently affected than others.

Distribution curve   A graph that is constructed from the frequencies of the values of a variable, for example, variable X.

DNA (deoxyribonucleic acid)   Found in the cells of humans and most other organisms, a nucleic acid that carries genetic information.

Dose-response assessment   The measurement of the relationship between the amount of exposure and the occurrence of unwanted health effects.

Dose-response curve   Graphical representation of the relationship between changes in the size of a dose or exposure and changes in response. This curve generally has an "S" shape.

Dose-response relationship   A type of correlative association between an exposure (e.g., dose of a toxic chemical) and effect (e.g., a biologic outcome).

Double-blind study (design)   Feature of a clinical trial in which neither the subject nor the experimenter is aware of the subject's group assignment in relation to control or treatment status.

E

Ecologic comparison study   Type of research design that assesses the correlation (association) between exposure rates and disease rates among different groups or populations over the same time period. The unit of analysis is the group.

Ecologic correlation   An association between two variables measured at the group level.

Ecologic fallacy   A misleading conclusion about the relationship between a factor and an outcome that occurs when the observed association obtained between study variables at the group level does not necessarily hold true at the individual level.

Emerging infectious disease   An infectious disease that has newly appeared in a population or that has been known for some time but is rapidly increasing in incidence or geographic range (e.g., hantaviral pulmonary syndrome found in the southwestern United States).

Endemic   Denotes a disease or infectious agent habitually present in a community, geographic area, or population group. Often an endemic disease maintains a low but continuous incidence.

Enteric protozoal parasites   Pathogenic single-celled microorganisms that can live in the intestinal tract; both giardiasis and cryptosporidiosis are diseases caused by these organisms.

Environment   Domain in which a disease-causing agent may exist, survive, or originate.

Environmental determinants   The sum of all influences that are not part of the host; it comprises physical, climatologic, biologic, social, and economic components.

Environmental epidemiology   The study of diseases and conditions (occurring in the population) that are linked to environmental factors.

Environmental influences   With regard to the causes of diseases, factors such as climate, geographic location, and water quality.

Epidemic   Occurrence in a community or region of cases of an illness, specific health-related behavior, or other health-related events clearly in excess of normal expectancy.

Epidemic curve   A graphic plotting of the distribution of cases by time of onset. A type of unimodal (having one mode) curve that aids in identifying the cause of a disease outbreak.

Epidemiologic transition   A shift in the pattern of morbidity and mortality from causes related primarily to infectious and communicable diseases to causes associated with chronic, degenerative diseases; is accompanied by demographic transition.

Epidemiologic triangle   A model that includes three major factors: agent, host, and environment; used to describe the etiology of infectious diseases.

Epidemiology   Concerned with the distribution and determinants of health and diseases, morbidity, injuries, disability, and mortality in populations. Epidemiologic studies are applied to the control of health problems in populations.

Essential public health services   Ten services subsumed under the three core functions of public health.

Estimation   The use of sample-based data to make conclusions about the population from which a sample has been selected.

Ethics   Norms for conduct that distinguish between acceptable and unacceptable behavior.

Ethics guidelines   A set of core values that guide practice in a field; for example, the set of guidelines developed by the American College of Epidemiology (ACE) for epidemiologists.

Evidence-based public health   The adoption of policies, laws, and programs that are supported by empirical data.

Experimental design (study)   Research design in which the investigator manipulates the study factor and randomly assigns subjects to exposed and nonexposed conditions.

Exposure assessment   The procedure that identifies populations exposed to the toxicant, describes their composition and size, and examines the roots, magnitudes, frequencies, and durations of such exposures.

Exposure-based cohort study   Compares cohorts with or without different exposures. A simple example is a cohort study with two exposure groups (exposed and not exposed).

Exposures   Contacts with disease-causing factors; the amounts of the factors that impinge upon a group or individuals.

External validity   Measure of the generalizability of the findings from the study population to the target population.

F

False negatives   Individuals who have been screened negative but truly have the condition.

False positives   Individuals who have been screened positive but do not have the condition.

Family recall bias   A type of bias that occurs when cases are more likely to remember the details of their family history than are controls (see Bias).

Fertility rate   See General fertility rate.

Fetal death rate (fetal mortality rate)   Number of fetal deaths after 20 weeks or more of gestation divided by the number of live births plus fetal deaths after 20 weeks or more of gestation during a year (expressed as rate per 1,000 live births plus fetal deaths).

Fomite   An inanimate object that carries infectious disease agents.

Forensic epidemiology   The use of epidemiological reasoning, knowledge, and methods in the investigation of public health problems that may have been caused by or associated with intentional and/or criminal acts.

G

Gene   A particular segment of a DNA (deoxyribonucleic acid) molecule on a chromosome that determines the nature of an inherited trait in an individual.

General fertility rate   Number of live births reported in an area during a given time interval divided by the number of women age 15 to 44 years in that area (expressed as rate per 1,000 women age 15–44 years).

Generation time   An interval of time between lodgment of an infectious agent in a host and the maximal communicability of the host.

Genetic epidemiology   Field of epidemiology concerned with inherited factors that influence risk of disease.

Genetic marker (of susceptibility)   A gene that may confer increased susceptibility to specific exposures.

Genetic screening   The use of genetic, clinical, and epidemiologic knowledge, reasoning, and techniques to detect genetic variants that have been demonstrated to place an individual at increased risk of a specific disease.

Germ theory of disease   A theory that links microorganisms to the causation of disease.

Global warming   The gradual increase in the earth's temperature over time.

Gold standard   A definitive diagnosis that has been determined by biopsy, surgery, autopsy, or other method and has been accepted as the standard.

H

Hawthorne effect   Participants' behavioral changes as a result of their knowledge of being in a research study.

Hazard   The inherent capability of an agent or a situation to have an adverse effect; a factor or exposure that may adversely affect health.

Hazard identification   Examines the evidence that associates exposure to an agent with its toxicity and produces a qualitative judgment about the strength of that evidence, whether it is derived from human epidemiologic research or extrapolated from laboratory animal data.

Health disparities   Differences in the occurrence of diseases and adverse health conditions in the population.

Health in All Policies   A collaborative approach to improving the health of all people by incorporating health considerations into decision making across sectors and policy areas.

Health policy   A policy that pertains to the health arena, for example, in dentistry, medicine, public health, or regarding provision of healthcare services.

Healthy People   A national collaborative effort that articulates science-derived objectives for advancing the health of Americans.

Healthy worker effect   Error linked to the observation that employed persons tend to have lower mortality rates than the general population; stems from the fact that good health is necessary for obtaining and maintaining employment (see Bias).

Herd immunity   Resistance of an entire community to an infectious disease due to the immunity of a large proportion of individuals in that community to the disease.

Histograms   Charts that are used to display the frequency distributions for grouped categories of a continuous variable.

Host   Person (or animal) who (that) has a lodgment of an infectious disease agent under natural conditions.

Hypothesis   Supposition tested by collecting facts that lead to its acceptance or rejection. Any conjecture cast in a form that will allow it to be tested and, possibly, refuted.

I

Infectious disease   A disease due to an infectious agent.

Immunity   A status usually associated with the presence of antibodies or cells having a specific action on a microorganism concerned with a particular infectious disease or on its toxin.

Inapparent (subclinical) infection   A type of infection that shows no clinical or obvious symptoms.

Incidence density   An incidence rate that is used when the time periods of observation of the members of a population (e.g., cohort) vary from person to person due to subject dropout and attrition. The numerator is the number of new cases of disease or other outcome during a time period divided by the total person-time of observation during the time period.

Incidence rate   Number of new cases of a disease or other condition in a population divided by the average population at risk over a time period times a multiplier (e.g., 100,000).

Incubation period   Time interval between invasion by an infectious agent and the appearance of the first signs or symptoms of disease.

Index case   In an epidemiologic investigation of a disease outbreak, the first case of disease to come to the attention of authorities (e.g., the initial case of Ebola virus).

Indirect transmission   Disease transmission by intermediary sources of infection, such as vehicles, droplet nuclei (particles), and vectors.

Infant mortality rate   Number of deaths among infants age 0 to 365 days during a year divided by the number of live births during the same year (expressed as the rate per 1,000 live births).

Infection   The entry and development or multiplication of an infectious agent in the body of persons or animals.

Infectious disease (communicable disease)   An illness due to a specific infectious agent or its toxic products that arises through transmission of that agent or its products from an infected person, animal, or reservoir to a susceptible host, either directly or indirectly through an intermediate plant or animal host, vector, or the inanimate environment.

Infectivity   Capacity of an agent to enter and multiply in a susceptible host and thus produce infection or disease.

Inference   The process of evolving from observations and axioms to generalizations.

Injury epidemiology   The study of the distribution and determinants of various types of injuries in the population.

Interdisciplinary science   A branch of knowledge that uses information from many fields.

Interquartile range (IQR)   A measure of the spread of a distribution that is the portion of a distribution between the first and third quartiles.

Interval estimate   A range of values that with a certain level of confidence contains the parameter.

Interval scale   A scale that consists of continuous data with equal intervals between points on the measurement scale and without a true zero point.

Internal validity   Degree to which a study has used methodologically sound procedures (e.g., assignment of subjects and use of reliable measurements).

Intervention study   An investigation involving intentional change in some aspect of the status of the subjects, e.g., introduction of a preventive or therapeutic regimen or an intervention designed to test a hypothesized relationship. Intervention studies include randomized controlled trials and community interventions.

Isolation   When persons who have a communicable disease are kept away from other persons for a period of time that corresponds generally to the interval when the disease is communicable.

L

Late fetal death rate   Number of fetal deaths after 28 weeks or more of gestation divided by the number of live births plus fetal deaths after 28 weeks or more of gestation during a year (expressed as rate per 1,000 live births plus late fetal deaths).

Latency   Time period between initial exposure to an agent and development of a measurable response. The latency period can range from a few seconds (in the case of acutely toxic agents) to several decades (in the case of some forms of cancer).

Life expectancy   Number of years that a person is expected to live, at any particular year.

Lifestyle   The choice of behaviors that affect how we live; these choices often are a function of social influences.

Lipoprotein panel Assesses total cholesterol as well as three types of blood lipids: low-density lipoprotein (LDL) cholesterol, high-density lipoprotein (HDL) cholesterol ("good" cholesterol), and triglycerides.

Longitudinal design A study design in which subjects are followed over an extended period of time.

M

Mammogram An X-ray image of the human breast.

Mass screening The application of screening tests to total population groups, regardless of their risk status.

Matched case-control study A type of study in which the cases and controls have been matched according to one or more criteria such as sex, age, race, or other variables.

Maternal mortality rate (Number of maternal deaths ascribed to childbirth divided by the number of live births) times 100,000 live births during a year.

Mean The arithmetic mean or average. It is a common measure of central tendency with many uses in epidemiology.

Mean deviation The average of the absolute values of the deviations of each observation about the mean.

Measure of central tendency A number that signifies a typical value of a group of numbers or of a distribution of numbers; also called a measure of location.

Measures of variation Range, midrange, mean deviation, and standard deviation.

Median The middle point of a set of numbers; the 50% point of continuous distributions. If a group of numbers is ranked from the smallest value to the highest value, the median is the point that demarcates the lower and upper half of the numbers.

Method of difference A situation in which all of the factors in two or more domains are the same except for a single factor.

Miasma An airborne toxic vapor composed of malodorous particles from decomposing fetid materials.

Miasmatic theory of disease An explanation for infectious diseases that held that disease was transmitted by a miasm, or cloud, that clung low on the surface of the earth.

Midrange The arithmetic mean of the highest and lowest values.

Mode The number occurring most frequently in a set or distribution of numbers; in a distribution curve of a variable, the most frequently occurring value of the variable.

Molecular epidemiology Field of epidemiology that uses biomarkers to establish exposure–disease associations.

Examples of biomarkers are serum levels of micronutrients and DNA fingerprints.

Morbidity Occurrence of an illness or illnesses in a population.

Mortality Occurrence of death in a population.

Multimodal curve A curve that has several peaks in the frequency of a condition.

Multivariate (multifactorial, multiple) causality The belief that a preponderance of the etiologies of diseases (particularly chronic diseases) involve more than one causal factor, e.g., the etiology of chronic diseases as well as infectious diseases usually involves multiple types of exposures and other risk factors.

Mutation A change in DNA that may adversely affect an organism.

N

Nanotechnology The manipulation of matter on a near-atomic scale [1 to 100 nanometers in length] to produce new structures, materials, and devices.

National Prevention Strategy An effort to improve the nation's level of health and well-being through four strategic directions and seven targeted priorities.

Nativity Place of origin (e.g., native born or foreign born) of an individual or his or her relatives.

Natural experiments Naturally occurring circumstances in which subsets of the population have different levels of exposure to a hypothesized causal factor in a situation resembling an actual experiment. The presence of persons in a particular group is typically nonrandom. Example: John Snow's natural experiment.

Natural history of disease The time course of disease from its beginning to its final clinical endpoints.

Nature of the data Source of the data (e.g., vital statistics, physician's records, or case registries.)

Necessary cause A factor whose presence is required for the occurrence of an effect.

Neonatal mortality rate Number of infant deaths among infants under 28 days of age divided by the number of live births during a year times 1,000 live births.

Nominal scales A type of qualitative scale that consists of categories that are not ordered.

Normal distribution Also called a Gaussian distribution, is a symmetrical distribution with several interesting properties that pertain to its central tendency and dispersion. Many human characteristics such as intelligence are normally distributed.

Null hypothesis A hypothesis of no difference in a population parameter among the groups being compared.

O

Observational science   A branch of knowledge that capitalizes on naturally occurring situations in order to study the occurrence of disease.

Observational study   A type of research design in which the investigator does not manipulate the study factor or use random assignment of subjects. There is careful measurement of the patterns of exposure and disease in a population in order to draw inferences about the distribution and etiology of diseases. Observational studies include cross-sectional, case-control, and cohort studies.

Occupational epidemiology   Among populations of workers, focuses on adverse health outcomes associated with the work environment.

Odds ratio   Measure of association between frequency of exposure and frequency of outcome used in case-control studies. The formula is (AD)/(BC), where A is the number of subjects who have the disease and have been exposed, B is the number who do not have the disease and have been exposed, C is the number who have the disease and have not been exposed, and D is the number who do not have the disease and have not been exposed.

Operationalization   Methods used to translate concepts used in research into actual measurements.

Operations research   A type of study of the placement of health services in a community and the optimum utilization of such services.

Ordinal scales   Scales that comprise categorical data that can be ordered (ranked data) but are still considered qualitative data.

Outcomes   Results that may arise from an exposure to a causal factor. Examples of outcomes in epidemiologic research are specific infectious diseases, disabling conditions, unintentional injuries, chronic diseases, and conditions associated with personal behavior and lifestyle.

Outliers   Extreme values that differ greatly from other values in the data set.

Overdiagnosis   The use of screening tests that lead to the detection of abnormalities that have little clinical significance.

P

Pandemic   An epidemic occurring worldwide, or over a very wide area, crossing international boundaries, and usually affecting a large number of people. A worldwide influenza pandemic is an example.

Parameter   A variable for describing a characteristic of a population, e.g., the average age of a population.

Parasitic disease   An infection caused by a parasite.

Passive immunity   Immunity that is acquired from antibodies produced by another person or animal.

Passive smoking (also, sidestream exposure to cigarette smoke)   Involuntary breathing of cigarette smoke by nonsmokers in an environment where cigarette smokers are present.

Pathogenesis   Process and mechanism of interaction of disease agent(s) with a host in causing disease. The period of pathogenesis occurs after the agent has interacted with a host. This situation can happen when a susceptible host comes into contact with a disease agent such as a virus or bacterium.

Percentage   A proportion that has been multiplied by 100.

Percentiles   Created by dividing a distribution into 100 parts. The pth percentile is the number for which p% of the data have values equal to or smaller than that number.

Perinatal mortality rate   Number of late fetal deaths after 28 weeks or more of gestation plus infant deaths within 7 days of birth divided by the number of live births plus the number of late fetal deaths during a year (expressed as rate per 1,000 live births and fetal deaths).

Period prevalence   All cases of a disease within a period of time. When expressed as a proportion, refers to the number of cases of illness during a time period divided by the average size of the population.

Pharmacoepidemiology   The study of the distribution and determinants of drug-related events in populations and the application of this study to efficacious treatment.

Phenylketonuria (PKU)   A condition marked by the inability to metabolize the amino acid phenylalanine; it is a genetic disorder that is associated with intellectual disability.

Pie chart   A circle that shows the proportion of cases according to several categories.

Point epidemic   Response of a group of people circumscribed in place to a common source of infection, contamination, or other etiologic factor to which they were exposed almost simultaneously.

Point estimate   A single value, e.g., sample mean, used to estimate a parameter.

Point prevalence   All cases of a disease, health condition, or deaths that exist at a particular point in time relative to a specific population from which the cases are derived.

Point source epidemic   A type of common-source epidemic that occurs when the exposure is brief and essentially simultaneous, and the resultant cases all develop within one incubation period of the disease.

Policy   A plan or course of action, as of a government, political party, or business, intended to influence and determine decisions, actions, and other matters.

Policy cycle   The distinct phases involved in the policy-making process.

Population   All the inhabitants of a given country or area considered together.

Population at risk   Those members of the population who are capable of developing a disease or condition.

Population-based cohort study   A type of cohort study that includes either an entire population or a representative sample of the population (see Cohort study).

Population risk difference   Difference between the incidence rate of disease in the nonexposed segment of the population and the overall incidence rate. It measures the benefit to the population derived by modifying a risk factor.

Portal of entry   Site where a disease agent enters the body; example: respiratory system (through inhalation).

Portal of exit   The site from which a disease agent leaves that person's body; portals of exit include respiratory passages, the alimentary canal, the genitourinary system, and skin lesions.

Postneonatal mortality rate   Number of infant deaths from 28 days to 365 days after birth divided by the number of live births minus neonatal deaths during a year (expressed as rate per 1,000 live births).

Posttraumatic stress disorder (PTSD)   An anxiety disorder that some people develop after seeing or living through an event that caused or threatened serious harm or death.

Power   The ability of a study to demonstrate an association or effect if one exists. Among the factors related to power are sample size and how large an effect is observed.

Predictive value (−)   A measure for those screened negative by the test; it is designated by the formula $d/(c + d)$; this is the probability that an individual who is screened negative does not have the disease.

Predictive value (+)   The proportion of individuals who are screened positive by the test and who actually have the disease.

Prepathogenesis   Period of time that precedes the interaction between an agent of disease and a host.

Prevalence   Number of existing cases of a disease or health condition in a population at some designated time.

Primary prevention   Activities designed to reduce the occurrence of disease and that occur during the period of prepathogenesis (i.e., before an agent interacts with a host).

Program evaluation   The determination of whether a community intervention program meets stated goals and is justified economically.

Prophylactic trial   A type of clinical trial designed to evaluate the effectiveness of a treatment or substance used to prevent disease. Examples are clinical trials to test vaccines and vitamin supplements.

Proportion   Fraction in which the numerator is a part of the denominator.

Proportional mortality ratio (PMR)   Number of deaths within a population due to a specific disease or cause divided by the total number of deaths in the population during a time period such as a year.

Prospective cohort study   A type of cohort study design that collects data on an exposure at the initiation (baseline) of a study and follows the population in order to observe the occurrence of health outcomes at some time in the future.

Protective factor   A circumstance or substance that provides a beneficial environment and makes a positive contribution to health.

Psychiatric epidemiology   Studies the incidence and prevalence of mental disorders according to variables such as age, sex, and social class; the discipline measures the frequency of occurrence of mental disorders and factors related to their etiology.

Public health surveillance   The systematic and continuous gathering of information about the occurrence of diseases and other health phenomena.

P value   An assessment that indicates the probability that the observed findings of a study could have occurred by chance alone.

Q

Qualitative data   Data that employ categories that do not have numerical values or rankings.

Quantitative data   Data reported as numerical quantities.

Quantification   The counting of cases of illness or other health outcomes.

Quarantine   When well persons who have been exposed to an infectious disease are prevented from interacting with those not exposed.

Quartiles   Subdivision of a distribution into units of 25% of the distribution.

Quasi-experimental study   Type of research design in which the investigator manipulates the study factor but does not assign subjects randomly to the exposed and nonexposed groups.

R

Randomization   A process whereby chance determines the subjects' likelihood of assignment to either an intervention group or a control group. Each subject has an equal probability of being assigned to either group.

Randomized controlled trial (RCT)   A clinical-epidemiologic experiment in which subjects are randomly allocated into groups, usually called *test* and *control* groups, to receive or not to receive a preventive or a therapeutic procedure or intervention.

Range   The difference between the highest (H) and lowest (L) value in a group of numbers.

Rate   A ratio that consists of a numerator and denominator in which time forms part of the denominator. Example: The crude death rate refers to the number of deaths in a given year (during the midpoint of the year) divided by the size of the reference population (expressed as rate per 100,000).

Ratio   Number obtained by dividing one quantity by another. A fraction (in its most general form) in which there is not necessarily any specified relationship between the numerator and denominator.

Ratio scale   A scale that retains the properties of an interval level scale and, in addition, has a true zero point.

Recall bias   A type of bias associated with the ability of the cases to remember an exposure more clearly than the controls.

Reference population   Group from which cases of a disease (or health-related phenomenon under study) have been taken; also refers to the group to which the results of a study may be generalized.

Registry   Centralized database for collection of information about a disease.

Relative risk   Ratio of the risk of disease or death among the exposed to the risk among the unexposed. The formula used (in cohort studies) is Relative risk = Incidence rate in the exposed/incidence rate in the unexposed.

Reliability (also, precision)   Ability of a measuring instrument to give consistent results on repeated trials.

Repeated measurement reliability   The degree of consistency between or among repeated measurements of the same individual on more than one occasion.

Reportable disease statistics   Statistics derived from diseases that physicians and other healthcare providers must report to government agencies according to legal statute. Such diseases are called reportable (notifiable) diseases.

Representativeness (also, external validity)   The degree to which the characteristics of the sample correspond to the characteristics of the population from which the sample was chosen; generalizability of the findings of an epidemiologic study to the population.

Reservoir   A place where infectious agents normally live and multiply; the reservoir can be human beings, animals, insects, soils, or plants.

Resistance (types: host, antibiotic)   *Host*: immunity of the host to an infectious disease agent. *Antibiotic*: resistance of bacteria to antibiotics.

Retrospective cohort study   Type of cohort study that uses historical data to determine exposure level at some time in the past; subsequently, follow-up measurements of occurrence(s) of disease between baseline and the present are taken.

Risk   The probability of an adverse or beneficial event in a defined population over a specified time interval.

Risk assessment   A process for identifying adverse consequences of exposures and their associated probability.

Risk characterization   Develops estimates of the number of excess unwarranted health events expected at different time intervals at each level of exposure.

Risk difference (see attributable risk and population risk difference)   Difference between the incidence rate of disease in the exposed group and the incidence rate of disease in the nonexposed group.

Risk factor   An exposure that is associated with a disease, morbidity, mortality, or another adverse health outcome.

Risk management   In environmental research with toxic substances, consists of actions taken to control exposures to toxic chemicals in the environment. Exposure standards, requirements for premarket testing, recalls of toxic products, and outright banning of very hazardous materials are among the actions that are used by governmental agencies to manage risk.

S

Sample   A subgroup that has been selected, using one of several methods, from the population (universe). Examples are simple random samples, systematic samples, stratified random samples, and convenience samples.

Sampling bias   The individuals who have been selected for the study are not representative of the population to which the epidemiologist would like to generalize the results of the research.

Sampling error   A type of error in random sampling that arises when values (statistics) obtained for a sample differ from the values (parameters) of the parent population.

Screening for disease   Presumptive identification of unrecognized disease or defects by the application of tests, examinations, or other procedures that can be administered rapidly.

Secondary prevention Intervention designed to reduce the progress of a disease after the agent interacts with the host; occurs during the period of pathogenesis.

Secular trends Gradual changes in disease frequency over long time periods.

Selection bias Bias in the estimated association or effect of an exposure on an outcome that arises from procedures used to select individuals into the study (see Bias).

Selective screening (also, targeted screening) The type of screening applied to high-risk groups such as those at risk for sexually transmitted diseases. Selective screening is likely to result in the greatest yield of true cases and to be the most economically productive form of screening (see Screening).

Sensitivity Ability of a test to correctly identify all screened individuals who actually have the disease for which screening is taking place.

Sex-linked disorder A disease conferred by abnormal genes carried on sex chromosomes. Example: hemophilia, which is caused by an abnormal gene carried on an X chromosome.

Sex ratio In demography, the number of males per 100 females.

Sex-specific rate The frequency of a disease in a sex group divided by the total number of persons within that sex group during a time period times a multiplier.

Sexually transmitted diseases (STDs) Infectious diseases and related conditions (such as crab lice) that can be spread by sexual contact. May also be called sexually transmitted infections (STIs).

Sewage epidemiology Monitoring levels of excreted drugs in the sewer system in order to assess the level of illicit drug use in the community.

Simple random sampling (SRS) The use of a random process to select a sample.

Skewed distribution A distribution that is asymmetric; it has a concentration of values on either the left or right side of the X-axis.

Snow, John (1813–1858) An English anesthesiologist who innovated several of the key epidemiologic methods that remain valid and in use today.

Social epidemiology The discipline that examines the social distribution and social determinants of states of health.

Social support Perceived emotional support that one receives from family members, friends, and others; may mediate against stress.

Socioeconomic status (SES) A measure that takes into account three interrelated dimensions: a person's income level, education level, and type of occupation. Some measures of SES use only one dimension such as income.

Spatial clustering Concentration of cases of a disease in a particular geographic area.

Specificity Ability of a test to identify nondiseased individuals who actually do not have a disease.

Specific rate Statistic referring to a particular subgroup of the population defined in terms of race, age, or sex; also may refer to the entire population but is specific for some single cause of death or illness.

Spontaneous generation A theory that postulated that simple life forms such as microorganisms could arise spontaneously from nonliving materials.

Standard deviation A measure used to quantify the degree of spread of a group of numbers.

Standard normal distribution A type of normal distribution with a mean of zero and a standard deviation of one unit.

Statistics Numbers that describe a sample, e.g., sample mean.

Statistical significance The assertion that the observed association is not likely to have occurred as a result of chance.

Stochastic process A process that incorporates some element of randomness. According to stochastic modeling, a cause is associated with an increased probability that an effect will happen.

Stratum A subgroup of a population; example: a racial or ethnic group. In stratified random sampling, some strata may be oversampled in order to obtain sufficient numbers of cases from those strata.

Stress A physical, chemical, or emotional factor that causes bodily or mental tension and may be a factor in disease causation.

Stressful life events Stressors (sources of stress) that arise from happenings such as job loss, financial problems, and death of a close family member. Include both positive events (e.g., birth of a child) and negative events.

Subclinical (also, inapparent) An infection that does not show obvious clinical signs or symptoms.

Sufficient cause A cause that is sufficient by itself to produce the effect.

Sufficient-component cause model A model that is constituted from a group of component causes, which can be diagrammed as a pie; also known as the causal pie model.

Surveillance Systematic collection, analysis, interpretation, dissemination, and consolidation of data pertaining to the occurrence of a specific disease.

Systematic sampling Sampling that uses a systematic procedure to select a sample of a fixed size from a sampling frame (a complete list of people who constitute the population).

T

Temporal clustering   Occurrence of health events that are related in time, such as the development of maternal postpartum depression a few days after a female gives birth.

Temporality   Timing of information about cause and effect; whether the information about cause and effect was assembled at the same time point or whether information about the cause was garnered before or after the information about the effect.

Tertiary prevention   Intervention that takes place during late pathogenesis and is designed to reduce the limitations of disability from disease.

Theories   General accounts of causal relationships between exposures and outcomes.

Therapeutic trial   A type of study designed to evaluate the effectiveness of a treatment in bringing about an improvement in a patient's health. An example is a trial that evaluates a new curative drug or a new surgical procedure.

Three core functions of public health   Assurance, assessment, and policy development.

Three levels of prevention   From the public health point of view, the three types of prevention (primary, secondary, and tertiary) that coincide with the periods of prepathogenesis and pathogenesis.

Threshold   Lowest dose (often of a toxic substance) at which a particular response may occur.

Toxicology   A discipline that examines the toxic effects of chemicals found in environmental venues such as the workplace.

Toxin   A material that is harmful to biologic systems and that is made by living organisms.

Trans fats   Fats that are manufactured through the process of hydrogenation, whereby hydrogen is added to vegetable oils.

True negatives   Individuals who have both been screened negative and do not have the condition.

True positives   Individuals who have both been screened positive and truly have the condition.

Tuskegee Study   An investigation of untreated syphilis among black men begun in 1932 that spanned 40 years with the purpose to record the natural history of syphilis in hopes of justifying treatment programs for blacks.

U

Unbiased   The average of the sample estimates over all possible samples is equal to the population parameter.

Universe   The total set of elements from which a sample is selected.

V

Vaccination (immunization)   Procedure in which a vaccine (a preparation that contains a killed or weakened pathogen) is introduced into the body to invoke an immune response against a disease-causing microbe, such as a virus or bacterium. Also called inoculation, immunization.

Vaccine-preventable diseases (VPDs)   Conditions that can be prevented by vaccination (immunization).

Validity (also, accuracy)   Ability of a measuring instrument to give a true measure (how well the instrument measures what it purports to measure).

Variable   Any quantity that can have different values across individuals or other study units.

Variance   A measure that quantifies the degree of variability in a set of numbers; the sample variance is denoted by s^2.

Vector   An animate, living insect or animal that is involved with the transmission of disease agents. Examples of vectors are arthropods (insects such as lice, flies, mosquitoes, and ticks) that bite their victims.

Vehicles   Contaminated, nonmoving objects involved with indirect transmission of disease; examples are fomites, unsanitary food, impure water, and infectious bodily fluids.

Virulence   Severity of the clinical manifestations of a disease.

Vital events   Deaths, births, marriages, divorces, and fetal deaths.

Vital statistics   Mortality and birth statistics maintained by government agencies.

Z

Zoonosis   An infection transmissible under natural conditions from vertebrate animals to humans.

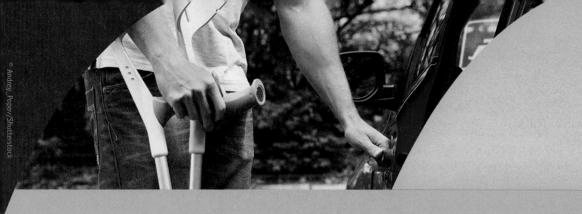

Index

Note: The letters 'f', and 't' following locators refer to figures, and tables.

E